NUTRITIONAL FLOW

NUTRITIONAL FLOW

Finding Whole Health with Functional Medicine

Roger James Simpson, MD

Amberlyn Simpson

Simpson Clinics

ISBN: 979-8-9870800-2-3 (Paperback)

Front cover image by Amberlyn Simpson.

Printed by IngramSpark in the United States of America.

First printing edition 2023.

Simpson Clinics
106 East C St.
North Platte, NE, 69101

www.simpsonclinics.com
www.nutritionalflow.com

NUTRITIONAL FLOW

Finding Whole Health with Functional Medicine

Roger James Simpson, MD

Amberlyn Simpson

Simpson Clinics

ISBN: 979-8-9870800-2-3 (Paperback)

Front cover image by Amberlyn Simpson.

Printed by IngramSpark in the United States of America.

First printing edition 2023.

Simpson Clinics
106 East C St.
North Platte, NE, 69101

www.simpsonclinics.com
www.nutritionalflow.com

CONTENTS

CONTENTS

3

Guiding Flow Away From Toxins and
Excess

The Paradigm of Flow Nutrition and Health

1

Flow Initiation

Have you ever spent years honing a craft or skill and found yourself in the midst of it, caught up in the moment where everything occurs naturally and in rhythm effortlessly? In the beginning of your journey, you may have been awkward, may have stumbled or struggled to comprehend the importance and necessity of the mundane or tiny details. But as your attention to the details passed into a proficiency or mastery of them, they were no longer a struggle to you and just occurred naturally. Any parent or teacher could tell you they have observed this in a young child learning to walk or in a student surpassing many intellectual milestones before finally getting the bigger picture and navigating gracefully within it.

These fluid ways of being are called flow states in Positive Psychology. In his book, *Flow: The Psychology of Optimal Experience*, Mihaly Csikszentmihalyi explains how athletes, chess players, musicians, songwriters, playwrights, and everyday people enter exhilarating states of being where everything flows like a beautiful stream or a sonnet. These creativity states do not come to the lazy or uninterested, but rather to those who have worked, struggled, are mindful, and passionate. Who can forget Michael Jordan floating and twisting effortlessly while hanging seemingly forever in space to make impossible shots against three or four defenders? Even when he was recovering from food poisoning in the finals of the 1997 NBA championship, he got off the bench and performed flawlessly flowing from one basket shot to another.

Many athletes striving for Olympic gold have hired coaches to teach them flow, balance, and rhythm. Some top industry executives go to flow camps or hire flow coaches to help them achieve super productive and creative work modes. According to Csikszentmihalyi, "The optimal state of inner experience is one in which there is *order in consciousness*. This happens when psychic energy—or attention—is invested in realistic goals, and when skills match the opportunities for action. The pursuit of a goal brings order in awareness because a person must concentrate attention on the task at hand and momentarily forget everything else."[1] It's a way of getting in the zone where everything progresses without the gnawing pressure of time being a distraction from what is occurring in the moment.

In this book, I will encourage using flow states to become proficient in preventive health and wellbeing as it is outlined by Functional Medicine. I will also take a more literal approach to flow by showing how the delicate flow and integration of the organs and tissues of the body can either work smoothly or become blocked when a person is unhealthy. I want to help people find their groove and have good nutrition become as effortless as a walk in the park. It will take some initial effort though, with a sincere desire to find and achieve wellness. The problem with American nutrition is that there is so much misinformation out there, it's hard to get to running when walking has never been fully understood yet alone mastered. When it comes to optimal nutrition, you must work hard initially to create your own nutritional flow state. Once this is achieved, mindful and well-prepared meals create light within, strength without, and an overall zest for life. This will give you the energy and foundation to reach all those other flow states you are pursuing in life so that you'll find it even more enlivened and full of rich experiences.

Much of allopathic, or mainstream, medicine doesn't consider the importance of flow states, self-reliance in health matters, and relationships in health maintenance. Luckily for us, Functional Medicine is becoming a more common healthcare paradigm in the US. It is a more holistic approach that focuses on disease prevention through life balance, mental and emotional health, and nutrition. It incorporates the use of progressive, alternative, and traditional medical approaches to healthcare treatments so that patients aren't over or under-medicated or subjected to unnecessary surgeries. It encourages more of a proactive relationship between the patient and their healthcare provider. With Nutritional Flow, I aim to give you the functional health tools and knowledge to become more of a team player with your doctor so that you spend less time in the doctor's office and more time enjoying your health elsewhere. Every health concept I draw from in this book is derived from Functional Medicine. I draw on the concept of flow states because I want you to view your health as a hobby that you work towards. One in which you find joy and personal fulfillment.

The daily practice of a nutritional flow state can create a balanced life that flows smoothly from one purposefully enriching activity to the next, not unlike a road trip on a smooth highway to a favorite beach. Unbalanced and unmindful nutrient intake, like that prescribed in the Standard American Diet (SAD), could be compared to a poorly maintained but main thoroughfare maligned with numerous potholes. The ride is chaotic and bumpy with frequent damage to the vehicle and passengers. It will eventually encourage a total wreck requiring extensive and costly repairs.

Many of the methods and ideas I offer in this book are already practiced in one form or another in countries that have been focusing on nutritional medicine and preventive health for centuries. The concept of flow can be applied to a mindset of optimal efficiency, but also to energy flows that can either be blocked or released. According to Traditional Chinese Medicine, the interior of the body will become disordered and healthy energy flows blocked by poor nutrition, toxins, and poor lifestyles. Good digestion and nutrient absorption are severely impacted when digestive flow is blocked. Many ancient cultures, with their traditional ways of eating still intact, incorporate foods that naturally maintain the ecosystem within the gut, help nourish good bacterial health, and fortify the stomach lining. Balanced flow nutritional advice is diametrically opposed to the chaotic eating habits of many Westerners. The five-minute-finger-food-fast meal eaten in cars and on the run is the opposite of the slow and relaxed eating of proper foods beautifully arranged on the dinner plate in a carefully planned, creative, and inspiring environment.

It's not possible for every meal to be served on the wedding china with a seven-hour prep time. But careful planning ahead and finding healthy patterns and habits can make enjoyable and healthy eating a reality. Simplifying our diet and eating more slowly are the subjects of two recent American books, *The Slow Down Diet* by Marc David and *The Instinct Diet* by Susan B. Roberts. The French have long been accustomed to eating in a more relaxed setting of minimal dissonance and simple beauty. Lately, the top Western restaurants, following old European and Chinese traditions, are creating sacred spaces of beauty for dining. When people feel good, when they let the meal be an experience to savor, and are surrounded by geometric beauty, they are on the road to healing numerous medical problems and preventing others.

The outdated trends are reversing with the Mayo Clinic Health Letter giving people access to self-help tools on improving everyday health through simple means. In Western Medicine, the sick come together at the same space, the hospital, the emergency room, the surgery center, or the doctor's office. In Germany, the family physicians do house calls for the majority of their day.[2] They see most of their patients in their own homes, in their family spaces observing the gestalt of the whole situation in one glance. This helps them see the whole problem so they can be more accurate in their health prescriptions. Here in the US, people dress up, drive through difficult traffic, find a parking space in a crowded parking lot, and wait in an emotionally sterile and packed waiting room. The busy environment makes it difficult for doctors to focus on relationship building. Being so far removed from our natural everyday experience and off the planet compared to a flow state, people feel helpless, trapped, caged, and anxious. My experience has been that nervous people create complications in surgery and treatment. Their greatest fears become realized as a twilight zone type of self-fulfilling prophecy. In my clinic, we spend a lot of time with creative guided imagery to help people enter a hypnotic flow state where the best outcomes are imagined and achieved. More important are the nutritional, physical, emotional, and mental flow states at home. They prevent disease or ill at ease patients. One example of negative thinking that enables worse outcomes is the occasional patient who fears the procedure and bleeding so much that they will get drunk the night before the surgery. This produces blood thinning and makes the operation difficult because of excessive bleeding.

In my practice, I see patients in the office as individuals divorced from their natural flow state which includes the spiritual and emotional layout of their home and family. They are often dressing, acting, and talking differently than they do at home and I am hard pressed to be as accurate in my assessments as would a German family physician. I must talk longer, ask more questions, and observe the patient more closely to glimpse these hidden health and disease secrets. Western Medicine is so sterile, lonely, and isolated. It looks at the body as a mechanical, chemical, and electrical machine run by a computer brain with connecting pumps and pulleys.

From the paradigm of Western Medicine, illness is a function of the breakdown of a single part that can be fixed in isolation from the rest of the body, soul, and family dynamics. The picture of functional health revolves around relationships and orientation to family, friends, coworkers, mother, father, and spirituality. This can also be applied to nutritional flow and relationship mapping to food. The word companion is built from two older words *com* meaning *with* and *pan* meaning *bread*. In other words, a companion was someone with whom you ate bread. So, there is a relationship occurring between the person, the food, and the people dining together that creates a meaningful whole.

There are many ways these relationships play out. In balancing a diet, the relationship between the foods themselves can have very different impacts on the body. That's where this concept of unity and flow comes to play. A diet needs to be balanced and complete as a whole. When I am counseling patients with hypoglycemia, I tell them to never eat a carb snack by itself. It should always be a whole grain food eaten with a quality protein and a vegetable all consumed in the same meal or snack.[3] I tell them to imagine a dinner plate divided into three parts with the three components present, and then to shrink the plate to the size of the snack. This should be eaten between meals to prevent hypoglycemic attacks. Flow state nutrition is all about relationships in time, space, and family with foods and food groups and how they are all combined to produce health.

Food as preventive medicine is such an ancient practice that its beginnings are lost in the midst of time. Both the Egyptians and Chinese were writing medical texts as early as 2700 B.C. to 3000 B.C. The alternative medicine ideas in this book draw mainly from Functional Medicine, but also partially from ancient Chinese Medicine techniques that arose from Chinese herbalism, acupuncture, massage, moxibustion, breathing exercises, and movement exercises that have blessed the world for centuries. I also encourage other forms of energy medicine, such as reiki, that historically came from Japan.

Mindfulness is an important aspect of thinking and being according to many Eastern philosophies and religions. Being mindful of what you are eating and balancing your food groups is the basis of the Polycystic Ovarian Syndrome (PCOS) diet and hypoglycemia diets. Eating mindlessly is asking for nutritional deficiencies and excesses. Marc David, in his book *The Slow Down Diet*, describes how one of his patients kicked the habit of eating fast food on the run. He asked the patient to chew his hamburger slowly and try to stretch the meal to fifteen minutes instead of two minutes. When the patient ate slowly, the hamburger tasted horrible. After that, he couldn't continue eating fast food.[4] Eating mindfully, thinking about the food you are eating and why you are eating it, and being grateful for the food and the nutrition it provides are all important for proper digestion and extraction of nutrients. For example, if I have been exposed to mercury and want my detox enzymes to deactivate it, I eat a small handful of brazil nuts. The body can use selenium, which is found in high amounts in brazil nuts, to bind mercury. I eat slowly and imagine my body absorbing the selenium so the mercury detox enzymes can use it to deactivate and neutralize the mercury.[5]

In this book, I will go into chelation methods and various ways to rid the body of toxic elements and metals. I also go in depth describing the various ways enzymes and antioxidants can be destroyed with improper food preparation methods. From there, I will uncover the complex relationships between certain foods and enzymes because one food containing certain enzymes can help digest another food for optimal nutrient absorption. There's an art to this that can be elegant when mastered. Balancing food colors is an important part of five-star cuisine. There are many books and culinary schools dedicated to this. Dr. Eric Braverman wrote about the dynamics of food color balance in his book, *A Younger You*. Chris Woollams also demonstrates this in *The Rainbow Diet: And How It Can Help You Beat Cancer*. Colorful plants have pigments to protect themselves from harmful UV sunlight radiation. These same antioxidant pigments help prevent aging which is an oxidation (rusting) process in the body.[6] So, while I will go into the microscopic reasons why certain foods and food preparation methods are ideal, I will also show how this leads to my theory of flow nutrition. Because with flow nutrition, learning the small details will lead to a mastery. And the mastery is elegant, colorful, flavorful, and in a word: enjoyable.

Our homes fill up with knickknacks, clutter, furniture, and mementos from times past. Creating flow states and spaces is about removing all the refuse and uncluttering our homes so that the energy, or chi, flows through them again and gives us vitality. Our homes should have a very beautiful, simple, and clean appearance. Flow nutrition is about removing all the toxic debris and detritus from our bodies and simplifying what we put into them in order to restore vitality. A simple, clean layout inside our homes is beautiful and calming to the spirit. The beauty arises from clean lines and simple elegance. Our bodies become more beautiful to look at and stay young longer when we simplify our nutrition and eat a rainbow of beautifully colored foods with pleasing shapes.

Flow nutrition is about mindfulness. We need to bring this mindfulness into what we are eating, how we eat, who we are eating with, the environment of the meal, what we wash ourselves with and put on our bodies, what we think and meditate on, and what we choose to do and say in our lives. Mindfulness is like a sonnet. In a good sonnet there is movement thematically in space, in time, in color, in sights, and sounds. There is an ending which sums up the whole of the existence of the sonnet. With proper mindful nutrition, the flow of vital energy is restored to flow freely in every direction for improved health. Mindless eating leads to disease and weight gain. So many of our toiletries have toxic chemicals, makeup contains lead, and many of our clothes have toxic dyes and formaldehyde fixing the dye in place. Our sleepwear contains antimony as a flame retardant, so do our couches and beds. Sudden Infant Death Syndrome (SIDS) has been linked to it in research studies.[7] When we are mindful of our nutritional and physical health milieu combined with toxin avoidance, we become healthier.

With a holistic and functional health mindset, we can see into the future by understanding where negative paths or behaviors can lead. From that point of view, we can perceive proper remedies for restoring the balance during out of sync or rough times. In much the same way, many astute doctors can predict the future of smokers, sugarholics, drug abusers, and emotionally unstable patients. What is more difficult to do, is to predict the future based on a particular set of genetics, the person's current health status, and what the person is eating. It's now possible to get genetic testing, CRI Genetics is a great resource, for many nutritionally related genes and to alter diets to avoid future diseases.[8] This testing has become cheaper lately and is powerful in helping to avoid disease later in life.

Our lives can become locked into bad prospects for people, relationships, health, emotions, gossip, arguments, lawsuits, sickness and pain, robbery, fire, bleeding, job losses, and imprisonment. Creating flow states in our lives is about discovering whether these locks against people or prosperity are present and how to remove them or neutralize them. From a nutritional perspective, we can also analyze health locks preventing good health and neutralize them with proper herbal treatments and medicinal food thereby unlocking happiness and good health.

This book is written for Americans and those in other countries who have an equally poisoned food supply and toxic environment. Balancing nutritional wisdom with an understanding of our own genetics, epigenetics, proteomics, enzyme expression, environmental toxins, poisonous pharmaceuticals, toxic non-food substances that have been creeping into processed foods over the last few decades, inflammation triggers, and day to day ups and downs is the heart of this book. All this is inspired by the practices of nutrition as preventive medicine passed down from ancestors and peoples around the globe.

Our bodies are temples and are highly ordered but living in today's world is all chaos. The sections that follow in this book will bring order out of chaos and create a harmonious qi flow state. We will focus on the true foundation of nutritious foods and what makes them different from American supermarket foods that are grown in sterile soils and contain minimal naturally occurring vitamins. We will focus on how to build a healthy diet following a functional health plan and from ancient nutritional wisdom. We will learn how to undo a lifetime of bad eating and even how to quickly reverse the ill effects of a single toxic meal. Once we are eating better, we will explore how to get the poison out, reduce inflammation and metal toxicity, and restore the bacterial health of the gut. And finally, we will explore the complexities of the mind and how we can harness its potential for good. *Nutritional Flow* will teach you how to open your body's pathways to accept healing nutrients and will set you on a lifelong journey of whole health prosperity.

2

When Is Stress Good and When Is It a Disease?

There is almost nothing that can imbalance us more than a severe stress reaction. When stress traps energies in various organs, we get disease. At that point, the qi is not flowing in our sacred internal spaces. Wherever it gets stuck, that organ suffers. Hans Selye was the first to investigate the widespread organ damage and atrophy in rats from the stress of being forcefully immobilized; akin to the human patient trapped in a bad job. He noted intense shrinkage of the thymus, lymph nodes, adrenal glands, and numerous stomach ulcers.[1] Robert Sapolsky documents the widespread human disease from unrelenting stress: addiction, cancer, shrinking the hippocampus, which is the seat of memory, decreased testosterone, depression, infertility, sleep disruption, gastrointestinal disease especially ulcers, decreased growth hormone secretion, decreased immunity, miscarriages, increased pain, atherosclerosis, cardiovascular disease, and decreased skeletal growth in children.[2]

Stress is becoming such a catchword these days that it would seem everyone went to Iraq or Afghanistan and was suffering post-traumatic stress disorder (PTSD). Maybe wartime stresses everyone more including those left behind and the ones who should feel more protected. The actual percentages of PTSD in the surviving firefighters of 9/11 are

8.6% at baseline and 11.1% three to four years later for a total of 15.5%.[3] Between 2003 and 2010, 7% of female and 4% of male troops were diagnosed with mental health conditions within one year after their first deployments to the Iraq and Afghanistan wars.[4] Vietnam veterans had more PTSD with about 19% reporting it.[5] It also occurs in portions of the general public who have experienced or witnessed traumatic and life altering events. The causes are multiple: rape, assault with severe beating, sexual assault, serious accident or injury, shooting or stabbing, sudden death of a family member or friend, witness to a killing, and natural disaster.[6] Lack of adequate sleep is an important factor in how severe PTSD becomes. Many people reach for a sleeping pill when in trouble. Few know the extensive psychology research on sleep enhancement with cognitive behavioral therapy (CBT).[7] So sometimes scheduling a regular therapy session can prevent calling on "mother's little helper" every night.

Putting a severe stress response into our bodies and keeping it there causes lack of sleep. Psychological stress is easier to handle when we sleep well. If we sleep poorly, we can end up feeling the world has come to an end over some little annoyance that becomes a major psychological stressor.[8] Later in this book, we will talk about how to get a good night's rest and begin to heal ourselves. Achieving a nutritional flow state requires the energy of a rested mind and body.

Back in my military days before ever attending medical school, I was a fire direction control officer at a Nike Hercules missile battery on the Sosan peninsula of South Korea. I could stand on a high mountain top that overlooked the Yellow Sea on three sides and see the many layers of rice paddies fading into the sea. Inside the control vans was all hell, and outside the most beautiful view. Down below, the main camp of Charley Battery was surrounded by a double perimeter barbwire fence. It was a dreary military isolation hundreds of miles from civilization, but many little things made life interesting there.

One novelty we encountered was the number of puppies that would magically show up in the fall. They were slipped under the fence by local rice farmers who lived in grass roofed huts nearby. All winter we would feed them table scraps and they would grow fat and happy by spring. In the spring, they would all vanish overnight. Inquiring around I found out that the Koreans ate dog meat in June to ward off the heat. They observed that dogs don't sweat. By eating dog meat *gaegogi* in the warm season, they believed they would acquire characteristics of the dog such as not sweating during the summer. The name for beef *bulgogi* was similar and soldiers in the camp would trick the new soldiers into ordering dog meat at the local restaurant.

This is how I was introduced to a recent scientific rediscovery of ancient wisdom. Xenohormesis is the acquiring of protection from everyday stress by eating plants that have been stressed by harsh environments. Plants that are eaten by bugs are stressed. Their roots thrive in soil full of fungus, bacteria, bugs, and viruses. Also, a large amount of ultraviolet light is trying to burn the plants. As the plants defend themselves, they make antioxidants, antibiotics, antivirals, antifungals, and natural pesticides. These substances are quite useful to us who must live in the same stressful world. Eating plants in a less processed way gives us this same protection from the poisonous world in which we also live.[9]

Eating fresh produce would be beneficial for Americans, only the plants we eat are spoiled-rotten children, coddled in every way and protected from all the stressors that make the natural plants so useful. Recent testing shows they are practically devoid of vitamins and antioxidants.[10] Add to that the over processing of most foods and one can easily see why our kids will be the first generation in the US to live fewer years on average than their parents.[11]

Coldwater fish need to prevent their blood from thickening so it circulates quickly to muscles and vital organs. This cold stress causes them to make more omega-3 fatty acids, like those found in fish oil, which thin the blood naturally. There have been conflicting studies about the long-term heart health benefits of consuming fish oil that have caused some doubt in the medical community.[12] But further studies have found those studies to have inherent flaws.[13] Most of the other drugs recommended by doctors for the thinning of blood cause numerous side effects, the most dangerous of which is severe internal bleeding. The drugs also cause depletion of crucial anti-aging vitamins.[14] Omega-3 fatty acids are a part of all animals that eat living grass. However, in the United States, most people are eating animals that are fattened up in feedlots with moldy corn flakes devoid of omega-3 fatty acids. There appears to be a preference for the corn-fed beef taste. The wild game taste of grass-fed beef is not what most people are used to.

Ancient cultures and cultures that are still in touch with their roots believe in the special powers of sustenance and life. The wedding cake of the Romans, for example, was made from sanctified wheat representing a deity and was broken over the head of the bride and bridegroom. They ate the pieces and the guests picked up the crumbs. The belief was that this brought the divine into their souls and marriage. This is what many ancient religions taught. They claimed that the properties of the divinely blessed substances people ate would become the properties of their own bodies.

In the United States, many people are eating hamburgers made from eight-year-old milk cow meat. The cow is so spent she cannot give milk. So, the tough meat that is already drained of life is ground up, flavored up with glutamate poisons to make it better tasting, partially cooked, then frozen, and cooked again.[15] If we eat it, our bodies assume the characteristics of the meat: we get inflammation (something the cow had in old age), our vitamins decline, and we age faster. Eating two hamburgers or more a week is associated with increased risk of leukemia.[16]

If we want to remove the stress from our bodies, we have to remove the toxic meats of stressed animals from our diets. We have to replace them with organic grass-fed animals. Then we have to replace toxic vegetables with properly stressed roots and vegetables grown in natural soil with modern organic farming techniques. We are walking a tightrope, stressed to the maximum by imbalance. We need to get off of the tightrope and walk barefoot on solid ground back to nature nutritionally so we can become nutritionally stress-free.

We must balance the energy within, the energy in our living spaces, and our inner world of thought and emotion. Balance is so critical to our survival, that the organ responsible for balance and equilibrium is one of the first organs to develop in the fetus. We are human and different partly because we balance standing up in contrast to most mammals. Finding nutritional flow will bring stability back into our lives. Making these healthier lifestyle choices will also bring wellness to our ecosystems as we are supporting ethically raised plants and animals.

3

Root Magic

Root Out the Bad

Roots live in the most toxic world imaginable. Soil is aerated by fungal filaments, or hyphae, holding the dirt clods apart so air, water, and other nutrients like dead bugs and dead plant material can penetrate the soil. Many viruses, bacteria, and toxins thrive in dirt. So how do the roots stay healthy in this mess? They make antioxidants, antifungals, antibacterials, antivirals, and anti-parasite nutraceuticals to fend off the constant attack. They have healthy skin cells that are not loaded with toxic fats (trans fat) like ours are. They have a lot of vitamins to help them stay healthy. They purify the water they take in. The plants themselves also purify the air we breathe and give it oxygen.

If we eat living roots, we eat this protection.[1] Cooking destroys a lot of this living medicine found naturally in roots. As we age, we lose our capacity to manufacture enough enzymes to make our bodies work. When we eat raw roots, they give us enzymes that seem to be divinely made to balance the enzymes we do not make anymore and to help us digest that particular plant's nutrients. In other words, the nutrients in the plant are associated with plant enzymes that help process the nutrients for our use. Unfortunately, any temperature above 104°F to 118°F destroys these enzymes. Some say that our stomach digestive enzymes and acid also destroy these enzymes, but research shows the opposite.[2]

And yet, we should chew each mouthful of food at least thirty times, and fifty times or more if it is meat. This slows down eating and helps mix salivary enzymes with the plant enzymes, so the food is partially digested before we fully ingest it.[3]

Plant enzymes are effective at low and high stomach acid levels whereas animal and human enzymes need high acid levels to be activated.[4] Many, if not most, people make less stomach acid as they grow older. According to Hiromi Shinya, the leading gastroenterologist of our times, "There is no such thing as too much stomach acid."[5] Adults also make fewer enzymes as they get older. After puberty, people make about 10% to 13% fewer enzymes each decade.[6] So, their already diminishing levels of digestive enzymes do not work as well because they are not "turned on" by high acid levels. But low stomach acid causes more reflux, so the poor patient thinks he or she has too much acid and takes antacids further lowering the digestive acid. So, in the end, we need all the help we can get from fresh or lightly cooked roots and herbs. They have the enzymes we lack internally that are effective in low acid levels in the stomach.[7]

Our kitchens bring hellfire and damnation to the nutrients in our food. We peel the potatoes and carrots. We cook the vitamins out of the roots. We take the tasty part of licorice root, anise, which has no health benefits, and mix sugar with it to make candy. We do the same with ginger ale, which used to be made from the fresh ginger root. We do the same with root beer, changing the formula of mixed roots into a batch of similar tasting test tube chemicals.

When our intestines are infected with parasites, we are prescribed toxic chemicals that poison our livers. This must now be a joke for parasites because they have since become resistant. The living roots have been in this parasitic battle for eons of time. They've been perfecting the game for much longer than our drug companies have. Certainly, it will seem like our generation was living in the Dark Ages a hundred years from now when the real science, that already exists now, breaks through the money-driven corporate media barrier.

Extensive literature has been written about our great need for the enzymes found in roots, fresh foods, and lightly cooked legumes. There are three thousand enzymes that run our metabolism. Our pancreases are much larger than the average animal, vegetarian, or carnivore. It's theorized that the reason for this is because we eat too much cooked food. In fact, a large Filipino autopsy of a series of 768 cadavers showed the pancreases to be 25% to 50% larger than those of Europeans. Filipinos typically ate cooked rice meals three times a day. Rice is a food devoid of the enzymes necessary to digest starch. So, the Filipinos' pancreases had to make more amylases and proteases to compensate for the dead food that was lacking enzymes.[8] All fresh meat contains cathepsin. So, when a lioness is tearing chunks of meat off of a fresh kill, she is consuming vast quantities of the very enzyme that is needed to digest that meat.[9] Each fresh or lightly cooked vegetable also contains all the enzymes necessary for digesting that food. This is one reason why fresh foods spoil so rapidly. Their enzymes auto-digest the fresh foods and cause spoilage making it easier to become infected with bacteria.

Omaha Steaks are softer, juicier, and easier to eat because they hang in refrigerators for thirty days. This allows the cathepsin, nature's natural enzymatic meat tenderizer, to work on the tough sinews and thereby soften them. Wok cooking sears the outside of meats and vegetables but doesn't give them an internal temperature high enough to destroy the enzymes necessary for digestion. Steaming vegetables softens the chewy outside without destroying the enzymes. Low temperature cooking below 115°F also preserves the enzymes, but it takes longer to cook the food.

Consuming cooked food puts a heavy burden on our bodies. Since there are few enzymes left in heavily cooked and over-processed food, we have a hard time making enough enzymes to compensate. In many cultures on the planet, the time lapse from loss of all the teeth to death is ten years. A toothless person now has to eat heavily cooked foods that are softer and easier to masticate without teeth. Since these foods are devoid of enzymes, the malnourished person has to make up for it with increased manufacture of enzymes from an older pancreas that is putting out fewer enzymes each year. Within a few short years, the person is dead from malnutrition. It's said that many of the elderly in the US die from malnutrition because they eat these types of food and have the same enzyme deficiency.[10] Access to dentistry in the US is helping people live longer if they manage to eat the right foods.

These enzymes in food and roots are not just for digestion. They are also used by the body to rid itself of foreign proteins, cancer cells, yeast, bacteria, and viruses.[11] So, an enzyme deficiency, whether inside us or the food, can promote disease. The pieces of the dead bacteria, yeast, and viruses that remain in the body after a person is healed must be cleaned out by these very same digestive enzymes.[12] Being deficient in enzymes causes these foreign proteins to accumulate in various places causing arthritis, discomfort, and pain.

So, the magic of roots is in their enzymes and nutrients. We need their antiviral, antibacterial, antifungal, and anticancer properties to balance the negative qi in our bodies. This brings us back into harmony within ourselves and with our environment. Flow nutrition is about educating and training ourselves to find the more efficient and enjoyable ways of achieving an artful balance through healthy living.

4

The Light of Life

Do you ever wonder how all the medicinal herbs were discovered to be beneficial in the first place? The oldest medical textbook we have evidence of was written by the ancient Egyptians in 1800 BC.[1] It's an herbal apothecary textbook that describes the treatment of various diseases with different herbs. Many of these herbs are still being used today. For example, a standard dose of white willow bark contains 60 mg to 120 mg of salicin. The salicin was acetylated by Bayer in Germany in the 1880s and became acetyl-salicylic acid, or ASA, or aspirin.[2] Over one-third of the drugs sold by drug companies today come from herbs that have been used by herbalists for centuries.[3]

In fact, many drug companies hire researchers to find new cures in old places such as the traditional healers of the Amazon jungle or the shamans and witch doctors of African nations. These herbalists are a dying breed. Pharmaceutical companies hire researchers to live with them or visit them often. The way the herb is prepared gives clues as to which one of the many elements in the herb is causing the desired effect. Each herb is either soaked, heated, or stewed with either lye, alcoholic beverages, or water. This brings out different chemicals and alters them. Lately, researchers have complained that instead of brewing up something like willow bark for over two hours, the traditional healers reach into their medicine cabinet filled with western medicines and take an aspirin. We are rapidly losing the age-old wisdom of the ancient healers and shamans.

So how did the first traditional healers figure out which herbs to use? So much of what is in a jungle or forest is toxic. Even everyday foods, like the leaves of rhubarb, are toxic. Even drought grass, which is too high in protein, is toxic for cows. These ancient healers closely observed nature and wild animals. They had a sensitivity for the different frequencies of the substances found in plants. If they were lacking some nutrient that causes a deficiency syndrome, their bodies would sense the substance vibrating at a particular frequency in some plant. As they prepared the plant, they could sense when the frequency disappeared. So, they would try a different way until they found one that worked. They watched sick animals to see what plants they ate.[4]

They observed bears as they would wake up from hibernation. The bears would have colons full of toxic material. They saw the bears eat only certain plants, like osha, which caused diarrhea and cleansed the bowels of the toxins.[5] The bears of the Rocky Mountains eat osha root (Ligusticum porteri) which grows wild throughout the region. It's related to *chuchupate*, an ancient Aztec name which means "bear medicine." Bears used it for courting rituals, chewed it up, spit it on their paws, and washed their faces and bodies with it. It has been found to have strong antiviral properties in addition to its superior bowel cleansing ability. Current studies of osha extract find that it has distinct antioxidant properties that can benefit humans in different capacities as well.[6] Since bears lack a caecum and do not have the ability to digest cellulose, they are at risk of starving during certain seasons. However, closely followed bears have been seen to eat deer scat and deer intestines left by other carnivores which are loaded with the cellulose enzyme to help them digest grass and other cellulose-rich plants. Is this a learned or instinctual action? And if it's an instinct, do we have a similar instinct to guide us to the nutrients and natural medicines we need?

Our bodies are full of light. Each cell has many microtubules which not only transmit light like lasers, but also transmit chemicals, proteins, and hormones.[7] The fiber optic fibers that run through intracellular space also transmit light. There are frequencies of radio waves, microwaves, and higher waves that transmit information between cells and inside of cells. Each organ has a fundamental frequency.[8] Hormones and vitamins have fundamental frequencies. These frequencies are enhanced by the background electromagnetic field of the earth called Schumann resonances. Each plant has the same microtubules. Each hormone and vitamin in the plant has its own fundamental frequency. Toxic metals and toxic substances have frequencies that interfere with the frequencies of our beneficial nutrients.[9] Since we communicate throughout our body with nerve conduction, chemical signaling, and electromagnetic radiation, we need to keep all the communications flowing freely. We are ingesting many things that poison these delicate communication pathways. We are being radiated with many frequencies that overwhelm the delicate magnetic field of the earth and block the background support for the natural biorhythmic frequencies. The field of medicine which studies this phenomenon is called energy medicine and the devices which supply missing frequencies or neutralize bad ones are called electroceutical devices.[10]

Drug companies would have us believe that their ten-billion-per-year blockbuster drug is a cure-all for whatever ails us. Some of their medicines are very necessary. This was proven when they created the COVID-19 vaccines to combat the coronavirus pandemic in such a short amount of time. However, it's not necessarily true that their effectiveness in emergencies translates well into long term effectiveness for the treatment of milder chronic diseases. Side effects are often worse than original symptoms. Examination of the top ten blockbuster drugs reveals that their method of action is to poison or block natural pathways in our bodies.[11] This is more about symptom relief rather than curing the fundamental cause of the symptom. The puke 'em and purge 'em doctors of the nineteenth century employed this methodology when using mercury to cure constipation and other diseases. They often killed their patients. With the fourth leading cause of death being properly prescribed medicines, we are not far from this archaic medical fallacy.[12]

Each of the top twenty-five drugs exhibits symptom relief at the expense of extremely harmful and long-term side effects.[13] For example, there is irrefutable evidence that long term daily use of aspirin, Motrin-like drugs, and Tylenol will eventually lead to kidney failure and dialysis.[14] Long term use of statins can cause muscle wasting, congestive heart failure, and mental decline. Long term use of antacids can cause increased bacterial colonization of the stomach, more reflux, poor calcium and vitamin absorption, and inadequate protein absorption.[15] This malnutrition causes many other diseases. Long term use of antidepressants alters the way the brain works, shrinks the brain, and creates lifetime dependency.[16] Long term use of antihypertensives creates nutritional deficiencies that worsen heart disease.[17] However, people can have a stroke or heart attack if hypertension is not well controlled or cured. Please see your doctor before stopping any drug for heart related illnesses.

These examples of the serious health consequences of long-term use of the top ten drugs prove that the true underlying cause of the disease, and the body's maladaptive response to fight the disease, are not even considered in the design of these drugs. An immediate physical reaction is required in the design of the drug. To accomplish this, well known pathways in the body are blocked by sledgehammer force drugs. This immediate effect is desirable if a doctor wants to immediately bring down malignant hypertension to prevent stroke. It's also useful if someone is in full blown schizophrenic delusion and is about to kill someone. It's also useful if a patient has a large bleeding ulcer. The use of these drugs in emergency situations is one of the great advances in allopathic medicine. However, it's not necessarily true that their effectiveness in emergencies translates well into long term effectiveness for the treatment of milder chronic diseases.[18]

Long term use of the top ten drugs exposes people to side effects that may be worse than the original disease and often results in a life expectancy no longer than the original disease would allow.[19] In recent studies, cholesterol lowering drugs resulted in an all-cause mortality which was the same as the control group. The disease-specific mortality was improved, in other words, fewer people died suddenly of heart attacks. However, more people by far died of suicide in the treatment group. So overall, the death rate was the same in both groups.[20] You cannot write off equal numbers on one hand as being a fluke while on the other hand say that these same numbers are very significant. But is suicide a side effect of statins? The answer is possibly yes. The mental decline, memory loss, and depression associated with statins, and also cholesterol deficient diets, play a big role in the increasing suicide rate among the elderly and in male populations globally.[21] But more studies are needed to establish this connection. Just looking at the big picture produces another question. If a person's life doesn't last longer in the treatment group compared to the control group, would the person rather live life without drug side effects and die suddenly or would he or she rather die a different way after suffering drug side effects such as memory loss for years?

So, when we look at natural treatments for chronic diseases, we quickly find that they are nutritional and lifestyle changes. Nutritional treatments have been around for a long time. In 300 BC, Hippocrates said that food is medicine. This is included in the Hippocratic Oath that doctors take.[22] If we understand energy medicine to be a part of this process, we see that sunlight falls on the earth, is absorbed by plants, and becomes a part of all living things. When we eat fresh food or food that has been minimally processed, such as two-minute steamed broccoli, we are eating light. The frequencies of the nutrients fill us with the spectrum of the rainbow. They replenish our light starved bodies and drive out the bad frequencies.[23] When our bodies are full of light, we are happy. In each country that has been studied from Norway to Chile, the farther someone is away from the equator and the less light they have in the winter, the more often depression occurs. The closer they are to the equator, the more often people experience happiness.[24] So, it is with food. The more light there is in our food due to its freshness, the more health benefit and happiness for us.

Illness can be seen from many different perspectives. The newest and the oldest one is that our sick bodies lack certain light frequencies that are found in certain foods and herbs. The light frequencies are also stimulated and replaced by acupuncture, accumassage, energy therapy, chiropractic, and other ancient healing modalities. Hippocrates also said to first, "do no harm."[25] Doesn't it make more sense to try proven and harmless alternatives over powerful sledgehammer drugs for the early stages of chronic diseases before they become life-threatening and irreversible? We find German scientists at the forefront of nutraceutical research studying the forty thousand different nutraceuticals in any given herb for their now scientifically verified beneficial effects on our health.[26]

Knowledge is the power to find your personal path towards wellness. Always look for professional help concerning grave health matters. But also trust your instincts once you have developed them to understand what is beneficial to you. You will feel a more complete and calmer wholeness inside when you are consuming and actually absorbing the nutrients you need from your diet. Does the food smell and taste savory and full of flavor? Does it have a vibrancy, a crispness, or texture even after being cooked? These subtle cues are both amazingly satisfying for your taste buds and for your health. The cherished Vietnamese Buddhist and Zen Master Thich Nhat Hanh brought the element of mindfulness to the realm of nutrition in his book, *Savor: Mindful Eating, Mindful Life*. He writes, "Mindfulness is the guiding light that already exists inside every one of us. Discover it. We beckon you to use it and let it illuminate your life in every moment. Living like this, you will find yourself savoring your life deeply. Not only will this help you achieve the healthy weight and well-being you seek; it will bring to surface life's rich abundance that is so often invisible to us."[27] The observation techniques that are instinctual in us can be brought forward when we calm the chatter in our brains and focus our energies on the present endeavor and moment. Flow nutrition's main aim to help you be your own hero and perhaps a guiding light to help others. Whether you prefer to call it mindfulness or getting into the flow of learning, being, and growing doesn't matter. What matters is that along this journey of life we find the integration and connectedness that enrich the human experience and brings out our best selves.

5

The Balance of Fire

Stress Masquerading as Disease

Stress alters the way our nerves and organs work. Hijacking our powerful nervous impulses for a primitive reflex to run away from danger, stress shuts down gut function, reproduction, memory, and frontal cortex. The qi of the mind, body, and spirit is blocked and not flowing properly. When stress hijacks our bodies, we feel the increased tension, power, and nervousness, but also the many wear and tear side effects of high stress hormones. Stress effectively shuts us out of our flow state. If we don't reign it in, all the other areas of balance in our lives and health will start to unravel and fall into disrepair.

In my younger years, when I was serving as a second lieutenant in the military, I spent many mornings in the motor pool where we kept all of our company vehicles. We had huge books full of checklists for everything from engine checks and brake checks to light checks and fluid checks. Gone were any ideas of jumping into the jeep without a thought of whether there was gas in the tank or not. There was always something broken and in need of repair. When we checked the battery cables to see if they were tight, we twisted them slightly. After a month or so, the battery cable would become loose from the checks and need to be tightened. This happened with almost everything we checked. At the time, we thought all the equipment was just a bunch of junk; always broken, always in need of repairs.

Later, when I was a major in the United States Army and serving as a doctor instead of an air defense officer, I was stationed at Fort Riley, Kansas. It was home to the Big Red One, First Division: a tank heavy division. The division was called up in Desert Storm and went to Kuwait. It was the main thrust division of the attack on Iraq. My tank friends who went came back to a victorious welcome. Everyone said the same thing. They were all amazed at how well the equipment worked. They traveled 300 miles in a short time, engaged the enemy tanks, and deployed all over Iraq without a single piece of equipment breaking down. The tanks that were always broken in the motor pool did not break down under the most rigorous and harsh conditions in the sands of Iraq.

Our bodies are like that. They like acute stress situations such as exercise. They are designed for challenges of every kind. They are very remarkable as multi-fuel engines. They are great at detoxing pollution. They are self-healing. When we sit around in our lazy-man recliners worrying about everything like we had Howard Hughes' bacteria phobia, checking every system, it all seems to be broken and dysfunctional. But if we give our brains and bodies something to do like exercising, gardening, crochet, playing musical instruments, crossword puzzles, Sudoku, or chess, they usually last a lot longer. Studies show prevention of Alzheimer's in patients who keep their brains active.[1] Men who work out regularly by weightlifting have 40% greater growth hormone, which is really a repair hormone, than those who do not. Their testosterone level nearly doubles fifteen minutes later.[2] Studies of women who exercise show their hormonal fluctuations flatten out. During menopause, there are several studies showing the same benefits of exercise as hormone replacement and postpartum depression has been effectively treated and reversed with exercise alone.[3] These people have a greater healthspan, or life without disease, than those who do not exercise. Those who meditate, pray, do yoga, tai chi, qigong, and other spiritual exercises live longer and happier lives.[4] Those who engage in many social activities with friends as they get older live happier and longer lives.[5] It seems like going and doing is better for tanks and humans than sitting and rusting in fear and despair.

A topic that is being extensively studied lately claims that eating a wide variety of whole plant foods helps our bodies in numerous ways. Some foods develop defensive poisons to ward off the animals who try to eat them. Our ancestors continued to eat the potentially poisonous plants. Their bodies developed detoxification chemical factories in their livers. The acute stress of eating the plant brought out mechanisms to handle the chronic stress of eating it all the time. These same detoxification pathways now help us detoxify the numerous plastic and chemical poisons in our lives.[6] One group of plants in particular called the Brassica family, or cruciferous vegetables, have glucosinolates and sulforaphanes. These chemicals rev up the detoxification pathways that prevent cancer caused by the poisonous chemicals in our lives.[7] So, eating them no longer poisons humans, but helps us be healthier. This plant family consists of broccoli, brussels sprouts, kale, cabbage, and more.

When we develop chronic stress of any kind, our bodies adapt to that stress in numerous ways so that we can continue to live and accomplish our life goals.[8] Some of these ways are beneficial[9] and some harmful.[10] If we remove the acute stress, our bodies return to normal operations using a mechanism called homeostasis.[11] If we workout too much or eat too large a meal, our bodies, when healthy, can return to normal operations after a few hours or days. If we get injured, it takes longer but usually everything returns back to normal. The maladaptive response to chronic stress is often called a disease in its own right.[12] Often this disease becomes the enemy rather than the underlying stress that caused it.[13] Treatments, both medicinal and surgical, trying to stop the maladaptive response often fail because they do not fix the underlying stress.[14] Many modern treatments are designed around destroying the function or removing the body part involved in the maladaptive response.

A good example of stress induced disease would be gastritis, heart-burn, or acid reflux. Poor food choices, poor eating habits, and stressful lives cause heartburn. Once people get it, they want an immediate cure. The stomach acid is blamed for the problem and every means is used to get rid of it. Tums, Rolaids, or worse yet, aluminum magnesium hydroxide are poured down the gullet. When those don't work, there are stronger acid blockers like Prilosec and Pepcid. It's not unusual that none of these medicines work very well. Weaker stomach acid causes symptoms when it's refluxed and causes even more aspiration than strong acids in those who are on antacid therapy.[15] Since many people aren't aware of this, they still go to doctors who prescribe the purple pill for the rest of their lives. And this is despite the fact that the original medical research studies, the FDA, and available drug prescription information all say that they are only to be taken for six weeks. When these medicines do not work, people are sent down the road of destroying the function of the organ itself.

When I was a surgeon in training, we would do highly selective vagotomies on difficult stomach ulcer patients. The intent of the operation was to open the belly and destroy the nerves that stimulated secretion of stomach acid. As an ENT specialist, I no longer perform such procedures. Yet recently one of my patients visited me because of problems arising from surgeries to stop acid function. She developed severe gastritis. She had the nerve function destroying vagotomy and she ended up with ulcers anyway. She then had another destructive operation to remove a portion of her stomach, called a partial gastrectomy. When that did not work, she had a gastric bypass. Each medication and each operation were designed to destroy the function or remove the offending organ. She became so malnourished she broke her back climbing the stairs. The osteoporosis that caused the spinal compression fracture was caused by lack of calcium absorption. The body needs stomach acid to ionize calcium so it can be absorbed.[16] So, destruction of one organ, the stomach, led directly to the destruction of another, the spine.

As I mentioned earlier, this kind of medicine is not far removed from the puke 'em and purge 'em doctors of the nineteenth century. They used mercury for constipation to induce diarrhea. Sometimes the mercury dose was so high it would cause necrosis of the bowel and kill the patient. They also used mercury for poor urination. It would destroy the filtering function of the kidney and the patient would urinate vast quantities of urine called dieresis. Eventually the patient would die of kidney failure.[17] We still have the same medical thinking today with the same outcomes. This fixation on the symptoms of a normal stress response leads to all kinds of medical and surgical therapies aimed at destroying the function of some organ.

There are numerous medicines designed to block the function of some body process. There are selective serotonin reuptake inhibitors blocking the normal recycling of serotonin keeping it longer in the area between nerve cells where it works. There are calcium channel blockers. There are acid blockers and pills that block prostaglandin synthesis. We have antihistamines and leukotriene inhibitors. There are numerous examples of medicines that block normal function and maladaptive responses. The side effects of most of these medicines are in many cases worse than the original disease.[18] From the surgical perspective, we have gallbladder removal, stomach removal, hysterectomies, tonsillectomies, and ovary removal. The idea is if the organ doesn't work right and medicines can't fix it, remove it. There are many other surgeries that do the same amount of destruction.

With all this, one might ask, what about a more natural remedy that doesn't destroy function? What about looking for the ultimate cause of the symptom? What about restoring natural function? What about preventing the disease in the first place? Returning to stomach acid, why do we need stomach acid at all? What normal body process are we destroying by reducing it or eliminating it medically and surgically? The answer is shocking for a nation addicted to antacids. We consume more meat than just about any other nation.[19] The body needs stomach acid to digest meat proteins properly. Without the acid, meat literally rots, putrefies with bacteria, in the stomach for hours while the body valiantly tries to make more acid to digest the meat and kill the bacteria.[20] The stomach is fighting a losing battle once antacids are poured into it. The pylorus, or valve at the bottom of the stomach, shuts down tightly to prevent this rotten mess from hitting the delicate intestines. The food, most of which was eaten in the evening, stays in the stomach while more and more food is added. Ice cream snacks at bedtime are common in this scenario. Milk temporarily calms the stomach pain, but more acid results thirty minutes later.

The person lies down to sleep only to have the distended stomach push open the lower esophageal sphincter. The sphincter cannot keep contracting for so long against so great a load and pressure. Like an overfull dam, the leak starts with a crack which causes pain in the delicate esophagus. With the powerful stomach muscles churning the food every second, the leak becomes a flood. If the person is exhausted from overwork or sleep apnea, he or she passes out before this happens. The flood of acid rises to the upper esophageal sphincter where pressure builds.

When asleep, the body's response is to tighten the throat muscles to help hold the acid back. Tightening of the throat muscles causes constriction of the airway as well as tightening of the upper sphincter. Constriction of the airway causes more sleep apnea and arousals when the person wakes up to take a deep breath. If the flood of pressure is too great for the upper esophageal sphincter, the acid breaks through and settles in the back of the throat pooling in front of the vacuum cleaner larynx or voice box (it really does look like a vacuum cleaner attachment). The acid is sucked into the windpipe and down into the lungs. When any acid reaches the vocal cords, they slam shut. The person can't sleep while struggling to take a breath with vigorous chest heaves called apnea spells. Sometimes this goes on too long and the brain gets starved for oxygen. When this happens, he or she wakes up choking for air.[21]

I have seen numerous patients through the years who have called 911 and been rushed to the hospital literally blue in the face and panicking from this process. The diagnosis is missed in the ER. Some are diagnosed with asthma and are given asthma medicines. Some turn pink on the way to the ER and are diagnosed with panic attacks and are given antipsychotics. One gentleman in his late thirties had been to the ER in the middle of the night at least five times before he saw me and got the appropriate diagnosis.

In children, this process is often misdiagnosed as asthma.[22] They wake up in the morning with tight airways from all the acid inhalations. Asthma medicines help but they are only treating the symptom and not the underlying cause. Most of the asthmatic children I see, however, have other causes for coughing and wheezing such as allergic asthma or airborne pollution. Most pediatricians and allergy doctors are now looking for this acid reflux in small children with difficult to treat asthma. Nowadays, ER doctors are getting smarter and I see fewer patient referrals from them for nighttime choking episodes.[23]

If overeating is one of the major causes of this problem, it would seem simpler to just eat smaller meals and fewer calories at night after 5:00 p.m. or 6:00 p.m. An average American meal needs five or six hours to leave the stomach. Eating late has numerous other adverse health effects such as obesity, insomnia, and the disruption of normal homeostatic biorhythms.[24]

So, are we ready to stop chemically and surgically destroying our body's natural stress responses? Or are we happy to lose a stomach, lose a healthy spine, be anxious from malnutrition, or get depressed in the unrelenting progress of man-made disease? Are we ready to get off the corporate money-making merry-go-round of fake diseases, fake drugs, and surgeries that don't always work? When are we going to stop calling symptoms of stress "disease?" Are we going to wake up before it's too late and fix the chronic stress in our lives?

Organizational behavior is the study of how organizations affect the people working in them and how the employees and management work together to make the company successful. One consultant I knew went to a company where the boss was a workaholic. He rewarded everyone who worked like he did, putting in long hours and staying intensely busy.

His company was failing and going bankrupt. So, he put more work on everyone to do more reporting. They had to do more call backs on previous customers. No one ordered. The stressed employees couldn't make a deal on the phone. Stress was in their voices and they failed to listen to the customer's needs. They displayed the same insensitivity towards the customers that their boss did to them. An organizational behavioral consultant was brought in who recommended that everyone get off work early at 4:30 p.m. and to not work on Saturdays. No work was allowed outside of business hours and no bosses could call workers at home anymore. Within weeks, the employees were rested, happy, and this carried over into calling old customers and the sales shot up. So, the old workaholic approach was less efficient. Longer work hours for salaried employees translated into fewer sales.

One way to de-stress is to take a long vacation with no major plans. It shouldn't be a workaholic vacation with numerous trips and things to do. Another is to empty your evening and weekends of all planned activities, hobbies, and commitments for three months. After the three months, add back one or two of the most important evening activities. Many people find they do not want to add anything. Another is to go to Hawaii for three weeks and find a stress reduction spa that specializes in reducing stress hormones.

So, are we going to work ourselves to death or are we going to get into the zone breezing easily through life like Michael Jordan at the top of his game? Do we have intense focus when needed, total confidence, and qi flowing dynamically? And then can we find the counterbalance to that engaged involvement and relax to restore ourselves when needed? Sometimes in those moments of mindful and relaxed stillness, we can discover the more important aspects of our health and life that need the most attention.

6

One Is the Best Number Around

We are entirely dependent on the environment in which we live and this gorgeous planet earth. What we put in our bodies helps determine whether or not we are able to thrive rather than just survive. The human body has adapted and evolved to thrive with specific nutrients found in certain plants, minerals, and animals. With flow nutrition, we can see how even one vitamin restores the harmonious flow of qi throughout an individual. Achieving a nutritional flow state is more of a journey than destination. It involves learning and slowly adding to a solid foundation of knowledge, skill, and awareness. It's important to not become overwhelmed by the process along the way. In this chapter, we will focus on building knowledge about how certain natural foods maintain the body's capacity to prevent disease and aging. We will also discuss how to use supplements to aid the body when someone is battling a severe deficiency or having trouble with access to the fresh and quality food sources needed for health maintenance. The key here is finding balance where possible and starting at the beginning, or root, of the nutrient deficiency.

Doctors and clinicians recognize different levels of nutrient deficiency. All deficiencies start in the subclinical phase. This is when a person is slowly using up their extra storage of a nutrient and there aren't any obvious symptoms. The clinical phase is when a named disease is identified through a history of symptoms, signs of the disease found in an exam, and vitamin-level testing to confirm it. There is a spectrum of disease studied in animals and some humans. The spectrum starts with the single vitamin deficient diet. This leads to the first biochemical signs of deficiency found in the urine and blood. It then grows in scale to the frankly overt clinical manifestations of the disease. When the deficiency causes an actual disease, it often requires large doses of the vitamin to restore function and get rid of the disease. Scurvy in sailors is an example of a single vitamin disease. The beriberi disease is a clinical diagnosis of thiamine or vitamin B1 deficiency.

Let's follow a few studies as they track the different stages of nutrient deficiency disease in animals and humans. In this case, we'll focus on thiamine deficiency. One of the main vitamins in our cells that is used for processing sugar is thiamin. Thiamin is needed to process carbohydrates into energy. Many people in the US are drinking large amounts of sugary caffeinated drinks or Starbucks coffees because they are exhausted from thiamin deficiency. Thiamin is chewed up during the processing of sugar. The more sugar you eat, the more rapidly you become thiamin deficient. The deficiency is common in people who consume a lot of sugar, carbohydrates, and alcohol. Our ancestors in 1850s ate one pound of sugar per year mostly in the form of honey and other natural sweeteners. Refined sugar didn't hit the market until later. The modern American consumes 160 pounds of sugar per year.

In stage 1 subclinical disease, thiamine is used up in the body and nothing is wasted. So, there is less of the vitamin found in the urine. In stage 2, there is impairment of the red blood cell transketolase enzyme which is a thiamine-dependent enzyme involved in the production of NADH. NADH is a mitochondrial energy molecule involved in burning sugar for energy.[1] Stage 3 is the beginnings of physiologic disease. This is where vague symptoms associated with thiamine deficiency appear such as loss of appetite, insomnia, irritability, and malaise. Since these symptoms are vague and universal in the elderly and other populations, a clinician would rarely think that a vitamin deficiency was in progress. If this stage is missed and allowed to progress, Wernicke's encephalopathy may result.[2] This is irreversible and leads to death.

A study of healthy European seventy to seventy-five-year-olds tracked their subclinical deficiencies of the vitamin B1 (thiamine), vitamin C, vitamin A, and vitamin B2 (riboflavin). Over the course of the ten-year study, health problems progressed in severity and the numbers of patients affected increased. Without the testing, no clinician would have found signs and symptoms of deficiency in these "normal," and otherwise healthy seventy-year-olds. Their insomnia would have been written off as normal for their age. This is not a matter of letting healthy people go, knowing that six percent of them may have crucial vitamin deficiencies. We can all live with subclinical vitamin deficiencies, but these elderly patients' health problems progressed in severity. So, the authors of the study recommended supplementation to prevent progressing to severe disease.[3]

Stage 4 thiamine deficiency produces named diseases that are evident on a careful clinical history and exam: intermittent claudication or cramps in the legs, polyneuritis, bradycardia, and peripheral edema. Stage 5 thiamine deficiency produces anatomical changes that are irreversible and lead to death: cardiac hypertrophy, degeneration of cerebellum which results in dizziness, movement disorders, emotional disturbances, visual distortions, arrhythmia, and heart failure.[4] This is when Wernicke's encephalopathy develops.[5] So, getting the balance right on nutrient intake is extremely important. Younger people can get away with cutting corners because they might be in the earlier subclinical stages of deficiency and have generally more robust health. But as the years progress of poor diet choices, these deficiencies can slowly erode their health.

Now that we've cleared up why nutrient balance is so important, let's look at the ways everyone can become proactive about their health and prevent these very preventable diseases. With all the hype and hyperbole surrounding vitamins and the many expensive vitamin systems being sold by pyramid schemes, I'm still amazed at how much healthier most people can get from buying a few bottles of cheap vitamins and taking them on a regular basis. I'm going simplify this as much as possible for you in memory of my first successes at vitamin therapy with my family. What follows is an introduction to and a run-down of simple treatments for those who don't have the time or money to prevent disease.

For a number of years, I owned a medium-sized health food store. Since people knew I owned it, they assumed at the beginning that I knew all about vitamins and supplements. I was often asked at my clinic or at church about what natural thing they could take for this or that disease. I didn't know much at first so I would tell them to take vitamin C or some other vitamin I had just read about. To my great surprise, they would run into me years later and tell me that my advice had cured them. I was always shocked because I didn't know much at that time. The more I learn, the more shocked I am by my early success. I had read *Vitamin C and the Common Cold* by Linus Pauling[6] during my first year in medical school in 1979. That first year we took biochemistry and organic chemistry. We learned from our teachers, a husband-and-wife team, that vitamin C was involved in numerous pathways in the body including the brain alertness neurotransmitter formation. Since I had slept through a lot of high school classes and wanted to stay awake for medical school, I decided to take 1000 mg four times a day. After that, I never had much illness during the four stressful years of medical school and five years of residency. I found out that Linus Pauling had been right.

During that first year of medical school, my wife had gotten sick. She had two small babies to take care of and she wanted something natural, so she went to a naturopath who ordered Shaklee vitamins. She had been a secretary for a Shaklee distributor. She recovered quickly. Before this time, I had never taken a vitamin and could not afford one. But vitamin C was cheap. In retrospect, I also got a lot of B vitamins in the homemade bread my wife always made for my medical school lunches. I couldn't afford cafeteria food, so she would make me two packed meals, one for lunch and one for dinner. During my residency, the other residents would come up and ask for one of my extra homemade sandwiches. I think my wife kept several residents alive for five years.

In 2000, I decided to remove a skylight from my roof. I had been trying unsuccessfully for years to get other roofers in town to fix it. After they had supposedly fixed it, I would repaint the ceiling, but it would always leak again. Finally, I decided to get rid of it but was put on a waiting list by two different companies. After four months, I gave up and took it out with the help of my sons. They had not done roofing like I had, and I was very worried about them falling off the roof. They seemed so cavalier and careless, running across the roof, running down the roof after a sliding hammer. I kept telling them to be careful. So later when I was climbing the sixteen-foot ladder to get up onto the twelve-foot roof ledge, I did not have a ladder spotter and the ladder slid out from under me as I stepped onto the roof. I fell thirteen feet onto concrete and shattered my heel. It took a long time to recover, and my business slowed down. This is when I bought a small health food store to make more money.

Shortly after that my sisters called and told me that our mother was becoming very forgetful and confused and would sit around doing nothing all day. I was worried she had Alzheimer's. So, I went to the vitamin store and took off the shelf some of the more affordable brands including Life Force and Nordic Naturals thinking anything was better than nothing. I sent her four bottles. She miraculously recovered and it put off cognitive decline for several years.[7] Whenever she ran out, she would become confused again. Later when we were remodeling the store, my fifty-year-old brother came to help with the remodel for several weeks. He did not look good either. He had lost his edge and was confused all the time. His eyes were dull and sunken in, his mouth hung open, and his skin looked sickly. I tried him on the same four bottles, and he swears they turned his life around. Now he looks totally different than the haggard and gaunt-looking man that shocked me ten years ago. The accident and owning the store influenced me to find ways to help friends and family so they could take care of their health on their own or in my absence.

Supplementation at home is a way to prevent disease and remedy minor illnesses before they become major health problems. Our difficulty lies in making sure that we are taking quality supplements in the right doses for the health issues we are trying to fix. The Canadian government hired a team of researchers headed by Lyle MacWilliam at NutriSearch to review all the new vitamins and supplements that had been discovered in the last fifty years. They were asked to come up with a list of necessary vitamins, their appropriate doses (RDA), and toxic doses. By the second edition of the book summarizing their research, they had listed forty-eight necessary nutrients and vitamins.[8] Most of these could all fit into one pill. Initially, they were also asked by their government to evaluate the 500 different multivitamins on the market from nearly 500 companies to see how they measured up to this optimal list.

The book relies on various reputable scientific studies and uses them to establish the standards by which to evaluate 1,433 standalone products (single pill dosing) and 179 combination products (multiple pill packets). The vitamins would get points for being close to the Canadian RDA and demerits for having toxic doses of vitamins A and iron.[9] I was shocked to see some of my favorite vitamin companies that had helped my family so much were in the bottom third of the rankings. I was most interested in the vitamins that had 90% or above of all the necessary vitamins and nutrients at the right doses. There were only a handful of companies that met those criteria.[10] Later in this chapter, I will list the supplements from his book that I personally recommend.

The other much needed analysis the company Nutrisearch offers is a thorough examination of the safety of nutritional supplements citing that in the decade of 1994-2004 only fourteen unintentional deaths in the US occurred and most were accidental infant consumption. They compare this to the deaths of 106,000 Americans in 1994 due to the adverse effects of properly prescribed and taken prescription medications.[11] Of the many vitamins and herbal supplements, there are only a few that people should monitor for cumulative toxicity. These include overconsumption of vitamin A at doses greater than 10,000 IU. For pregnant women, they should preferably supplement with beta-carotene or consume lower than 5,000 IU. With iron, most fatalities have occurred in accidental overdoses of young children so monitoring or locking up chewable children's tablets is recommended. Among herbal supplements, care should be taken when consuming Ma-huang (ephedra), kava, berberine, lobelia, fox glove (digitalis), and mistletoe.[12]

The biggest health threat comes not from the substance of the herbs or nutrients but from the ways in which they are manufactured and processed. The FDA and Health Canada have inspections for pharmaceutical and food companies that will give products a stamp of good manufacturing practice (GMP) if they fit certain potency and purity standards. You can find these Canadian products in the American market although the US has no such system in place to authenticate supplement claims of proper manufacturing. The FDA regulates food and pharmaceuticals and has, in recent years, begun the process of doing the same for supplements.

In fact, part of what propagates the myth that supplementation and herbal remedies aren't effective is that they are produced with substandard materials. For example, for most of the last century, Americans have been consuming Parthenium integrifolium, also known as wild quinine or Missouri snakeroot, in place of Echinacea as it was labeled on the bottle. Another switch up occurred with ginseng as Americans were given American ginseng called Panax quinquefolius in place of Panax ginseng.

Why do we need vitamins in the first place? Why can't we just eat good food? The problem is that so much of our pretty produce and boxed or canned food have very few vitamins anymore. They are taken out by cooking and processing. Some of them, much less than forty-eight, are added back in.[13] A good rule of thumb for deciding which foods would be most nutritious for our families is that if there is a FDA approved health claim on the box, don't believe it or buy it. Fresh, whole foods do not need FDA approval to be healthy for us. Processed foods are unhealthy, and companies are always seeking ways to advertise that they are healthy. Their products have not been studied in research or double-blind studies to see if their health claims are true, but their processed ingredients have.[14] Oat bran is supposedly good for our hearts. So, health claims about it appear on all sorts of boxes. The actual comparison studies have been performed by independent researchers. Real oatmeal that takes ten minutes to cook helps us lose weight, whereas instant oatmeal can cause a three-pound weight gain over one month. Whole foods are better for us than processed foods.[15] Since we can't get away from processed foods entirely, supplements may be helpful. They are especially helpful if we are sicker than the average person we know.

So, if we are to take one vitamin when sick or running out the door in the morning, what would that be? As I said earlier that vitamin would be vitamin C. A while back, there was a conference on Vitamin C and cancer. Researchers from around the world presented numerous scientific papers confirming what Linus Pauling had said twenty years earlier. Linus Pauling won two Nobel Prizes, and almost discovered DNA which is related to his first Nobel Prize, the discovery of the alpha helix, and founded the Linus Pauling Institute which still produces high quality vitamin research today.

Vitamin C is an antioxidant. Think of it as a smoke evacuator. We need oxygen and sugar to start our internal fire in order to make heat and chemical energy for our bodies. The smoke from that fire in the mitochondria is free radical oxygen. The antioxidants evacuate this oxidized smoke from our cells so that it will not damage the delicate membranes and DNA of our cells.[16] The RDA for vitamin C was studied in the early part of the twentieth century. Limes prevented scurvy on Chinese sailing ships 600 years ago only to be rediscovered by European sailors 265 years later.[17] So, the early studies on vitamin C were to find the minimum dose to prevent scurvy which was 10 mg. The researchers were generous when they proposed six times that amount for the RDA.[18] However, there are a lot of pathways in our bodies that depend on vitamin C other than the collagenase enzyme that builds the protein backbone of our bones. And what are the RDAs for vitamin C for each of these enzymes? We don't know. Only the scurvy prevention doses have been studied. It turns out that we do not have to study them individually because we have other ways of knowing the right dose.

Too much vitamin C and will cause diarrhea and loss of potassium. Too little vitamin C and the mitochondria is poisoned with the oxygen radicals the vitamin C was supposed to remove. This causes people to age faster. Vitamin C hydroxylates the amino acids proline and lysine which are then made into protocollagen and then collagen which is the backbone matrix of bone onto which calcium is placed. This is precisely how scurvy is prevented. Vitamin C deficiency affects the dopamine to norepinephrine conversion since it's the cofactor that catalyzes that reaction. Without it, people get fatigued easily and have less alertness. The immune system depends on vitamin C to make peroxide through the catalase enzyme. Too little vitamin C dependent peroxide production results in an immune system that can't kill viruses. Vitamin C also is an important cofactor in the synthesis of carnitine which helps us lose weight by exercising.

All the organisms that have mitochondria on the planet use vitamin C as an antioxidant. Almost all mammals make vitamin C in their livers out of the glucose that is stored there. Only four mammals lack the enzyme necessary for vitamin C production: humans, monkeys, fruit bats, and guinea pigs.[19] Monkeys are used for research. A sick monkey can ruin an expensive research study, not to mention the budget of the researcher. So, the RDA for a 150-pound monkey, which has 98% of our human genes in its cells, has been a hot research area in the past. Researchers studied monkeys in the wild to see what they ate and how much of it. They measured the vitamin C content and then added it to the research monkeys' daily chow. They tried lesser amounts and got sick monkeys. That amount is 1,750 mg to 3,500 mg a day.[20] The trouble with vitamin C is that it leaves the body so quickly. It's water soluble and comes out in the urine. The other problem is that the body gets used to however much vitamin C is consumed on average.

If humans take no vitamin C supplements and don't have enough of it in their diets, they get used to not having it. Our bodies work hard to maintain constant but low levels of it. If we take high levels, our twenty enzymes that use vitamin C get used to those levels and increase their use of it. After that, if we miss a dose of vitamin C, these same enzymes working at a faster pace use it all up and we end up with less than if we had never taken it in the first place. Then we get sick. This is why the numerous human studies of vitamin C do not show much of an effect. Many were poorly designed and did not account for the biochemistry peculiarities of vitamin C.[21] The moral of all this is: if you can't take vitamin C on a regular schedule, don't take monkey doses of it. You will get sick when you miss doses. Take the RDA or less than 250 mg. If you want to take monkey doses, take long-acting time release vitamin C in its ester form and never forget a dose. If you do forget a dose, you will probably be more tired than usual that day and get sick two weeks later. It's also better to divide higher dose vitamin C into multiple doses. If you have food allergies and gut problems, the timed-release vitamin C may not be well absorbed. If you take too much vitamin C you might get diarrhea as a side effect. Also, men whose bodies make oxalate kidney stones have to be careful taking vitamin C in the form of supplemental ascorbic acid. Studies have shown them to have safer results from eating more foods naturally high in vitamin C if they want to improve their dietary intake.[22]

You might ask how much vitamin C the other mammals make in their livers. How much do they make when they are sick? Goats will eat anything and everything, kind of like humans. So, studies were done to see how their bodies reacted when exposed to viral illnesses. Their bodies took all the sugar in their livers and turned it into vitamin C because vitamin C is made from sugar. The first day they were sick, they made 100,000 mg of vitamin C. Their illness did not last too long because vitamin C is antiviral, and it turns on human and mammal interferon production.[23] When we get a virus, the body makes interferon to prevent the virus from spreading to other cells. Interferon locks up the other cells and keeps the virus out. Goats that weigh 150 pounds and are not sick make about 13,000 mg a day of vitamin C.[24] Guinea pigs, who can't make vitamin C, have an RDA that would be the equivalent of 10,000 mg a day if they weighed the same as humans. If we took that much, we would be healthier in one way, but get diarrhea, malabsorption, and get sick in other ways.

So, what about those who are sick, debilitated, over forty, and those taking lots of prescription medicines who think they might need some extra vitamins. Which one should they take? If someone wants to take just one multivitamin pill a day, which one should it be? This is where it's important to sort company hype from fact and rely on nutrition researchers, industry standards, and certifications. It always helps if the vitamin potency is analyzed by an independent lab. For example, vitamin D toxicity has resulted from a lack of an independent lab verification of vitamin potency.

Lyle MacWilliam, the Canadian vitamin researcher, lists eighteen health areas where vitamins have the role of supporting normal function: antioxidant support, lipotropic (fat) factors, liver health, metabolic health (insulin/sugar support), mineral absorption, bone health, phenols, ocular health, glycation (sugar protein) control, heart health, gamma tocopherol (vitamin E), bioactivity of vitamin E, methylation support (coronary heart protection), inflammation control, and bioflavonoid profile, potency, and completeness.[25] To these I would add growth hormone support, endothelial function support, intestinal lining support, blood brain barrier factors, mitochondrial support, skin health, kidney health, liver detox, and anti-aging SIRT1 gene support.[26]

I'm sticking with MacWilliam's categories in this section of the book instead of my personal expanded list. There are only a handful of multivitamins of over a thousand global brands he's researched that he gives his "NutriSearch Medal of Achievement" ratings. They are based on the optimal levels of dozens of vitamins, nutrients, phytochemicals, and antioxidants from Canadian research derived RDAs. He gives a platinum rating to the multi-vitamin Blueberry Health Sciences Essentials Premium III. His diamond ratings go to Blueberry Health Sciences Essentials Premium, Blueberry Health Sciences Essentials Premium II, DHelix Nutrition Alliance DNA Essentials, and Nutricleotide Health Nutricleotide Factors. He gives gold ratings to Douglas Labs Ultra Preventive X, Douglas Labs Ultra Preventive Easy Swallow, Rejuvenation Science Maximum Vitality, and Rejuvenation Science Maximum Vitality ESP. And lastly, he gives a silver rating to AOR Multi Basics 3.[27] His newest edition is a bit of a rewrite from previous editions as he explores more cutting-edge research into antioxidants and their role in pumping up cell's "heavy guns" that help keep us healthy.

Since many of these top-rated vitamins have six or more single pills to be taken in divided doses throughout the day, compliance may be an issue with busy or elderly patients. So, I recommend for the people who are only able to take one or two pills daily Rejuvenation Science's Maximum Vitality which is cheap at around thirty dollars with one pill being taken twice daily. The other, which I sold in my former health food store Happy Heart Specialty Foods, was Source Naturals' Life Force Multiple which is one pill taken twice daily for around twenty dollars a bottle. These two have the highest rating for twice-a-day pills and have the cheapest cost. Long term use is better guaranteed with the ease of access making them more beneficial than the higher priced multi-pill awarded varieties mentioned above. One way to get the best of both worlds is to take the higher priced alternatives when you are sick and switch to the lower priced brands when well.

After all this is said and done, there is a balanced approach to vitamin taking if you consider the flow of your daily life and the nutritional structure of your habitual diet. The best sources of vitamins and nutrients comes from lightly processed foods that are either lightly cooked or fresh when consumed. How you supplement your diet depends on whether or not you have the time, money, or resources to obtain all the nutrients you need. For example, if you don't eat grass-fed beef that is mostly hormone-free and never raised in a feedlot and don't eat fish twice a week, then you'll need to supplement your diet with fish oil pills. Pills I commonly recommended to patients and family members are Norwegian cold water fish oil pills from a high-quality brand and CoQ10 for those with heart disease, fatigue, and multiple heart medications which deplete CoQ10.[28]

Next, consider where you live. If you live in the northern half of the US and you don't tan in the summer, you will need vitamin D supplements.[29] This is especially true during the winter. If you are eating a lot of fresh broccoli or cauliflower that is lightly steamed or cooked in a wok, you probably don't need vitamin A supplements. If you are taking vitamin C supplements, it's best to consume them with fruits and vegetables.

You also need to consider your genetic likelihood for inheriting various diseases and your current health problems when deciding on which vitamins to take. For example, if you have Northern European ancestry and there is cancer, heart disease, cleft palate, or spina bifida in your immediate family, you need to take a special form of folic acid. The folic acid you want to take is the 5-MTHF variety.[30] Obviously, women trying to conceive and expectant mothers should be taking prenatal vitamins that contain this as well.

If you have memory problems or Alzheimer's runs in your family, you need vitamin B12 supplementation. Families with a history of heart disease should be taking niacin. If you are prone to migraines, you need to be taking mega-doses of all B vitamins, especially B1 and B2. If hip fractures and osteoporosis run in the family, you'll need more vitamin K2 and vitamin D3. Calcium hydroxyapatite is also very beneficial and highly absorbable by bones. If you have lots of allergies, skin rashes, dry and flaky skin, gut issues, frequent viral colds, you need vitamin A. The best source is beta-carotene from actual fruits and veggies. You can find it in apricots, kale, peaches, papaya, spinach, oranges, tomatoes, red peppers, pumpkins, guava, and cantaloupe.

Over the past years, vitamin E has been broken down and defined more specifically into eight different varieties of gamma tocopherols and tocotrienols that are also considered to be antioxidants. The best way to get health benefits from these tocols is to eat them in their natural form from seed oils and nuts. Gamma tocopherol is commonly found in canola, corn, camelina, linseed, soybean, and walnut oils. They have been found to promote stroke healing, lower the risk of heart disease, improve insulin sensitivity, protect brain circuitry, and prevent bone loss. It's important to note that previously alpha tocopherols were promoted to be the best form of vitamin E, but recent research has established gamma tocopherol to be the most beneficial for the body as it helps prevent prostate and other cancers, reduces stroke and cardiovascular mortality, and is anti-inflammatory.[31]

It should be noted that in most cases, a healthy individual with a balanced lifestyle and minimal family diseases who is eating a fresh and varied diet will not need to be overly concerned with supplements. In fact, it's better to gain nutrients from the foods themselves as they have cofactors that actually help you absorb the beneficial elements better. It should also be noted that obtaining vitamin D3 from fortified milk is not enough for even healthy people. However, while it's important to not overdose on supplement pills and vitamins, people who are concerned with their health should investigate what would be beneficial for disease prevention or overall health maintenance and supplement strategically. One vitamin pill is better than many vitamins. Some patients are taking thirty or more different vitamins for different reasons. Looking at their bottles, which I have done, I can find five or six bottles with nearly the same ingredients. Adding up the single vitamins for all thirty, I find them taking toxic doses of some and not enough of others. The B vitamins like to be in a ratio with one another. So does zinc and copper at 25 to 1 and calcium and magnesium at 2 to 1.

So, a simpler vitamin program is not only easier and cheaper, but safer. It's important to periodically go through your cabinet and get rid of expired or duplicate vitamins. Consider a powerful single pill multivitamin that has been tested for lead, purity, and potency that doesn't have toxic doses of ingredients and has been tested by outside laboratories to have the amounts listed accurately on the label. If it seems hard to sort out, see a holistic health practitioner, get a consultation with a nutritionist, see an anti-aging doctor, see a chiropractic wellness center, or an acupuncturist who knows nutrition.

7

The Antioxidant Agony

How We Rust from Within

When I was stationed in Korea for fourteen months, I often saw the Korean flag with its yin-yang symbol of red fire and blue water colors. The symbol is surrounded by four of the eight trigram symbols of the bagua which is an essential part of feng shui. I even learned how to speak a little Korean, along with learning the alphabet, and reading street signs. At the time, I didn't know much about the ancient wisdom of the symbol in the middle of that beautiful flag. Every day, I looked down from the top of a tall mountain to the Yellow Sea and saw a sharp demarcation of coastline separating the yang land and yin water. The wind blew over the mountain giving us breathtaking views and sunsets.

Not unlike the ever separate but intertwined symbol of yin-yang, our body parts and functions are classified into oily compartments and watery compartments. In allopathic medicine, most antibiotics are water-based and don't clear out the oily compartments where some pathogens prefer to hide. Naturopaths know this and use oregano oil and other oil-based therapies to clear the pathogens out of the oily parts, lymphatics, cell membranes, etc., of the body. Ignoring the oily compartments of the body leads to long treatment courses and failure of otherwise smart and effective scientific treatment paradigms.

The same goes true for antioxidants. There is a lot of hype about antioxidants in the popular media but they are never classified in the oily (lipophilic) and watery (hydrophilic) categories. So, there is a yin-yang perspective to antioxidants too. They are both necessary, and there needs to be a balance between the two. It's also necessary to have a balance between oxidation and reduction of oxidation (redox) by antioxidants. These are two separate processes with particularly essential functions in the body. For example, too many antioxidants can cause disease just as too few can cause disease.[1] Flow nutrition is all about balance and harmony. So how do we balance oxidation with redox antioxidants?

When people fast, or take a break from eating, they oxidize. This is therapeutic. It's also harmful when carried to extremes. Everyone except those who are pregnant, children, and the frail should fast once a month to clean all the toxins out of their bodies. Everyone fasts overnight while sleeping and breaks their fast over breakfast, hopefully with nutritionally balanced food full of antioxidants, to put out the oxidation of fasting. A whole new paradigm of intermittent fasting has become popular for weight-loss and overall calorie reduction.[2] These diets recommend stopping eating earlier in the day to extend the nighttime fast to twelve or sixteen hours. Some diets also encourage doing this for just a few days a week. The important thing is to incorporate it into the flow of daily life so that there is balance. Care should be taken so that it does not slip into extreme fasting, or in worst case scenario, anorexia.

When someone fasts, the oxidation forces the body to make more of its own antioxidants than usual. This helps remove poisonous toxins and heavy metals from the body, as well as excess hormones. People make lipophilic antioxidants and hydrophilic antioxidants in excess while they fast. They make protein-like antioxidants in their bodies when they eat high quality protein. This is turned into amino acids which are made into albumin in the liver. Albumin is a major antioxidant in the system, recently becoming a hot new research topic for many scientists.[3]

So why do people have to eat antioxidants if the body makes so many on its own? Why do they have to eat raw and steamed vegetables to get the enzymes that help their bodies process food if their bodies are already making the same or similar enzymes? Living in a toxic world, overconsuming lifeless dead food, drinking water with fluoride, toxic metals, and trihalomethanes, and breathing air filled with toxic gases and particulates puts a huge demand on natural enzyme defenses. They are overwhelmed, the enzymes depleted, the oxidation exceeds the natural redox antioxidant capacity and people literally rust inside like metal oxidizing in the rain. This oxidative damage to DNA, lipids, and proteins leads to heart disease, cancer, arteriosclerosis, diabetes mellitus, metabolic syndrome, Alzheimer's, fatty liver degeneration, and ethanol damage to the body and liver, and it promotes rapid aging.[4]

Bad food oxidizes the body even more. And yet, good food aids its antioxidant defenses. Oxidized albumin does the opposite causing diseases. Whereas the naturally antioxidant albumin, which carries antioxidant thiols and reduces metals, prevents disease. Oxidized albumin is found in cooked egg whites that once, when raw, had ovalbumin, a perfect protein that is a perfect antioxidant. When the egg is cooked, the protein is so badly damaged by heating that it loses its ability to trigger food allergy reactions.[5] Oxidized albumin is also found in pasteurized milk that once had lactalbumin, part of whey protein, that was full of antioxidant capacity.[6] Pasteurization destroys whey. So bad food, overly processed food, has the opposite effect of good and fresh food in the body. The two types of food may even look the same as they do with raw milk and pasteurized milk. But they do not taste the same and do not have the same health effect in the body.

In the United States, we tend to live yang lives full of frenetic energy that are completely unbalanced by the contemplative and relaxed yin. We consume Starbucks coffee with 320 mg of caffeine, three times the caffeine of a regular cup of coffee, drink lots of energy drinks with high caffeine doses, and take pep pills. We get up early and hit the gym outrunning, out-lifting, and out-exercising all previous generations. We're falling subject to over-training syndrome without even knowing what it is or how to treat it. Then we eat a very fast-food breakfast on the fly from the gym to the office in the car listening to audiobooks, all the while getting road rage and cussing at traffic. Then we enter the Machiavellian world of the modern workforce where we face gladiators whose only goal is to kill us: bosses from above jealous of our successes and threatened by them, subordinates from below trying to make us look bad so they can take our jobs, our fellow employees from the side, and lastly, waylaid by backstabbing from them all. Then we rush home, only to rush to the kid's frenetic life of soccer, gymnastics, football, taekwondo, etc. Then we rush over to friends, then start our take home-work or worse yet, go to a second or third job to help pay the mortgage on a house too big for our budget, and then rush home, and lay awake, wired and tired and unable to sleep without alcohol or Ambien, or worse yet, Xanax and Zoloft.

Everyone in Shakespeare's scenes knew what a yang life led to: early death, unnatural and sickly skinniness, consumption (Tuberculosis), plotting, scheming, and backstabbing. "It is not these well-fed long-haired men that I fear," said Julius Caesar, "but the pale and the hungry-looking."[7] Yin is sleep, water, relaxation, and harmony with the environment. Yang is all fire and destruction if untamed by yin. Severe, unrelenting oxidation is the Rosemary's child of the workaholic American life. Dipping into the yin water of relaxing, refreshing sleep, and nurturing our toxic bodies with the right antioxidants restores the balance of the yin-yang that lives at the heart of the South Korean flag. Achieving this type of balance leads toward the nutritional flow state. So much of this way of life requires paying attention and finding a mindful state of being. Armed with knowledge and skill, we can then use our senses as a guide to gravitate toward the healthiest options for us and to avoid the unhealthy or toxic paths.

Oxygen is poison. Plants, plankton, trees, and weeds get rid of it as fast as they can. They burn carbon dioxide from which, at the least, they produce sugar out of the carbon and release oxygen for people to breathe. This process occurs in their leaves and not their bodies. The thin leaves are porous which allows the oxygen to leave more quickly. If the leaf dies, the plant makes a new one the following year. They make many antioxidants to protect themselves from this process of handling the hot potato oxygen.[8] When people eat raw plants, they get some of these important antioxidants.

Like plants, humans must handle oxygen with care as we use it. When we burn oxygen deep in our bodies, we create an oxidative crisis. If unquenched by the proper antioxidants, the free radical oxygen damages our mitochondrial DNA. Fortunately, our own body makes many powerful antioxidants that are used here in the mitochondrial fires. But unfortunately for those who eat poorly, they must get other critically important ones, like vitamin C, that the body cannot make from food.

When we burn oxygen and sugar in the fires of our mitochondria, we make smoke there. It's called reactive oxygen species or ROS. Our nerves, heart, muscles, arteries, mitochondria, and mitochondrial DNA can be severely damaged by this smoke. The damage is so severe that, if unchecked by antioxidant vitamins and our own antioxidant enzyme systems, many serious diseases develop over time. Among these are coronary heart disease, cancer, cataracts, age-related macular degeneration, and neuronal diseases such as Parkinson's, Lou Gehrig's, and Alzheimer's.[9] So, we have several enzyme systems to help extinguish these fires. One of them is superoxide dismutase or SOD. It's dependent on vitamin C and other vitamins for proper functioning. If you want to be healthy, you can either increase the vitamins or reduce the ROS production.[10]

We usually make enough of our own antioxidants to prevent disease with the added help from those we get from plants. However, when we get older, we do not make as many of our own powerful antioxidants as we did when younger, and therefore, we rust faster.[11] The FDA does not recognize all these antioxidants as necessary supplements. Many researchers believe that vitamins can only be defined as the compounds that are vital to life and are not made by the body.[12] However, when we age, we lose the ability to make many other vital nutrients like CoQ10, the enzymes superoxide dismutase (SOD), and catalase. Many people in medicine believe that humans age because we are genetically programmed to age. The loss of vitamins and vital nutrients is believed to be a necessary part of aging. Others believe we age because of the loss of these vital nutrients that were formerly made in abundance.[13] Therefore, all these vital nutrients should be recommended with RDAs representing youthful levels. RDAs were originally created to prevent serious diseases like Rickets: a bone disease caused by the lack of vitamin D. We need new RDAs for optimal wellness, preventive health, and nutritional flow.

However, there are many more symptoms and signs of nutritional deficiency for each vitamin that do not disappear till much higher doses are administered daily. Some vitamins are toxic at higher doses, so there is a therapeutic window where too little is harmful and too much is harmful.[14] One way to sort this out is to do a functional vitamin assay to see how much of what a person eats and what supplement is actually being absorbed by the body and which particular vitamin is still lacking.[15] There are RDA's for only fourteen vitamins and fifteen minerals.[16] There aren't any RDAs for self-made antioxidants that decline with age. At least in Canada several researchers recognize all of these declining natural antioxidants and have given them minimum RDAs or recommended daily allowances. They even helped the consumer with MacWilliam's book, mentioned in the earlier chapter, that rates all the vitamin pills available worldwide against their golden standard RDAs for the essential nutrients.[17]

There are two major compartments in the body needing free radical protection from oxidation or rusting from within. One is the fluid compartment consisting of blood and intracellular fluids, the other is the oilier tissue compartment consisting of lymphatics and the protective cellular membranes that separate the cells from one another. Correspondingly, there are two antioxidant systems to remove the reactive oxygen species (ROS) from the body. The water-soluble antioxidants are vitamin C, glutathione, lipoic acid, and uric acid. The lipid or fat-soluble antioxidants are vitamin E, carotenoids such as beta-carotene and vitamin A, and ubiquinol or CoQ10. To get an idea of the relative density of these antioxidants and thus their relative importance, you only need to look at their concentrations in tissues and fluids. Glutathione has the highest concentration at 6400 micromole/Kg. Next is uric acid at 1600, vitamin C at 260, and CoQ10 at 200 micromoles/Kg.

Glutathione and uric acid cannot be taken as supplements. The body has to manufacture them. N-acetyl cysteine and two other amino acids combine to make glutathione. Purines give rise to uric acid. So, the most abundant and critical antioxidants are manufactured from food substances in our bodies. Disease, aging, and stress deplete these two substantially. A German study on total flavonoid antioxidants in the average German meal was 11.5 mg of flavanols from European fruits and vegetables, black tea, and wine. In this study, other epidemiological studies were reviewed showing a decrease of heart attacks and cancer risk with flavonoid consumption.[18]

Categorizing antioxidants is not easy. There are so many of them and most of the literature is outdated to point that they only share information about a few of them. So much of internet tripe on antioxidants comes from parroting the older literature to push this or that new-fangled antioxidant to make a marketing guru, who knows nothing about antioxidants, rich at the public's expense and loss of health. To be specific, antioxidants can be organized by their basic chemical structure. They are categorized by whether they are lipophilic or hydrophilic and by whether they are endogenous, made in our bodies, or exogenous, consumed as food or supplements.

Some minerals are antioxidants like iodide salts which are found in heavy concentrations in sea kelp.[19] Zinc is involved in many antioxidant enzymes[20] such as CuZn-SOD (SOD1).[21] Manganese is involved in a redox enzyme Mn-SOD (SOD2).[22] And importantly, selenium is the necessary activating mineral for one of the most powerful antioxidant enzymes glutathione peroxidase.[23] In order to help you keep track of the many different antioxidants that are beneficial to you, I'm including a detailed categorization chart below:

Categories of Antioxidants

Hormone Antioxidants	Melatonin[24]
Protein Antioxidants	Superoxide Dismutase (SOD), Glutathione Peroxidase (GPX), Ferritin, Ceruloplasmin, Bilirubin, and Albumin
Lipophilic Antioxidants	Vitamin E, Retinoic Acid (Vitamin A), Beta Carotene, Alpha Carotene, Lutein, and Lycopene
Hydrophilic Antioxidants	Vitamin C, Uric Acid, Glutathione, and Superoxide Dismutase
Hydrophilic and Lipophilic (Both)	Alpha Lipoic Acid
Self-Made (Autologous) Antioxidants	Albumin, Glutathione, Superoxide Dismutase, Glutathione Peroxidase, Ceruloplasmin, Ferritin, and Uric Acid.
Plant Derived (Exogenous) Antioxidants in Food	Vitamin C (Ascorbic Acid), Vitamin E (Tocopherols and Tocotrienols), Vitamin A (Retinoic Acid), Carotenoids like Alpha and Beta Carotene, Lutein, Lycopene, etc., Flavonoids and Phenolic Flavonoids, Non-Flavonoid Phenolics, Terpenoids, etc.

We should understand our wonderful bodies and all the natural antioxidants they make in abundance for nearly every need. If we don't, we'll inevitably dry up and burn from within. The fires of Mount Doom oxidation will eventually erupt into the darkness of aging. We need to be strategic in administering these nutrients rather than pouring useless and overhyped vitamins on an out-of-control fire. Using a flow nutrition approach to diet will help you increase your antioxidant capacity to put out these fires. Colorful foods, balanced proportions of quality and lightly processed proteins, natural and fresh oils, lightly cooked vegetables, whole grains, nuts, and a small helping of fruit will create complete balance without much worry or thought. In the following section, I will help you build a diet to include these essential nutrients that prime your body for deep cleansing and increased flow.

8

The Hype and Hawking of Miracle Vitamins

Snake oil salesmen hawked their worthless wares to unsuspecting Americans near the end of the nineteenth century. If a scientist said that frog tongues cured an upset stomach, the salesmen would buy frog tongues, mix them with vodka, and hawk their latest cure to the unsuspecting public. Testimonials were the glue that held this shaky enterprise together. Paid helpers would be in the audience saying to those nearby that they had been cured of this or that by the patent medicine. Unhealthy people were desperate to try anything that worked. The placebo effect would show an improvement in 35% of the people who tried the medicine. This guaranteed that enough people would be cured in order to ensure that the fallacious promotion achieved a life of its own with large groups of devotees.[1]

We are bombarded by the health claims of so many modern snake oil salesmen in every form of media. This creates a lot of confusion for the unsuspecting patient. The placebo effect will help some of these patients. So, the deception perpetuates itself. Particularly egregious sales are those made by pyramid marketing schemes. With our aging population of sick and wealthy retirees, there are a lot of customers for the fast pitch sales with glossy advertisements, titillating informercials, and numerous testimonials. Once they purchase the product, they are asked to sell it to their friends. If 35% of those purchasing the product are improved by the placebo effect, then the scheme is bound to make money for those at the top of the pyramid, but the rest are not so fortunate.[2]

For example, mangos have a chemical called mangosteen which is a powerful antioxidant. It has been promoted as a wonder cure by modern snake oil salesmen. There are literally hundreds of antioxidants in plants that help prevent aging, heart disease, and cancer. It's often better to eat them as the whole plant rather than as extractions mixed with liquor-like additives to sweeten the desire for modern nutraceuticals.[3] There are many different companies currently marketing mangosteen. Their methods of production and marketing begin with making a typical product from scratch. They can't sell the raw extract because it tastes bitter like many other antioxidants do. So, they mix a little pear juice, raspberry juice, blueberry juice, and cheapest of all, apple juice to the small amount of mangosteen bought from the supplier at dirt cheap prices. Now it tastes sweet and delicious and the scientific studies will show that mangosteen is a great antioxidant. They pass it around to their friends who end up loving the taste of something that is supposedly so healthy. Now they have testimonials. They hire a top marketing firm that helps them bottle it in expensive looking bottles and use modern marketing techniques that are known to work very well. They test market it to find the highest price that will sell. Then they bundle it in boxes of four or six and have monthly shipments that arrive on schedule thanks to credit card authorization. Then there are discounts for the sales reps if they get others to buy it directly from them or from the company. They get kickbacks if they make good sales and they get bonuses, vacations, and free cars if they are really successful.

When I was visiting the home of an elderly patient, I noticed some mangosteen bottles in her house and refrigerator. Four bottles cost almost three hundred dollars. I used to sell much cheaper bottles in my health food store that have the same ingredients. I also sold bottles of mangosteen pills that are guaranteed to have much more active mangosteen per pill. The health food store bottles sell for twenty-two dollars and probably have more active mangosteen in them than the four bottles of mangosteen fruit juice my patient bought.

There are other problems with fruit juice being the main ingredient of these snake oil products. There is a current explosion of obesity and diabetes in this country. Fruit juice is composed of fructose, glucose, and sucrose in varying amounts.[4] The sugar in these fruit juice products can raise blood sugar dangerously, especially if a person consumes one or two ounces of it daily along with all the other sugary products one consumes.[5] Each kind of sugar induces insulin resistance in a different way.[6] The fructose is converted to fat in the liver more so than glucose and is a leading cause of insulin resistance and obesity in the US among teenagers who consume soft drinks.[7] The sucrose and glucose sugar spikes after the consumption of fruit juice releases insulin which can cause low blood sugar. Over time, too much fruit juice, fructose, and glucose can cause insulin resistance and hyperinsulinemia. Insulin is an inflammatory hormone. When it's overexpressed, insulin causes many symptoms including mental fogginess, fatigue, increased pain, and dizziness. That wouldn't be so bad but hyperinsulinemia, insulin resistance, causes many diseases such as the group of diseases called metabolic syndrome which include abdominal obesity, coronary artery disease, hypertension, elevated cholesterol, proinflammatory state, prothrombotic state, and insulin resistance or glucose intolerance.[8] The overexpression of insulin causes our sugars to fall and the emergency response to this is to secrete adrenalin and cortisol which raise blood sugar and also cause hypertension, anxiety, and nervousness. Fruit juices promote yeast overgrowth in our intestines. The yeast release mycotoxins that poison the liver and brain. People feel lousy when there is too much fruit juice and yeast in their intestines.[9]

The promotion of one antioxidant over others causes problems. Our bodies need a lot of certain antioxidants that are crucial for removing the waste ash of the energy production fires in the mitochondria. The other antioxidants are helpful but not crucial to our survival. If we do not have enough of the essential antioxidants, no amount of these other useful ones will do anything for us. Our bodies even manufacture a lot of these essential antioxidants, although the levels decline with age causing numerous diseases.[10] If we are going to spend any money at all, we should buy high quality vegetables and some fruits. If we have any money left over, we should buy the vitamins and antioxidants that our body critically needs but doesn't make itself. We can even get tested to see if our bodies are functionally lacking in any of these critical nutrients. A few notable testing sources can be found online from Genova Diagnostics with their NutrEval test and SpectraCell's Micronutrient test.[11] We can even have our overall antioxidant capacity tested before and after changing our diet to see if we are eating enough vegetables.

Flax seed is another example of a product that companies hype with scientific findings. We see numerous examples of flax seed products on the market. Most of them are cereals with refined carbohydrates that cause more diabetes problems. However, it's true that flaxseed is good for us. It contains omega-3 essential fatty acids. Diets are often lacking in this essential nutrient. Fish oil, which is high in omega-3, is recommended by the American Heart Association for protecting the heart and preventing and treating heart disease.[12] Some people cannot tolerate fish oil because they get upset stomachs and burp up a rancid fish taste from cheap fish oil pills. These people can usually tolerate flax seed oil. The only problem is that if their diet is heavy in rancid oils and vegetable oils that have a lot of omega-6 in them, they will have trouble converting the omega-3 into DHA which the brain needs for proper functioning.[13] DHA is already present in fish oil and is ready to be incorporated into the lining of the brain cells.[14]

Is the flax seed in heavily promoted breakfast cereal products enough or of sufficient quality after processing to improve our health? The simple answer is that some amount is better than none. But if you want a cheaper more reliable source, buy organic flax seed from the health food store. In its whole seed form, we cannot absorb the omega-3.[15] Since it's hard to crush with teeth, we can buy a small twelve-dollar coffee grinder which we can also use to grind other healthy spices, grind up a tablespoon, and put it on our breakfast meal. It tastes good when fresh and is better for us. If that is too much of a hassle, we can buy it already ground in the health food store. It will be less fresh and less useful, but better than the inflammatory oils like corn oil that Americans are so used to.[16] If we are eating healthy already and wonder if we need flax seed in the first place, we can get our omega-3/omega-6 ratio tested with the aforementioned NutrEval test from Genova Diagnostics.[17] We can then eat more omega-3 foods and supplements and test again to see if we need to consume more or cut back on our omega-6 oils and foods.

A good rule of thumb is to go for the original product (in this case fresh-ground flax seed) that is scientifically promoted, eat it in its freshest and most unprocessed state, and balance the diet with many different vegetables, fruits, and small quantities of lean meats. In this way, we can be proactive about our health by laying out a simple and intuitive plan for healthy eating. We need to get away from the deceptive hype and hawking of miracle vitamins and fruit juices by the modern snake oil salesmen. They will only distract and block us from achieving our desired nutritional flow state.

Designing a Healthy Diet

9

Fractured Food Groups

Like the cartoon *Shrek* with its contorted fairy tales, our basic food groups are so fractured they are comically tragic. They are altered chemically and nutritionally from the original foods our ancestors ate. This is evidenced by a study of the immigration patterns of Asians to the US. They were found to move to Asian communities where they purchased and prepared the same foods they had eaten in their original countries. However, they were not as healthy as the relatives they left behind. They often gained weight and developed heart disease. It was found that the traditional foods they had eaten in their home countries were modified or fractured in the US from the original foods they had eaten previously. For example, the identical plant food grown in chemicalized sterile American soil had almost none of the vitamins and minerals found in the same plant food grown in Asia.[1]

Numerous studies show that the supposedly healthy original four basic food groups were unhealthy to begin with.[2] The first two groups: dairy/eggs and meat/fowl/fish emphasize excessive animal protein intake. After years of congressionally funded elementary school miseducation, our protein consumption has skyrocketed to 30% more than other nations. As a result, a study of the Standard American Diet showed 33% more calcium loss in the group remaining on the high protein diet versus those who were instructed how to eat the right amount of it.[3] The author of the *South Beach Diet*, cardiologist Dr. Arthur

Agatston, set up a research foundation to study the effects of healthier diets in elementary schools. One study, Healthier Options for Public Schoolchildren (HOPS), has spent over 20 million dollars on just one of their studies that helps children grow gardens and aids schools with providing healthier meals. The children lost weight on the diet, but often cheat with bad food brought from home in lunch bags.[4]

Our Big Macs, super-sized everything, and "all you can eat" buffets have brought us cheap meat by the wagonload. Our ancestors could not consume the vast quantities of meat and dairy that we do because it was money and labor intensive to do so. Only kings and queens could afford it and they had all the modern diseases we do including gout, arthritis, osteoporosis, and infertility. The original food group guidelines were sponsored by the meat and dairy lobbyists. Following the original guidelines from the 1960s will cause acidosis from excessive meat and dairy consumption. The least harmful thing that acidosis can do is strip the calcium out of your bones and cause hip fractures which is one of the leading causes of death for women, exceeding that of breast cancer.[5]

Does milk cause bone loss? Pasteurized milk causes bone loss according to a study funded by the Dairy Institute. The more milk that was consumed, the more calcium was lost in the urine.[6] The Nurses Fit study of 73,000 women found that excess teenage consumption of milk was associated with increased hip fractures later in life. This scientific study comes to the opposite conclusion of the advertising campaign by the milk lobby. Milk destroys bones in reality and does not build bones as advertised.[7]

One of the more current models of the food pyramid, or the "My Plate" model the USDA endorses, now shows five food groups with fruits and vegetables being in separate groups and the vegetable group has been enlarged. The grains group has been reduced from the original, but is still largely represented. The problem with this model is that it is largely deceptive. The reality of what people are actually eating when they think they are following this model is actually quite different. A few examples are listed below:

1. Fractured fats and oils (grocery store oils and margarines stripped of vitamins B6, E, magnesium, antioxidants, and more)
2. High meat diets from animals bred to have abnormal essential fatty acids and high chemical overload (antibiotics, hormones, pesticides)
3. Purified sugar or fermented sugars (alcohol)[8]
4. Broken or refined grains (again stripped of many nutrients to improve shelf life)

This new food pyramid represents over half of what we eat. For many, it's all they eat. It's not unusual for a baby to get half its calories from sugared artificially flavored fruit juices and the other half from overcooked pasteurized milk formulas. It's not unusual for a college student to survive on Diet Coke, candy, Twinkies, Big Macs, and alcohol. A hundred years ago, a typical poor college student would spend what little money they had on a loaf of bread and a brick of cheese. These freshly sourced foods, even though low in diverse nutrient content, in many cases is a much healthier way to eat when compared to heavily processed and artificial foods. In the next chapter, we take a closer look at how the everyday and casual consumption of unhealthy and unnatural foods can ruin a perfectly good day.

10

You're Only as Good as Your
Last Meal

With more food being eaten out than ever before, the possibility of health issues arising from this type of consumption also increases. Restaurants use microwaves extensively to thaw frozen food before cooking it. It has been shown that microwaves do not cook evenly by overheating foods and creating Frankenstein-like proteins. And simultaneously they under-heat the superbugs allowing them to survive.[1] Hopefully the further hot surface cooking will be complete and kill the surviving bugs. But according to the final analysis for home or restaurant cooking, the FDA statistics indicate this is not happening. Foodborne diseases are suspected to cause 76 million illnesses, 325,000 hospitalizations, and 5,200 deaths each year with 20% of these numbers being clearly documented pathogens.[2] In the following sections, the focus will be on how improperly prepared and low-quality foods affect your overall health and well-being. It is important to listen to your body because it is constantly informing you of the internal balance, or imbalance, of the system.

Part 1: Why You Feel Lousy After Eating Fast Food

When you feel ill after a fast-food meal, it's usually not due to pathogens. It's usually a combination of nutritional excesses, rancid fat, toxins, rancid protein, and food additive poisoning. You will also feel lousy because of nutritional deficiencies created by unnatural sugars and the overall imbalance of the nutrients that affect the processes of the body. This is what happens to the body after eating fast food:

Too much animal protein causes acidosis and subsequent bone loss, gout, and ketosis.[3] Excess protein is broken down into sugars by our bodies and stored as fat. High meat diets cause heart disease and weight gain.

Too much sugar causes hyperglycemia, reactive advanced glycation end products (RAGE), oxidosis, mitochondrial nutrient deficiencies, and hyperinsulinemia which triggers polycystic ovary syndrome (PCOS). High sugar diets, the average being 1.5 cups of sugar a day in various commercially prepared foods, can cause reactive hypoglycemia, hyperactivity in children, and mood swings in adults. Since glucose and vitamin C are on a seesaw, high sugar causes failure of vitamin C to be absorbed into the cell (vitamin C uses the same door into cells that sugar does). High sugar intake also causes immune system dysfunction because vitamin C is depleted in macrophages. They use it through the catalase reaction to create hydrogen peroxide which is used to kill cancer, viruses, and other pathogens.[4]

Too many vegetable oils cause a mismatch between omega-3, omega-6, and omega-9 fatty acids. Omega-6 fatty acid excess causes more inflammation by tying up the enzymes that convert omega-3 fatty acids into anti-inflammatory prostaglandins which are as powerful as aspirin or other powerful painkillers.[5]

Too much rancid fat causes heartburn, acid reflux, and esophagitis while hurting the rest of the body with oxidation and inflammation.[6] For example, rancid or oxidized Omega-6 fatty acids found in commercial food, fast food, and microwave food cause inflammation.

Too much trans-fat causes membrane instability in our brain, cerebral dysfunction, weight gain, and cancer.[7]

Too many food additives cause headaches, brain cell loss, weight gain, rashes, and ill feelings.[8]

Too many diet drinks and caffeinated drinks cause hypertension, insomnia, long term weight gain, and numerous other problems.[9]

Too many rich foods, protein, and sugar cause constipation, colon cancer, and higher estrogen levels in men and women.[10]

Too few vegetables in a fast-food diet causes potassium and magnesium deficiency which can lead to muscle cramps.[11]

Part 2: How to Reverse Fast Food Rotten Feelings

Occasionally someone will eat poorly and feel lousy afterwards. People are much like computers in this regard. If you put nonsense code into a computer, drivel and nonsense come out. If toxic food goes in, how can anyone expect to feel anything but toxic later? The usual treatment for feeling lousy after a meal would be to take antacids, aspirin, acetaminophen, or ibuprofen. However, the last three are toxic and the first one causes protein malabsorption, calcium and mineral loss, and putrefaction of animal proteins in the gut. When a liver is poisoned by toxic food, the last thing the body needs is a liver poison like Tylenol that makes the problem worse. The liver has a lot of work to do after a healthy meal. It can get clogged with overwhelmingly high volumes of toxic food that it can't detox fast enough thereby jeopardizing that person's health. Adding medicines that require large amounts of liver enzymes to detoxify to this dicey situation is asking for trouble. The kidneys don't like this double whammy either. Here are a few ways to reverse the effects of overconsumption of bad food without causing new symptoms and diseases that need further medications:

Overconsumption of protein can overwhelm the fewer digestive enzymes people make as they get older. If they splurge on that steak, they should eat lots of fresh fruits and vegetables a half hour prior to the steak. This will ensure that the plant enzymes are in the gut prior to the protein. They relieve the shortage of pancreatic enzymes caused by aging, malnutrition, and disease. This can also be done in reverse by eating plant derived enzymes that are pH independent after a meal. Plant enzymes help digest a stomach full of protein that is already lacking acid and enzymes.[12] If a person chews slowly and carefully thirty to seventy times a mouthful instead of gobbling food, the saliva is mixed thoroughly with very small particles for quicker pre-digestion and greater exposure to stomach acids and enzymes.[13] Chomping food leads to large chunks of protein that rot in the gut instead of disassembling quickly into highly absorbable amino acids. Human and animal digestive enzymes such as pancreatic enzymes are pH dependent. In other words, they need high acid levels to function, which most people don't have as they age.

The most common cause of acid reflux is not an overabundance of stomach acid, but a lack of stomach acid that causes the lower esophageal sphincter to relax too much.[14] Most elderly wrongly believe that they make too much stomach acid when the opposite is true. Insufficient stomach acid causes the lower esophageal sphincter to relax and even weak acid will go up the esophagus and burn it. People have a tendency to eat a large volume of food and liquids during a meal. This puts too much pressure on a weak sphincter and overwhelms what little acid the body can make. Plant enzymes are not pH dependent and do well in low stomach acid environments. Some companies like Enzymedica make products that have multiple and distinct plant enzymes which chop up food proteins into many little pieces. This helps disassemble the food and hide the evidence from an allergic person's immune system.

Acidosis reversal can be accomplished by eating raw vegetables or taking magnesium glycinate, tri-salts, Swedish Bitters, and if you don't have any of the above, you can use lots of neutral pH or alkaline water two hours after the meal. You can also use Rolaids which has calcium and magnesium in it to alkalinize or reverse the acidosis.[15]

Omega-6 imbalance can be reversed with one and a half ounces (a handful) of fresh walnuts. They are rich in omega-3 fatty acids and the handful of walnuts represents the minimum daily requirement for omega-3 fatty acids in the first place. Grass-fed beef (no feedlot exposure), wild game, ocean fish, and free-range eggs have omega-3 in them. The quickest natural reversal of this stomach distress comes with walnuts or 1000 mg of Norwegian fish oil or krill oil capsules.[16]

Rancid omega-6 overconsumption can be reversed with essential fresh omega-6 in fresh nuts. The quickest way is to take capsules of essential oils such as evening primrose oil, borage seed oil, black current oil, or pumpkin seed oil.[17]

Overconsumption of sugar in a single meal such as a snack of only sugary donuts can be partially reversed with vitamin C in high doses which balances the glucose load with the ascorbic acid load.[18] When you eat a lot of sugar, a good first line treatment would be to eat a plate of broccoli or cauliflower which have a lot of vitamin C in them. This will compete with the sugar for entry into your cells. The broccoli restores the balance. For prediabetics, something stronger like Bitter Melon pills or cinnamon can help lower blood sugar safely. They help quell the insulin surge that a bad meal causes and prevent reactive hypoglycemia from occurring later.

Glutamate, NutraSweet, and other excitotoxins found in hydrolyzed foods, autolysed foods, and barley malt can be partially reversed by eating more protein. Slurping on diet drinks all day long on an empty stomach causes serious neuronal toxicity. Diet drinks eaten with meals cause less neurotoxicity because animal protein may offset some of the toxicity. However, drinking diet drinks with meals has been shown to cause overconsumption of calories in the meals and eventual weight gain. So it would be better to avoid them or replace them with healthier options.[19]

Trans fats can be chased out with eggs which have choline, lecithin and phosphatidylcholine. All three substances come in pills if you want to have a quick meal fix.[20] Trans fats have been proven to distort cell membranes including brain cell membranes. This can lead to increased depression and increased cognitive decline and Alzheimer's risk in the elderly. The main health risk is the more commonly known increase in coronary heart disease.[21]

Too much sugar and protein causing constipation can be reversed by eating a handful of prunes, several Fibercon tablets, or psyllium husk powder. The better way is to eat raw cruciferous vegetables later by the handful.[22]

Too many sugar calories cause insulin release. The quickest way to reverse the donut sugar/insulin surge is to eat protein right away like a piece of chicken, turkey, or even a one-inch cube of cheese. After a while it will become habit never to eat a carb snack without protein to negate the insulin. When a person consumes protein, glucagon is released and it raises the blood sugar. Insulin is released when a person consumes carbohydrates and it lowers blood sugar. If the portions are balanced between carbs and protein, the net effect is no change in blood sugar and no change in the way that person feels.[23]

As for eating out, there are some suggestions for eating healthier. The top five healthiest chain restaurants are Panera Bread, Jason's Deli, Au Bon Pain, Noodles and Co., and Corner Bakery Cafe. Raw food restaurants with low temperature cooking to preserve the enzymes are the latest health food trend.[24] Whole Foods has a deli that provides some healthy choices. The National Restaurant Association brochure on "Putting Nutrition at the Center of the Plate" has some suggestions as well. The brochure states that "menu items listed as 'healthy' grew by 65% between Q2 2009 and Q2 2010."[25] So the public is demanding healthier choices in restaurants which in turn are responding to public preferences.

Some people find it hard to eat healthy and are eating poorly night after night. So this recommended treatment may not work as well as desired. It will help. So the best thing for those who want to change but are having difficulty, is to try one stress free day a week to eat healthy. After a while you can try every third day or twice a week to eat healthy.

Then go on to eating right every other day. Finally, you can eat healthy five days a week. The weekend will be a party to look forward to. At this point many will find they feel so lousy on weekends that they start to eat healthy there too. At that point, an occasional bad meal with a friend can easily be reversed with the techniques listed above.

Eating a plate of broccoli after a huge triple chocolate dessert may seem like punishment for some, but it works. After a while, it becomes easier to eat only three teaspoons of the dessert to minimize the damage and a few broccoli spears will do. The overall goal with nutritional flow is to be mindful of how the things you consume may be affecting you and then to adjust in a realistic way for the stage of development that you are in. If you are in the early stages of overhauling a health and diet plan, small adjustments to establish eventual positive habits are a realistic place to start. So, in a nutshell, we want to replace bad food with good nutrition and, where not possible, drown out the bad with properly matched good food.

11

Fake the Food and Fake Your Health

In Feng shui, chi flow is crucial to the overall healthy feeling of a home. Objects or structures that clash with the environment, impede movement, block light, or encourage mold and infestations represent the negative chi that will block the healthy feeling of a home. In terms of flow nutrition, the negative chi takes the form of toxins, ingredients, or poisons that do not belong in a healthy body. The goal with nutritional flow is to find that zone where awareness, focus, and eventually effortlessness lead to overall feelings and manifestations of wellbeing. When we use the term toxins, it generally refers to things that are immediately recognized by the body as elements that do not belong. Often the body responds with an allergic reaction. The body will go into crisis mode to contain or eliminate these negative intruders. The problem is that the more toxins that overload the system, the harder it becomes for the body to protect itself. The body begins storing the toxins in the liver, in fatty tissues, the thyroid, or the toxins simply act like a monkey wrench in an organ causing it to reduce productivity or produce cancers. In this chapter, we will put a magnifying glass up to these objects that do not belong to discover exactly how they destroy the health of an otherwise perfect body.

Part 1: Faking the Flavor

After the US signed the armistice to end the war with Japan, their navy ships docked next to the Japanese fleet. US sailors visited the Japanese ships frequently. When the American cooks went over, they were very curious to see what the Japanese Navy fed their sailors. They used similar ingredients in stews, but the taste was so much better. When the Japanese cooks were salting their soup, they dumped a lot of a white powder from a shaker into the mix. The American cooks noticed an immediate improvement in taste. They brought the powder home where it caught the attention of Campbell's soup. In Japan it was called Ajinmoto and in the US it was marketed as Accent. Campbell's soup formed the Glutamate Association, a group of companies dedicated to the promotion of widespread use of MSG (Monosodium Glutamate) as a flavor enhancer.[1] It's now hard to eat anything premade, in a restaurant, or from a premixed box in the grocery store that does not have MSG or one of its numerous imitators going by different names. The FDA has declared that it's natural, therefore does not have to be listed separately, but can be listed as "Natural Flavors."[2]

The Japanese promoted MSG as a flavor enhancer, saying that it gives a fifth taste sensation called umami. It gives the brain the pleasurable sensation that is necessary to tell it when protein is being consumed and how much. Humans need about three ounces of high-quality protein a day to be healthy. MSG tricks the brain into thinking that it's getting protein. MSG is one of the twenty-two amino acids found as building blocks in protein. In order to save energy and space, the amino acid glutamate is the protein sensor for the brain. It is also one of the neurotransmitters in the brain representing 60% of the neurons in the brain with glutamate receptors.[3] This makes it highly addictive because it makes the brain more alert. It has been added to cigarettes in a different form to make them more addictive.[4] And it has also been added to the majority of foods to ensure the overconsumption of those foods with larger serving sizes which leads to bigger profits.

When I was in medical school, students were taught that the tongue only senses sweet, salty, sour, and bitter. All the other flavors came from the added sense of smell. So when people lose their smell from a cold, flu, or a head injury, they lose most of their taste. Smokers lose their smell and taste too. Unfortunately, vegetables have little taste to begin with and children don't have a developed sense of smell till after puberty. That is why smokers and children do not reach for vegetables as often and why they prefer salty and sweet foods.

None of this would be so bad if glutamate were just another flavor enhancer like black pepper. But it is not. It can overexcite brain neurons and kill them. It causes hyperactivity in children and the need for drugs like Ritalin to control their behavior in school. It also causes sleep disturbance in teenagers. Lack of sleep has led to widespread emotional problems in teenagers which leads to doctors prescribing more Prozac.[5] Children do not have Ritalin and Prozac deficiencies.[6] The only way to cure a problem is to look at the root causes of diseases and fix those before the disease becomes uncontrollable. An important primal cause of their health problems is the overconsumption of free glutamic acid, something that nature never intended to be free. It should be joined with other amino acids in short segments so that its toxicity is neutralized till the brain and other tissues need it.[7] Obviously, the overconsumption of addictive MSG laced foods has led to the obesity epidemic in children requiring more drugs to lower blood sugar and cholesterol.

While all this seems bad enough, Senomyx, a company which supplies all the major food and soda companies with flavor enhancers, developed an aspartame and MSG enhancer from fetal kidney cells. So an abortion clinic fetus from the 1970's generated a kidney cell line which has been used to develop modifiers for our taste buds to make them more sensitive to MSG and aspartame (Nutrasweet). Since this allows for a reduction in MSG and aspartame content in food, the major food processors and soda companies licensed the technology for widespread use in their products. There are numerous patents and patent applications on file protecting this trade secret and the FDA has given the fetal cell

additive a GRAS rating (Generally Recognized As Safe).[8] These fetal stem cell products don't just leave the body after digestion. People are actually being genetically modified by them to enhance or change their taste buds to respond more strongly to umami and sweet tastes as well as the other taste sensations. There are grave ethical questions about this flavor technology. Modifying our taste buds without our knowledge and not doing seventy-year studies to see if it might cause overeating and obesity and obesity-related diseases in humans is a tragedy waiting to happen. It's bad enough that genetically engineered (GE) ingredients are present in nearly 80% of all processed foods[9] and the recent studies from Europe show that there is cauliflower mosaic viral DNA in all GMO foods[10] (these type of studies are banned in the US by our federal government). When the viral DNA inserts itself into our DNA, are we now being spliced into a new creature or a modern-day Frankenstein's creation? The mad geniuses who invented this technology are profiting off of dangerous and largely hidden science to make more money for food companies which in turn are owned by tobacco corporations.[11]

Part 2: Faking the Fat

Another fake food, "chemicalized fat," is mass produced in the USA. Trans fat is an elusive, yet ubiquitous ingredient in the American food supply. Despite new labeling laws, it's difficult to find it on food labels because the government has watered down the labeling requirements under intense pressure from large food corporation lobbyists. It's added to cakes, cookies, pies, muffins, nearly all fast-food products, french fries, sandwiches, frozen dinners, salad dressings, margarine, and even specialty ice creams. It's found in 40% of all the supermarket foods.[12]

Back in 1911, Proctor and Gamble tried to introduce lard into the market but couldn't get it cheaply enough from the slaughterhouses to make a profit. So they turned to a German chemist who had a brilliant invention, hydrogenated vegetable oil, which cost a lot less to produce and sell. By the time the cholesterol studies came out fifty years after its introduction into the food supply, two-thirds of all the oils consumed in America were coming from hydrogenated vegetable oil. Crisco rapidly took over the market and by 1960 had all but replaced butter and lard in American cooking. For decades it was promoted as the better alternative to animal fat such as butter, lard, and fatty meats. Yet all the while, the rise of heart disease mirrored the rise of trans-fat consumption from 1913 to the 1950s. By this time, the American Heart Association was claiming the existence of an epidemic of heart disease from unknown causes.

Doctors began publishing studies suggesting these trans-fat oils were possibly behind the sudden rise in heart attacks.[13] They were saying that it causes the good cholesterol to decrease and the bad cholesterol to increase.[14] Numerous studies have shown that trans-fat causes more heart and health problems than any of the animal fats. In response to this, the propaganda machine of Proctor and Gamble and Fleischmann's went into overdrive blaming butter and lard, both saturated fats, for heart disease. So much corporate sponsored research was done that the tide of public opinion, enamored with scientists of the Sputnik age, was turned against healthy fats and toward the unhealthiest fat ever invented. Great profit and corporate greed were at play due to the fact that vegetable shortening, and later margarine, were very cheap to produce and could be sold for a little less than lard and butter which were expensive to produce. Then the pharmaceutical industry saw a profit in this false science of cholesterol causing heart disease. Numerous poorly designed and completely bogus scientific studies were put forward to say a vital nutrient such as cholesterol was the cause of heart disease.[15] Before trans fat was invented, heart disease was hardly noted in any of the thousands of autopsies done in the world every year.[16]

Olestra is one of the fake fats invented in this fat-free boom. Potato chips fried with Olestra lowered the amount of fat absorbed by the body. But when the absorption of fat is prevented, it has to leave the body somehow intact. This caused numerous side effects, some of them rather unpleasant. The loose stools and diarrhea would have been tolerated, but the anal leakage or dripping of fat without a bowel movement was the intolerable side effect. One report stated in 1997, "The anal oil leakage symptoms were observed in this study (3% to 9% incidence range above background), as well as other changes in elimination. . . . Underwear spotting was statistically significant in one of two low level consumer groups at a 5% incidence above background."[17] Ironically, this fake fat can bond with other toxic fats in the gut and can be used to eliminate them although there are healthier, and more pleasant, ways of achieving this.

The body has ways of storing sugar as glycogen and fat. This stored energy can be retrieved for later use. However, fat storage does not release sugar. Exercise and starvation are the only way it can be burned in the mitochondria. Starvation is not a good way to burn fat. It turns on the body's energy saving systems and fewer calories are burned with the same exercise. Exercise, if done properly, can burn fat very well. People need to avoid excessive, exhausting exercise because it can put them into a mitochondrial exhaustion state called overtraining syndrome.[18] At this point, the mitochondria will have trouble making ATP, our main energy molecule.[19]

Since persistent organic pollutants (POPs) are fatty toxins, they are stored in our fat and other fatty tissues like our brains. But they cannot be burned in the mitochondria like the fat storage from overeating sugar, fructose, and natural fats. POPs have been found to increase the risk of diabetes.[20] The reason why POPs are called persistent is because they have a half-life of between eleven and fifteen years. So if a person's body is full of toxins, it will take approximately five half-lives or an entire life for them to disappear on their own. And all this provided that the tank is not being filled daily with fast food and restaurant fish.

POPs are dioxins, PCBs in transformers, chlorinated pesticides such as DDT, DDE, and chlordanes (termite treatments), weed treatments for lawns, and halogenated flame retardants found in children's clothing, beds, couches, chairs, and drapes. So families are surrounded by these toxins and they absorb them from physical contact, inhalation, and consuming them in polluted water, fast food, farmed fish, and sardines.[21]

It is possible to detox ourselves, but we will have to change our diets and continue the treatment for several years. There are several ways to get rid of these sticky toxins that cause obesity and diabetes:

1. Eating seven Olestra potato chips a day for two years. This will cause extremely uncomfortable side effects and may not be the best for health.[22]
2. A more natural solution would be to eat a slow cooked brown rice, chlorella, and green tea extract dish.[23]
3. Avoid salmon and other fish like carp, catfish, and tilapia because the vast majority of them are grown in fish farms. These fish are fed fish derived products full of PCBs and POPs. Avoid fresh-water fish from rivers and lakes such as the Great Lakes. Avoid non-organic meats and dairy products.[24]

Refined oils are not as bad as trans-fat but are lacking all the vitamins that were stripped out and sold to the health food stores for supplements. People need a variety of natural oils in the forms found in nature. Most people know to limit the amount of white sugar and white flour they eat, but it doesn't dawn on them that processed oils are the equivalent. Some people will call them white oils referring to the fact that they've been refined and stripped of nutritional value. As noted elsewhere in this book, even the standard organic olive oil you buy at Whole Foods doesn't contain the plentiful amount of antioxidants as the more expensive, yet freshly processed, olive oil. To get the health claims of olive oil, it must be processed into oil the same day it's harvested from the olive tree. Always look for a processed date on olive oil bottles if you want the health benefit.[25]

The other fake fat is the hydrogenated soybean oil. Soybeans in general cause gastrointestinal distress. Apparently, the inhabitants of East Asia knew this from thousands of years of experimentation. They eventually decided to only eat fermented soybeans since the fermentation removed the part that caused problems. Miso and tofu are fermented soy products used in small amounts as condiments. But Agra Business needed soybeans for another reason. They needed to plant soybeans in the corn fields to replenish nitrogen cheaply. The plant has a rhizome made of fungi that take nitrogen from the air and put it into the plant and soil. All plants need nitrogen. So this saved the expense of nitrogen fertilizer. Every so many years instead of nitrogen demanding corn, soybeans were planted. They were not very useful in the beginning except for animal feed and nitrogen replacement in the soil. But big Agra Business started looking for ways to make even more money off of soybeans. They couldn't get regular people to eat them because of gastrointestinal side effects. So they decided to push vegetarianism and put them into health food stores and talked the yuppies into buying them for health reasons.[26]

Soy milk was pushed as a replacement in formulas for children with milk allergies. Soon they were making more money than ever off of soybeans. The rich thought it was an imported delicacy. The poor saw the rich eating it and began imitating them. The only problem was side effects. The beans caused gas and lots of it. So they hydrolyzed the soybean and got rid of that problem. But then, soybeans are rich in glutamate which doesn't cause many problems as long as it's bound to other amino acids and released slowly by the body as needed. The hydrolyzed soybeans had glutamate in its free form, separate from other amino acids. In its free form, it readily absorbs into the brain and there is taken up by 60% of the neurons and excites them as never before. So much so that it kills them. It's one of the neurotransmitters, kind of like taking speed till your brain is mush. It triggers migraines and asthma attacks in susceptible patients.[27] They would never know from the healthcare world that their flare-ups are from these hydrolyzed proteins found in many foods these days. European watchdog governments have banned many of these MSG analogues for use in food.[28] They also cause increased cravings for the food that stimulates the brain to the point of illness, thus increasing revenue for the food companies.

It should be mentioned that soymilk also causes hormonal imbalances in young male infants. It stunts their growth because of the estrogenic side effects of an estrogen-like molecule in soy called genistein.[29] It's quite helpful for menstrual problems and menopause to harmonize the female system. Yet it is quite dangerous to male infants, boys, and men who are experiencing decreased testicle size, lower sperm counts, and lower testosterone levels than ever in US history.[30]

In the 1980s, the soybean was becoming a cash crop for all of the above reasons. But an even bigger money-maker was around the corner. Soybean oil was promoted to all the restaurants to replace lard for frying french fries.[31] It was cheaper and supposedly healthier than lard which we had all been told was the cause of heart disease, not the Crisco which had replaced most of the butter and lard fifty years earlier. Crisco and soybean oil have one nasty thing in common. They are both hydrogenated vegetable oils. Hydrogenated vegetable oils have 50% trans-fat by weight. Trans-fat has now recently been blamed for numerous health problems from heart disease and neurological disease to cancer. Since the bad press has surfaced over trans-fat, the fastfood market has been quietly replacing hydrogenated soybean oil for non-hydrogenated vegetable oil. But for thirty or more years soybean oil with its trans-fat had been the mainstay of french fries. It was another fake oil with a fake promise that destroyed our health and made millions for Agra Business.

Part 3: Faking the Water

Nothing is more enchanting than a waterfall dancing at your feet on the Wonderland Trail thousands of feet up Mt. Rainier. Your senses are enlivened with a cool breeze on a hot sunny day. Wildflower kaleidoscope colors are all around. The irregular pulsating sounds of a Riverdance staccato fills the air as the taste buds are about to experience ecologic ecstasy. Pure water, a unique and indescribable joy, trickles down the face, and refreshes the gullet. The earth's earlier inhabitants used to breathe the air of the gods on high, drink from Pyrenean Springs, and live in the luxury of Eden.

Nowadays, much of the water consumed in the US comes in plastic from faraway places that are rarely inspirational. Some would cause revulsion if seen. It's likely Cincinnati River water, with a modicum of sanitizing, sold as spring water with faded pictures of a mountain.[32] The public is being deceived into thinking they are getting something of greater worth than tap water with all its chemicals. The new water makes the kingmakers richer, but us poorer in pocket and health. It's hyped with fancy names like intelligent water, energy water, or nutrient water with a tenth of a cent of vitamins in it. The names are numerous, the deception is ingenious. Of the unpolluted springs left, many have been stolen from the local landholders. The water on the surface, the real spring water, is bypassed by pipes drilled deep into the underground aquifer. The water is pumped out by the trillions of gallons draining the local lakes and creeks dry. All the companies have to do is mix a few more chemicals and it turns into someone's favorite soda or seltzer. Over half the water consumed in the USA comes from a can or bottle. The energy wasted by corporate greed to double charge the American people for supposedly healthy water is incalculable.[33]

The waste of these bottles is creating vast islands of plastic in the Pacific Ocean that will take decades to break down but never fully disintegrate and will poison the waters and fish further. The trucking and shipping of bottled water poisons the air. These plastic bottles are also polluting the rivers of our bodies because each one contains small plastic particles that release BPA xenoestrogens into the bloodstream. Following this trend of taxing people for being thirsty, the next big thing will probably be pure air parlors, like the oxygen parlors in Japan, where people are charged just to get a breath of fresh air. It seems that what was once free is now exploitable. The rich are becoming richer through their buying up and cornering of the market of basic necessities. You could argue that tap water is unhealthy and cite all the studies that are used to scare people into buying water that in some instances is no less toxic. But the bottled water trend is not good for humans or the beautiful planet we've inherited. We are not going to leave it as we found it for our descendants.

Part 4: Faking the Salt

Modern table salt, whether labeled as such or as sea salt, comes from the chemical industry. It's purposely heated to high temperatures, treated with minerals and chemicals to keep it from caking or clumping, and often contains cyanide and aluminum.[34] This salt is also bleached by adding excess chloride to the mixture in order to remove the trace minerals that make real sea salt brown. They refine it further in a 1,200°F furnace that creates unnaturally hard salt. It takes the body eight precious water molecules to crack the diamond-like crystal created in the fires of a modern Mount Doom. Energy and water are lost in the process. This alien salt is everywhere. It's in water softeners, in rock salt, in shakers, in prepackaged store-bought food, and in restaurant food.[35]

No wonder it raises blood pressure. Ancient salt, now found only in a few places on the planet and is sometimes called Celtic Sea Salt, contains many trace minerals necessary for health and a hefty dose of magnesium which all lower blood pressure.[36] Himalayan salt is gaining in popularity. It is pure being harvested from ancient seabeds undisturbed by pollution.

Part 5: Faking the Protein

The last chapter itemized the raw food nutrients that should be flowing into each and every one of the body's cells. Most of them are essential, some can be made from scratch if the body is healthy, others are needed in toxic or diseased states, and some can be recycled.

This chapter demonstrates how these pristine nutrients are modified beyond recognition by the modern food industry. Nutrition, as taught to hospital, government, and corporate nutritionists in their master's degree programs, has changed little in a hundred years. To them, a calorie is a calorie and a fat calorie is a fat calorie no matter how altered or toxic it has become. A protein serving is a protein serving no matter how indigestible it has become, and a carbohydrate is a carbohydrate no matter how likely it is to cause insulin resistance. So when planning school or hospital menus, tables are used for balancing fat, carbohydrates, and proteins. These tables do not differentiate between the quality of the fat, carb, or protein. To do so would expose the sham of the food industry. Since the food industry controls research, publication, and training of nutritionists, the data is corrupted in order to conceal the fact that food is no longer as raw or real as far as the body perceives it. Some researchers are trying to get beyond the1940s studies to establish the differences between essential amino acids versus "dispensable amino acids." The unnecessary amino acids would not cause a problem or deficiency if lost in food processing.[37]

The same kind of misguided thinking has been rampant in the medical community where all types of fats are called by the same name in many of the medical studies on fat and heart disease. When the studies were first done, the toxic fat called hydrogenated vegetable oil was responsible for 90% of the fat consumption in America. But the original studies did not differentiate between this toxic fat, butter, or lard. Since the studies showed a correlation between heart disease and fat in general, it was wrongly believed that butter and lard caused heart disease. This led to campaigns to further reduce butter consumption in favor of the supposedly safer margarine which is 40% to 50% hydrogenated vegetable oil. Obviously, heart disease did not decline but went up after this. So labeling all fats under the same name made a dietician's job easier, but led to serious medical problems for everyone else.

What was once a proven scientific fact about fat is now one of medical sciences biggest blunders. Trans-fat is so toxic that it's required to be stated on a label if there is more than 500 mg per serving. Many food manufacturers simply change the serving size on the label so they don't have to change the product. They simply change the label to read "Trans Fat 0g." These products still have trans-fat but the public is unaware that they are being poisoned by it. You might think this is an exaggeration and that no food company would lie about something so life-threatening. Most food companies are owned by tobacco companies that lied to the public for years about how safe tobacco was and used fake or manipulated studies to back them up.

So in regards to the health food store or companies claiming to have healthy foods with healthy ingredients, can their labels be trusted? It turns out that many of them have been using GMO corn and other GMO foods in their products.[38] The outcry was so bad over this news, that one of them said they would label the GMO foods in a couple of years.

What about foods cooked at home? Does cooking destroy the quality of food? It seems that people are more addicted to their taste bud fulfillment than the common sense of eating responsibly. It seems like every new menu in the restaurant is loaded with sugar, toxic fat, burnt meat, or Cajun seasonings loaded with MSG. It tastes good but often leaves people feeling so bad they have to poison themselves with other medicines to squash the miserable gastric symptoms.

To understand exactly how dangerous these burnt meats affect health, it's helpful to understand what they do to the body after being eaten. There is a folding structure for proteins similar to a folding chair or a folded new shirt still in the bag. Some proteins are folded four times and are called quaternaries. This delicate structure is greatly affected by food processing such as heating, cooling, mechanical stirring and beating, hydrostatic pressure, and ionizing radiation. Current FDA laws and the Codex Alimentarius from UN treaties require radiation of food produced on farms. Shipped food bought off of the internet is subject to radiation from scanners looking for bombs. Food proteins are denatured or altered by acids and bases added while cooking, interactions with metals in the food itself, cooking pans, high salt concentrations, organic solvents, chemicals, and colorings. Denaturation or change in structure is often an irreversible process.

Some of the undesirable denaturation processes are the destruction of enzymes that help metabolize food in the body, the exposing of peptide bonds in the protein to chemical degradation, the altering of water retention properties amongst many others. Food processing causes chemical degradation of proteins by several known reactions. Everyone from the corporation to the middleman, to the consumer is happy. But the human body is not tricked into health by fake proteins that have degraded essential amino acids. The body can't make the essential amino acids. So if they are not in the fake food, a deficiency disease results.[39]

Imagine what would happen if you threw bleach on a beautiful nature painting. It would not only destroy the painting, but cause harm if it splashed on clothes, the wall, or other people. Processed food is often treated to alkali, a harsh alternative to bleach, high heat, and high pressure. Not only is the natural quality of food destroyed but we are also destroyed. This even extends to those for whom we cooked or bought food for as they are harmed as well.

Overcooking food creates many anti-nutritional factors that ruin our health and prevent proper absorption of critical minerals and amino acids. The food lacks vitality, life force, and energy and causes the same reaction in us. Poor growth in infants and children, bad gastrointestinal tract problems, and dysfunctional immune systems are just some of the many problems with processed foods. The worst effects are seen in mono food diets consumed by babies, teenage boys, and the elderly. Obviously, a well-rounded diet rich in lightly processed natural foods would overcome the effects of an occasional bad processed food or fast-food meal. These anti-nutritional factors are studied extensively in order to improve the diets of American meat animals which include chicken, turkey, hogs, and cattle. There are many ways to eradicate the anti-nutritional aspects of their diet in order to achieve maximum healthy weight gain in the animals. With human nutrition, however, there are studies showing how these anti-nutritional factors are created, but not much is being done to actually improve the quality of food in the US.

Many natural foods are hard to eat because of anti-germination enzymes that prevent seeds from sprouting till conditions are right. They also contain pesticides that prevent animals and insects from eating them. So when we do not prepare these foods right, we are poisoned and have our digestive enzymes blocked. Everyone knows that to cook raw beans you have to soak them overnight to get them to properly begin to sprout or they will have to face gastrointestinal distress. Fermentation, sprouting, hulling, and many other techniques are used to get rid of enzyme inhibitors traditionally. Lately, modern food manufacturers are using high pressure, high heat, and alkali treatments in addition to the previous.

Modern human food processing is not focused on growing healthy children and maintaining health in adults, but rather it seems to only care about making the product taste so good that it will sell more and increase stock prices. Thus modern food processing with high heat, high pressure, extrusion, mechanical grinding, and alkali treatments create a large number of anti-nutritional factors that destroy our health and ability to absorb minerals and high quality essential amino acids from unadulterated proteins.

These Frankenstein food anti-nutritional factors are trypsin inhibitors, phytates, tannins, excessive DNA nucleotides, Maillard reaction products (MRPs), D-aminos, and lysinoalanine (LAL).[40] Trypsin inhibitors are found in soy, peas and beans, cereals, potatoes, and tomatoes. Fortunately, they are inactivated by food processing unlike many other anti-nutritional factors. Unfortunately, they are still present at high levels in adult soy beverages, lower levels in infant formulas, and somehow end up making people sick when soy is added to tuna salad. They cause loss of digestive enzymes, poor growth in infants, and poor repair in adults. Another major problem is that they cause the pancreas to enlarge by making more digestive enzymes to replace the destroyed ones.[41]

Tannins are enzyme inhibitors and resist food processing. In rich countries, people avoid foods that have them. However, in poor countries, these foods are staples and are the leading cause of malnutrition since the tannins prevent absorption of vital amino acids. They protect grains against insects, birds, and fungus. But they make us sick. Found in sorghum, a drought resistant grain popular in poor countries, beans, peas, and millet, they can bind up to twelve times their weight in protein. They can cause parotid gland enlargement as well as the protein malnourishment called kwashiorkor.[42]

Phytic acid is found in seeds, grains, nuts, and legumes. It chelates or binds essential minerals like magnesium, calcium, sodium, potassium, and zinc. When it binds minerals, it deactivates digestive enzymes that depend on the minerals so people don't absorb essential amino acids. Like tannins it resists destruction, but unlike tannins, it's found in many foods in developed countries as well as poor countries.[43]

Maillard reaction products (MRP) are made by a caramelization process producing caramel from milk and sugar or browning meat with sugar rubs. High MRP causes 50% of the protein in a food to be lost. Liquid infant formulas have high MRP when compared to powder infant formulas which have low MRP. Males aged eleven through fourteen often have mono food diets consisting of a few high MRP foods in the fast foods and snacks they eat. They can have stunted growth because of it. Dairy foods, eggs, and cereals are most susceptible to Maillard reactions when processed. Lysine, an essential amino acid for immune health and muscle is deactivated by this food processing into lactuloselysine which has no benefit to health.[44] So why do people intentionally cause MRP formation in their precious foods? Because it tastes and looks better! It sells more. To make up for the loss of lysine in milk, biscuits, bread, and pasta, health food stores sell lots of super lysine to help the now dysfunctional immune system.

Almost every molecule on the planet comes in two forms which are mirror images of each other. One left-handed and one right-handed. Our bodies are almost all left-handed and raw foods are mostly left-handed. However, when food is processed, it becomes right-handed which is useless to us. These products are called D-amino acids in contrast to L-amino acids. The D-aminos cause malabsorption of protein and protein indigestibility. They are created by high temperature and pressure in food processing. For example, raw milk has the lowest level of D-aspartic acid which is a fake amino acid. High levels of D-aspartic acid are found in milk powder, kefir, evaporated milk, yogurt, infant formulas, heated soy, bacon, crackers, Mexican pancakes, and corn cakes.[45]

Another product of food processing is a fake amino acid combination called lysinoalanine (LAL). Like phytic acid, it can bind minerals such as calcium, iron, zinc, and copper. This causes numerous health problems as mentioned earlier with phytic acid. The other toxic effects are decreased lysine, cysteine, threonine, decreased protein digestibility, and severe kidney damage. The safe dose is less than two hundred parts per million. Yet many high temperature cooked foods have five to ten times more than that especially liquid infant formulas, sausage, chicken, and eggs.[46]

Gout and kidney stones are caused by consuming foods high in nucleic acids. Although there are a lot of natural foods that people have to avoid with these medical conditions, modern day food processing is making food choices worse for these patients. Brewer's yeast and other food yeasts are added to many processed foods to make them taste better. Unfortunately, they are very high in nucleic acids.[47]

As you can see, natural foods cause disease if not prepared properly. However, the biggest problem is high temperature cooking that creates Frankenfood and many anti-nutritional factors that destroy health from every direction. So moving from the overall structure of food proteins, we can zero in on what happens to the many essential and conditionally essential amino acids as the food is processed. Heat treatment of foods creates abnormal reaction products which have been studied and are used as markers to see how much the amino acids in protein, especially lysine, have been degraded. The Maillard reaction products

(MRPs) are furosine, N(epsilon)-carboxymethyllsine (CML), hydrox-ymethylfurfural, pyrraline, pentosidine, and pronyl-lysine. Of these furosine has the highest concentration followed by CML, pyrraline, and pentosidine. Furosine shows up with mild degradation. The others have more severe heat and Maillard reaction degradation. Since lysine is an essential amino acid and is so easily destroyed by the Maillard heat reaction in cooking, its loss is troubling. It's even more distressing when you learn that the many proteins the body makes depend on lysine as a rate limiting step. Without lysine, you can't build the many necessary functional parts of the body including muscles and tendons.[48]

Even fermentation of foods creates biogenic amines in sometimes toxic amounts. The enzymes in the supposedly friendly bacteria make the toxic amino acids such as tyramine in aged cheese which causes migraines and asthma attacks in susceptible people. You can utilize biogenic amines in normal metabolic pathways, so in one sense they are functional. But if you consume too many, they can create illness. It's not unusual for a wine and cheese snack to create toxicity from high levels of tyramine and histamine in wine, and others such as putrescine, cadaverine, phenethylamine and tryptamine. Tyramine has been found to cause pathogenic bacteria to adhere to the intestinal mucosa and cause disease. The presence of alcohol and medicinal drugs in the gut at the same time in large doses of biogenic amines causes systemic absorption right into the blood where they trigger release of adrenaline and noradrenanline, increase cardiac output, cause tachycardia, raise blood sugar levels, and hypertension. They also cause increased gastric acid and stomach pain.[49]

But looking at baby formulas which depend on a single over processed protein source, the deficiency of lysine becomes tragic. For several months, lysine deficient baby formulas are all the baby eats.[50] An easy way to see how much the food has been degraded is to analyze the lysine levels compared to furosine which represents the amount of inactivated lysine. Some formulas for infants and protein drinks for older hospital patients had more inactivated lysine than lysine, suggesting considerable heat damage. So the dietician makes rounds in the hospital consulting on patients who are wasting away and prescribes a diet of six cans of adult protein formula a day. However, according to a research study, the adult formula may not have enough lysine to reverse the wasting disease state.[51]

So for thirty-six years I have done major cancer surgery on patients who were cachectic or super thin from liver disease and alcoholism. If they did not eat enough real food, they were losing bone, muscle, and had abnormally low albumin levels. If their albumin was less than 1.8 compared 4.0 as normal, they had a 50% chance of a serious complication from the six-hour surgery, such as pneumonia, graft necrosis, and fistula. When we tried to cure the complication we consulted the dietician, who recommended six cans of adult formula daily. They had trouble getting even four cans down. So they lost even more weight and the fistulas did not resolve with repeated surgery until we got the albumin up to 3.2. In retrospect, this recent study shows why we had so much trouble getting the albumin up before, during, and after surgery. The adult liquid meal replacement drinks were missing lysine, a critical amino acid for muscle, bone, and tissue repair. So the recommended dose to supplement when consuming adult meal in a can or if you are eating too much fast food and over-processed package food is 1000 mg to 3000 mg of L-Lysine. It is also recommended to supplement with vitamin C in divided doses two or three times a day.

The Mallaird Reaction Products (MRPs) also destroy tryptophan which is the amino acid that is a precursor to the hormone that makes you feel good called serotonin. They deplete zinc, which is necessary for two hundred enzymatic processes in the body, and copper which is also critical.[52] Methionine and cysteine are also lost with food processing, thereby reducing the digestibility of the protein.[53]

Many normal amino acids in their free form (not part of a complete protein) are added to food for various desirable effects. For example, glutamate is added to give food a pleasant umami or meaty taste. Glutamate has been extensively studied for ill effects in humans in its free form. Everyone knows it better as MSG or monosodium glutamate. A recent study showed adding free amino acids one by one to a standard protein diet for rats caused stunting of their growth. Alanine was the only essential amino acid that caused no growth retardation. The rest varied from 8% to 79% with only 3 below 25%. So weanling rats do not tolerate free amino acids very well. In fact, 5% cysteine in the diet caused deaths.[54]

As mentioned in the last chapter tyrosine is the precursor to all the brain neurotransmitters for alertness: epinephrine, norepinephrine, dopamine, and L-dopa. It is also the precursor to thyroid hormones. For these reasons, it can be used as an antidepressant. What is little known about tyrosine is that it's degraded by food processing into a toxic amino acid called tyramine. Although it can't cross the blood brain barrier like tyrosine, it nonetheless causes migraines. For years I have counseled migrainers to avoid foods rich in tyramine like aged cheese, beer, sauerkraut, chocolate, soy sauce, soybean derivatives like miso and tofu, teriyaki sauce, and tempeh.[55] In fact any spoiled, smoked, pickled, fermented, marinated, or aged protein from any source, animal, fish or plant can have its tyrosine converted to tyramine.

Tyramine can cause hypertension. It should not be eaten with mono-amine oxidase inhibitors (MAOIs) because it creates a hypertensive crisis. So making food tastier by aging and fermentation can cause health problems in humans. Since so much of our food is processed, mixed, cooked, frozen, and recooked, amino acids like tyrosine suffer degradation into toxic amino acids as a result. It's unfortunate that many of the things that are done to food to make food tastier causes illness later.

Cadavarine is the decarboxylation or rotting of the amino acid L-Lysine. As seen in the last chapter, L-Lysine is critical for health, depleted by modern food processing, and is missing from corn and all corn products. Lysine deficiency causes widespread disease and frequent viral outbreaks. What is even more harmful than not getting enough of it in our fast over-processed food diet, is getting its rotting byproduct, cadaverine. Cadaverine stinks like rotting cadavers and that is why it is given its name. To keep rancid food from stinking, many additives are put in it to improve taste and smell. These additives are for the most part harmful as well. So we are fed rancid food loaded up with more toxic additives to make it seem to taste normal or better than normal. Welcome to the Alice-in-Wonderland food megalopolis where nothing is real or as it seems to be. Cadaverine is toxic and, at high doses, kills rats.[56]

One of the food products people are commonly eating is pink slime. The food industry calls it "boneless lean beef trimmings." After store bought meat is trimmed and presentable, it goes to the market shelf pretty and tasty but wrapped in toxic phthalate plastic to keep it fresh looking. The meat trimmings used to be sent to animal feed. Now they are centrifuged with heat to separate fat and meat slime, bleached with ammonia to get rid of the bacteria that make cadaverine by putrefaction, then mixed with hamburger and other meats as a cheap extender, making it cheaper for fast food companies. The FDA allows up to 25% of this former dog food in our hamburger without fines or labeling.[57] I have patients in Nebraska where they can get a side of beef from the local slaughterhouse ground up as hamburger. If they eat this natural (not organic) fresh hamburger they have no headaches. If they eat a restaurant or fast food hamburger they get severe migraines. They have asked me what the difference was between the two. I would suspect that bleaching with ammonia or citric acid alters the amino acids and causes toxic byproducts.

Putrascine is the decarboxylation rotting of the amino acid ornithine. Putrascine has a rotten flesh taste and smell. Like cadaverine, it's the byproduct of rotting flesh, or commercial food grade meat that has had a chance to rot from too high a temperature after slaughtering. Essential amino acid studies suggest that the three nonessential amino acids ornithine, citrulline, and arginine are really essential in some cases of dysbiosis and gut dysfunction. They can all be converted one to another through the urea cycle. So having ornithine destroyed by over processing rancid food causes a depletion of a very critical amino acid arginine. Weightlifters use arginine to improve blood flow to muscles and enhance natural growth hormone secretion. Both are also needed for brain blood flow and preventing Alzheimer's and vascular dementia.

Putrascine also attacks and uses up SAMe (S-adenosyl methionine) which is critical for regulating brain neurotransmitters, methylation pathways that detox chemicals in the liver, and the production of glutathione, the main antioxidant made by the human body for the prevention of modern diseases.[58] SAMe converts putrescine into two more toxic substances, spermidine and then spermine.[59] SAMe has been studied extensively worldwide by scientists and is used for depression, liver disease, and osteoarthritis.[60] If you lose too much SAMe from eating rancid food, and not enough nutritious food loaded with folate, methionine, and B6, then the DNA methylation pathway breaks down and the chromosomes become unstable and cause mutations, cancer, and disease.

Homocysteine, a toxic amino acid, is elevated in SAMe deficient patients. Homocystinuria or elevated homocysteine causes heart disease according to numerous studies.[61] While eating rotten flesh, people get sick short term from food poisoning and by eating over processed food. They get sick in numerous ways from toxic amino acids that are rotten forms of the ones people need to be healthy.

Some amino acids don't work as well by themselves, they have to be in a complete protein or segment of the amino acid chain of a protein. The body wants nature's balance and not the test tube balance found in many body-building protein drinks. Indigenous natives of Central and South America combine ingredients by adding whole proteins together to get the combined amino acids. So lysine needs to be combined with other amino acids in order for it to be absorbed and processed correctly in the body.Corn, wheat flour, and white rice are lysine deficient. A corn/gluten diet for farmed rainbow trout caused weight loss correctable by adding lysine.[62] Vegetarians have a very healthy diet, but it's usually deficient or low in lysine and iron.[63]

Lysine helps the energy cycle in our mitochondria in a very important way. Some weightlifters supplement with L-carnitine to boost their energy and burn fat. It turns out that Lysine is the precursor to L-carnitine. Without enough good L-Lysine, you don't make enough L-carnitine. Without L-carnitine, the fatty acid shuttle of fats into the mitochondria to be burned as fuel does not take place. So fatigue and weight gain ensue.

Not only do people need more L-carnitine, they also need more than just a supplement called L-Lysine, its precursor. Many people take L-Lysine for cold sores. It works for that. But nature is picky in what it wants for making L-carnitine. It needs a special form of L-Lysine called trimethyllysine found only in certain proteins. The free form amino acid L-Lysine will not suffice. Once again, the numerous health problems caused by eating nothing but poor food cannot not be alleviated by taking supplements. Nature cannot be fooled. Whole health needs whole foods in their most natural and least processed state.

What many food manufacturers do to increase the supposed quality of health food store snack bars is to add hydrolyzed soy protein. Normally, the corn, wheat, and rice flour that are used in these bars are all Lysine deficient. So to make a complete protein for better health, soy flour is added. Only raw soy flour causes gas and digestive issues. The Chinese got around this gas problem by fermenting the soy. But in America it's hydrolyzed into separate amino acids and added to food. But now it has at least two toxic aminos in their free form, glutamate and aspartic acid, and the wrong form of lysine in its free form that will not be available to make L-Carnitine. So that health food bar is looking less healthy by the minute. The proteins that have only lysine and not trimethyllysine have to use our limited and precious SAMe to methylate lysine so that it can become L-carnitine.[64] So the loss of SAMe to correct poor food choices causes people to become poor methylators by having more heart disease and cancer. Without trimethylisine, a person would have fatigue and weight gain because of limited production of its final product, L-Carnitine, the fat burner.

Part 6: Faking the Sugar

So after all the years of hype, everyone began to realize that they were gaining weight instead of losing it. Currently, the same process of deception is being carried on with sugar free foods, drinks, and gum. The new craze of fat free and carb free diets often end up to be full of chemicals that actually harm dieters and cause them to gain weight. People are ever in search of something sweet that doesn't make them fat, but they are increasingly disappointed with the reality that they have been deceived by the crass commercialization of a once precious food. People often become dependent on addictive "fun foods." Life is not fun without them. Everyone in the commercials appear to be enjoying themselves. And yet, our very essence is tied up in what we eat. We become what we eat.

Numerous scientific studies are showing sugar-free foods trick the body in a nasty way. Being deceived, the body punishes the eater by causing the consumer to gain weight and eat more food at the meal paired with a sugar-free drink than if they had drunk a sugared soda.[65] Sugar-free drinks have long been used by college students, dieters, and obese patients trying to lose weight. That is why they are used. The original study with saccharin showed that college students who drank soft drinks with saccharin sweetener in them ate less food in the twenty-four hours after the soft drink. The study was replicated with aspartame years later and the opposite effect was noticed, the college students consumed more sugar in the twenty-four hours after a diet soft drink. Males were more affected than females.[66] This is in contrast to animal studies that showed saccharin causes increased food intake.[67]

But what is worse about these zero calorie deceptions is the fact that they are poisons made from poison. They cause numerous side effects. Aspartame had the most calls to the FDA about toxic side effects in 1988 of any food additive, exceeding 80% of the calls.[68] A full 10% of the weight of aspartame is methanol. Methanol is well known to cause liver toxicity and death. I even had a patient last month who consumed large quantities of diet Gatorade and had elevated liver enzymes. No one can say that methanol is good for the body. The other ingredients of aspartame, phenylalanine and aspartic acid cause problems too but the scientific literature is full of biased industry studies. PKU babies have to avoid aspartame because of the phenylalanine. Free form aspartic acid causes the same holes in the brain that MSG does according to studies by Dr. John Olney since it has the same exitotoxic effect as MSG on the N-methyl D-aspartate receptors (NMDA).[69] He went on to postulate that it caused the increase in brain tumors noticed by neurosurgeons a couple years after aspartame was approved by the FDA.[70] This aspartame/cancer connection was later confirmed by an Italian researcher in rats.[71]

The food and soft drink companies are nonetheless losing the public relations battle with aspartame despite winning the scientific study battle with hundreds of positive studies in contrast to the few negative studies. Lately they have been reducing the amount of aspartame in food and beverages by adding other fake sweeteners like acesulfame and sucralose, both of which have been proven to be toxic. Acesulfame has impurities like methylene chloride, a known carcinogen, and has raised concerns in many scientists.[72] Sucralose has three chloride molecules on it and its manufacturer got sued by the real sugar industry because they claimed it was made from sugar.[73] The manufacturer was able to persuade FDA approval by explaining away all the rat studies showing multi-organ toxicities.[74] Chlorine is a known thyroid poison by mimicking iodine and displacing it. The animal studies showed decrease in thyroid hormone with sucralose.[75] There are many other artificial sweeteners like neotame, cyclamate, and alitame. Most of these do not have enough research to draw conclusions as to their safety.

But a bigger issue is the sweet tooth modern consumers have all developed. Americans are consuming one cup of real sugar a day, and many milligrams of artificial sweeteners daily. People are expecting and demanding sugar in foods that were never meant to be sweet. Nature has been changed from four seasons to only summer. One day everyone will regret the endless Sugar Daddy summer and the health problems it invariably brings.

High fructose corn syrup is another Frankenstein food that unnaturally disrupts the processes of the body. It was invented in the US as a cheap replacement for sugar. Due to government subsidies and price supports, corn syrup was a cheaper alternative. It soon became the preferred sugar replacement. The initial push came when Nixon wanted to get more farm votes in the late 60s and early 70s. He found a way to get them by pushing for more consumption of high fructose corn syrup. Since it was made from corn, the government program meant more corn could be planted and sold for higher profit. This would appease the farm lobby and get more votes. Decades later, corn syrup is being consumed more often than sugar.[76]

This all might be a happily-ever-after story except for the fact that it has been one of the leading causes of obesity in America. Fructose is found in fruit and supposedly does not make a big demand on insulin like glucose does. Because of this, fructose has been used in foods promoted for use in diabetic diets as a replacement for glucose which requires large amounts of the insulin that diabetics are already lacking. Unfortunately, this simplistic thinking sidesteps the larger health risks.

For starters, the fructose in high fructose corn syrup is not the same fructose that is found in fruit. It has been exposed to high temperatures and other processing that makes it different and harder for the body to use. The only thing the body can do with it is store it as fat.[77] The latest research shows that this kind of fat is very toxic causing inflammation and secreting hormones that cause breast cancer.[78] The inflammation caused by the oxidized fat causes heart disease, insulin resistance, more diabetes, more hip fractures and knee problems, and severe arthritis.[79]

Studies are continually being done to find out how much high fructose corn syrup is being consumed by the average American per year since it was introduced decades ago in the 70s. Recently, yearly intake is at forty-two pounds and the average daily consumption is two hundred calories of high fructose corn syrup. Most of this comes from soft drinks. Since these are unnecessary calories, every ten days someone would consume enough to gain an extra pound. Many of my patients who have quit drinking soft drinks have lost thirty pounds in one year, which is the equivalent of the calories missing from ridding the diet of high fructose corn syrup. The fake sugar in high fructose corn syrup (HFCS) soft drinks not only causes obesity in children and teenagers, but also causes decreased natural vitamin D3 production. Numerous studies show calcium bone loss in teenage girls and older women drinking HFCS soft drinks. They had an increase in brittle bones and increased bone fractures.[80] A recent study by Veronique Douard, et al., found that HFCS causes induction of the 24-hydroxylase enzyme CYP24A1 which makes a fake vitamin D3 called 24,25(OH)2D3. This fake vitamin D lowers real vitamin D levels and causes numerous problems. In the study, they found decreased bone mineralization and stunted growth, decreased absorption of calcium from intestines, and decreased reuptake of calcium from wasted urine.[81] Faking real glucose in favor of fructose causes numerous vitamin D deficiency diseases in humans by faking the vitamin D3.

So diets with unnecessarily excessive proportions of fake sugar, fake flavor, fake water, fake fat, fake salt, and fake proteins cause severe imbalances in the metabolic pathways and influence many of our modern disease plagues. As with a well-designed and furnished home, the more you collect unnecessary objects, the more the home needs to be cleaned and maintained. Upon applying the magnifying glass to the dark corners of the body, we find that many consumers eating the foods and drinks readily available in US supermarkets and restaurants could probably be featured in the popular reality show Hoarders. Flow nutrition will declutter this pretty but dysfunctional house built upon consumption and will restore proper healthy balance between real food and real food nutrients.

12

Harmonizing Real Food for Real Health

In a symphony, the harmonization of so many different instruments makes the cacophony not only tolerable, but sublime. When the body's many different instruments are in tune and following the lead of the conductor, the internal song radiates outward and harmonizes with the symphony of the ecosystem, planet, and universe. Rarely can one element be separated without affecting this completely mysterious and encompassing music. This is the essence of finding a flow state. With a thoughtful ordering of many different natural foods, each with their own fundamental frequencies of light, you can achieve a shimmering aura of wellness and wholeness unrivaled in this toxic world. This chapter will outline these essential players in your diet and give you the sheet music for creating your own masterpiece.

Part 1: Real Sugar (Essential Sugars)

Eating eight servings of fruits and vegetables per day is not only recommended by leading nutritionists and the American Heart Association, but also is included in the government FDA guidelines. Following these standards will provide all the essential sugars needed for healthy balance. These essential sugars are also called biological sugars, good sugars, saccharides, and monosaccharides.

If they are so essential, why are so many people unfamiliar with most of them? Most people know the fake sugars by name, but this isn't necessarily the case with the essential sugars. They are glucose, galactose, fucose, mannose, glucosamine, galactosamine, neuraminic acid, and xylose. Apparently, sucrose (table sugar), sorbitol, mannitol, stevia, and fructose (soft drink sugar) aren't on this list. Also missing are the fake sugars aspartame, Sucralose, saccharin, and neotame.

Healthy people need each of the essential sugars balanced for the many different pathways in their bodies. One of the principal actions of the immune system is the ability to differentiate between its own cells and foreign cells, viral proteins sitting on the cells, bacteria, fungi, and parasites. Military training involves purposely placing friendly targets side by side, behind, or in front of enemy targets. Quick thinking gets rid of the bad guys and preserves the friendlies. The immune system has to do the same thing every millisecond and it cannot make mistakes. When too many friendlies are attacked mistakenly by the immune system, the war is lost and the diseases resulting are called autoimmune disease or thyroiditis, systemic lupus erythematosus, and rheumatoid arthritis. The essential sugars are bound to proteins in the body called glycoproteins. Each person makes his or her own unique sugar chains that latch on to the body's proteins. In much the same way horse jockeys use the same colors but with different patterns to differentiate themselves and their horses from the other jockeys and horse farms, so everyone has a different order for the eight essential sugars attached to our proteins on every cell and structure in their bodies. This order is recognized by the immune system and the body's cells are left undisturbed. But what if someone eats a diet of only sucrose, saccharin, Sucralose, and aspartame. The fake sugars cannot fit into this glycoprotein sugar chain.

And how does the average American who only eats 1.5 servings of vegetables a day get enough of each of the essential sugars to make correct sugar chains on every cell? Is this why there are 30% of Americans with autoimmune disease with the incidence growing each year? If you compare this to the jockey's scarf with a pattern of red, blue, green, yellow, orange, and purple stripes, the average American loom only weaves red, blue, and the occasional yellow. Can they make a distinctive scarf that identifies the jockey in the mud of the race? Probably not. So people lose their health fighting their own immune systems, an enemy more powerful than themselves.

Some other important glycoproteins which need these essential sugars are MHA (major histocompatibility antigens), thyroid stimulating hormone, luteinizing hormone, follicle stimulating hormone, structural proteins such as connective tissue, transferrin, mucins, ceruloplasmin, glycoprotein IIb/IIIa for enhancing platelet activity such as stickiness, collagens, and antibodies. So having the manufacture of glycoproteins breakdown because of non-availability of essential sugars in a fast-food diet is a health disaster of serious proportions.

Achieving a nutritional flow with essential sugars is as easy as shopping for colorful vegetables and fruits in the grocery store seeking a wide variety of colors to consume each week. Obviously, we should eat more vegetables by 4:1 than fruits.

Part 2: Real Fat

Americans have not only gotten fatter, but also deficient in the essential fats needed to be healthy. This has been happening ever since fat became public enemy number one while the real criminal, trans fat, was promoted as healthy. Research studies show 80% of Americans are deficient in essential lipids and every last one of them are fat. So they are completely imbalanced from a lipid perspective. Frenzied, fast-paced eating leads to consuming too much of the wrong lipids, too many toxic lipids, and not enough of the essential lipids. Thus the craze for conjugated linolenic acid (CLA) which is just one of the essential lipids missing in the average American diet. It's promoted as a weight loss pill because it helps restore lipid balance which is crucial for weight loss.

When people consume excess sugars and carbohydrates compared to their activity needs, the sugars are turned into fats. When they need sugar for their brains to work, they cannot convert the fat back into sugar. Fat can only be burned in the muscles, and then, only after the body has burned through the stored glucose (glycogen) in the muscles and liver.[1] So people get low blood sugar and have to over-consume carbohydrates to get their blood and brain sugar levels up to get rid of the foggy thinking. This only exacerbates the problem.

The following charts show the categories of fats we consume:

MONOUNSATURATED FAT
(best to worst)

Extra Virgin Olive Oil *(A stamped production date on the bottle ensures its anti-inflammatory properties are preserved)*

Sunflower Oil

Macadamia Oil

Chicken Fat

Turkey Fat

Goose Fat

Duck Fat

Canola Oil *(Canadian rapeseed oil with low erucic acid)*

Safflower Oil

Peanut Oil *(inflammatory and allergy issues)*

Lard *(slaughterhouse fat from beef, sometimes partially hydrogenated)*

POLYUNSATURATED FAT

Omega-3 Fatty Acids
(best to worst, but they're all good)

Docosahexaenoic Acid (DHA): Fish Oil *(brain health)*

Eicosapentaenoic Acid (EPA): Fish Oil *(anti-inflammatory)*

Alpha-Linolenic Acid (ALA): Flax Seed Oil *(linseed)*[2]

Omega-6 Fatty Acids
(best to worst)

Dihomo-Gamma-Linolenic Acid (DGLA)

Gamma-Linolenic Acid (GLA): Black Current Oil, Borage Oil, Evening Primrose Oil

Linoleic Acid (LA): Sunflower Oil, Safflower Oil, Corn Oil *(inflammatory fat, GMO, pesticide residues)*, Cotton Oil *(GMO, pesticide residues)*, Soybean Oil *(inflammatory, GMO, pesticide residues)*

Omega-9 Fatty Acids

Oleic Acid

Elaidic Acid

Gondoic Acid

Mead Acid

Erucic Acid

Nervonic Acid

(Your fat cells make Omega-9, but it is also found in foods such as olive oil, almond oil, walnuts, animal fat, fish, and avocado)[3]

Cis Fat (*polyunsaturated vegetable oils in their healthy natural state before processing, i.e., hydrogenation*)

Trans Fat (*is extremely toxic—all vegetable oils like those below of the omega 6 variety become trans fat when they are partially dehydrogenated*)

SATURATED FATS
(best to worst)

Extra Virgin Coconut Oil

Cocoa Butter

Nutmeg Butter

Palm Fat

Dairy Fat *(cream—inflammatory, often contains an inflammatory protein-casein)*

Tallow *(fat from animals—inflammatory)*

Stearines

Interesterified Fat *(FDA has ok'd the terms "high stearate" and "stearic rich fats" to mask the identity of this ingredient—a fake fat with side effects similar to or worse than trans fats)*[4]

From the above lists, you can see multiple fat possibilities for a healthy diet or an unhealthy one. Eating carbohydrates for breakfast causes low blood sugar and hunger an hour or two later. Eating essential fats along with high quality protein gives a feeling of fullness that can last for hours because fat is filling. Simple carbohydrates dig a hole in the appetite that can never be filled or satisfied. The Mediterranean diet is rich in real olive oil which prevents sudden death from heart attacks even in the face of obesity, diabetes, coronary artery disease, and dyslipidemia. Because it has a powerful anti-inflammatory effect on our coronaries, it prevents unstable plaque rupture.[5] Extra virgin coconut oil can replace the trans-fat and has the opposite effect on our coronaries, it calms down inflammation like extra virgin olive oil. One way to test olive oil for purity is to place it in the refrigerator for three days. If it solidifies, then it's real olive oil. If it's still liquid, then it has been cut with vegetable oil and will not provide the same health benefit (the FDA allows the adding of vegetable oil to olive oil without requiring the corporations to label it). Also, to get the most amount of antioxidants, buying olive oil that was processed the same day it was picked it crucial. Bottles that have a processing date stamped on them guarantee the higher antioxidant count.[6] Eating a lot of vegetables gets the rest of the essential oils. Flax seed ground up is rich in omega-3 fatty acids like fish oil and is anti-inflammatory. Evening Primrose oil is loaded with oils that balance fats. Borage and Black currant oils have Gamma-Linolenic Acid (GLA).

Consuming a wide variety of fatty acids is more important than eating just one all the time. Balance is better than any single oil. People can get sick from using just one of them all the time. A nutritional flow state is best achieved with beauty, simplicity, order, and appropriate variety.

Part 3: Real Salt

We live in a watery planet that is two-thirds salt water and three percent fresh water. Whatever a modern doctor may say about salt, it used to be worth more than gold. If salt has lost its savor, it's good for nothing. Wars were fought over salt anciently. All that is left of this vast salt gathering empire of merchants is Celtic sea salt. It truly was a pearl of great price. Rare, beautiful, healthy, tasteful, invigorating, and as modern science has shown, can lower blood pressure. Since people have gotten away from eating real sea salt harvested from clay ponds at the ocean's edge, they are losing the trace minerals that kept their ancestors healthy.

So where does the salt craving come from in the first place? According to Traditional Chinese Medicine (TCM), salt is stimulating and is a yang food. When people are tired, run down, exhausted, or weak, they are in a yin state. The TCM way to correct this is with yang foods, of which salt is one.[7] Modern nutritional science in America and elsewhere has shown that mineralized salt, like Celtic Sea Salt, is important for adrenal function, health, and healing.[8] Natural sea salt breaks down easily in the body. Having a high concentration of magnesium, Celtic sea salt relaxes the smooth muscles around blood vessels and thereby lowers blood pressure. It also has trace minerals like chromium and vanadium which help us balance blood sugar and prevents diabetes. The selenium in it can bind mercury and other toxins and neutralize them.[9]

Since over-worked, over-anxious, and sleepless Americans are in a state of adrenal exhaustion, they need the healing powers of ancient salt. Anciently and in Ireland today, it was dried out of the sea in clay ponds which imparted minerals from the clay and captured the mineral essence of the sea. These minerals heal the adrenal gland. Usually, a person with adrenal exhaustion would consume vast quantities of caffeine for energy, further exhausting themselves, but also raising their blood pressure in the process. They would also eat a lot of chemicalized salt in salty snack foods that they crave which would also raise their blood pressure.[10] So there is more to the story of salt than meets the tongue.

Part 4: Real Fiber

After my experience on the slopes of Mt. Rainier, I can still imagine a crystal creek flowing beautifully down the mountain side through fields of delicate and wild mountain flowers shimmering in the breeze. In contrast to this, a blocked creek from a dam quickly turns muddy brown, with a stagnant, stinky rotten flesh smell. Molds grow, moss grows, algae blooms in waters devoid of oxygen. Sometimes the fish die and are replaced by species that love muddy waters.

So it is with the gut. Although most people wouldn't consider it to be "beautiful," the digestive tract is like a stream through the body. With a nursed baby, the milk comes in and then it goes out of the body with a fairly predictable timing and outcome. There is a continuous flow. No blockages, no stagnation, or unfriendly bacteria. It could be compared to a veritable river of life running through the infant giving proper nourishment for a rapidly growing body. Life in the food and friendly bacterial life in the gut creates a healthy balance.

However, this baby grows up into a toxic food world very quickly. Eating sugary, moldy food and fruit juices far removed from nature. With fake fats and toxic fake proteins, the gut gets blocked by too much sugar and too little fiber. Fiber creates the flow. Fiber is in the flowing long cell walls of growing plants. It prevents disease and blockages. When youth and adults are subject to continuous constipation over the years, they get colon cancer. The rate of this occurring is climbing because of toxic food and blocked flow.

There are three fibers everyone should be eating: insoluble fiber found in the plant cell wall called cellulose, soluble fiber like pectins and gums, and lignins which give wood structure and water transport. The structure of the woody stems and trunks is ordered by these fibers allowing for the free flow of life-giving water to all parts of the highly ordered living plant structure. When people consume fibers of all types, they get the energy of the plant flowing through their desert-like desiccated bodies bringing life-giving water to the toxic gut, recreating the crystal creek flow, and removing the artificial dams that stagnate. Each fiber type has its benefits and disadvantages. The proper balance of types is necessary for health. So when a person goes to the pharmacy and gets a fiber pill, he or she is getting one type of fiber and will be unbalanced as a result.

The insoluble fibers like cellulose are indigestible and provide bulk to the stool. They are not fermented by gut bacteria and do not cause gas. Soluble fibers are fermented (eaten) by gut bacteria and can cause gas, an undesirable side effect. I tell my patients that they can either have constipation without soluble fiber or occasional intestinal gas as a side effect of eating it. They also have to be careful about what types of foods they are eating. They can't have their cake and eat it too. Cake constipates while veggie fibers produce proper motility and may cause odorless gas.

Recently, the international community that created the Codex Alimentarius, a new global type of FDA, proposed a definition of dietary fiber that included function as well as a description. They propose that dietary fiber is that which "includes all non-digestible carbohydrate polymers with a degree of polymerization of three or more as dietary fiber with the proviso that they show health benefits."[11]

Researchers at the Ninth Vahouny Fiber Symposium were surveyed on the benefits of fiber and over 80% of the seventy-five respondents said that fiber had at least the following four benefits:

1. Reduction in total and/or LDL cholesterol
2. Reduction in postprandial blood sugar and insulin
3. Increased stool bulk and/or less constipation
4. Fermentability by colonic bacteria

Over 30% of respondents felt that there was enough scientific proof to expand the list to include:

1. Reduced hypertension
2. Positive influence on friendly gut bacteria
3. Weight loss and loss of fat deposits

Part 5: Real Proteins (Amino Acids)

We wear a coat of many colors in the bodies we live in. Each protein is composed of several dozen amino acids, each one providing its own life-giving power. We need all of the essential amino acids and some of the non-essential ones when we are ill and cannot readily make them ourselves from the other amino acids. When we eat foods with a wide diversity of unmodified natural amino acids in their proper sequence in the food proteins, we put on our coat of many colors and it shimmers with beauty. Our skin, hair, nails, and bones shine with luster and are flexing with power.

Each of the building blocks of protein, each amino acid, has a specific function in the body. Blood sugar regulators are L-glycine, L-glutamine, and L-taurine. The immune boosters are N-acetylcysteine and L-lyseine. The mood enhancers are L-tryptophan, L-theanine, and GABA (Gamma-Aminobutyric Acid). For muscle building in the elderly, branched chain amino acids are recommended. Beta-alanine is also helpful for the elderly. Pain relief comes from DL-Phenylalanine (DLPA). Vascular support requires L-arginine. Amino acids build the brain and body. A harmonized body needs the right amino acids (protein building blocks) entering the right sacred spaces in our bodies through the right portals so that proper body system construction and remodeling can take place. Muscle building for the elderly is accomplished by supplementing with the branched chain amino acids such as leucine, isoleucine and valine. Pain relief is provided by supplementation with DL-Phenylalanine (DLPA). And finally, growth and repair rely heavily on the L-arginine effect on the manufacture and release of growth hormone.

Now with this broad overview in place, we can zoom in on the individual amino acids to see the different effects they have on each compartment of our bodies. We will visualize the balancing of each amino acid listed below:

Alanine

Our connective tissue is made from alanine. Muscles derive energy from amino acids through the glucose alanine cycle. Alanine stimulates the immune system. Animal-based sources include dairy and dairy products, eggs, meat, and fish. Plant-based sources include watercress, soy, beans, asparagus, spinach, seeds of watermelon, lentils, and cauliflower.

Arginine

Used by body builders because of its natural ability to raise growth hormone levels, arginine also helps children and the elderly who need both growth and repair, the essential functions of growth hormone. Arginine also increases endothelial function acting like a fuel source to the cells that line blood vessels, helping them to be more flexible, lowering blood pressure naturally, and increasing blood flow to the muscles. It also increases T-lymphocyte response and sperm cell counts. It's a precursor to creatine, another supplement used by body builders to increase muscle mass and muscle energy molecules. Being a precursor to GABA, arginine elevates our happy mood naturally. Animal-based sources include turkey, pork loin, chicken, and dairy. Plant-based sources include pumpkin seeds, soybeans, peanuts, spirulina, chickpeas, and lentils.

Aspartic Acid

Muscles turn carbohydrates to energy with the help of aspartic acid. It helps build immunoglobulins for fighting infection and reduces ammonia waste in our muscles after exercise. Animal-based sources include Alaska native halibut, orange roughy, tilapia, eggs, and tuna. Plant-rich sources include swamp cabbage, soy protein, seaweed, spirulina, and bamboo shoots.

Cysteine

Cysteine is the precursor to glutathione, which is made in the liver in abundance to help detoxify all the poisons we eat, breathe, and put on our bodies as personal care products. Cysteine also stimulates white blood cell activity. Animal-based sources include pork chops, beef, lean chicken breast, tuna, yogurt, swiss cheese, and eggs. Plant-based sources include lentils, oatmeal, and sunflower seeds.

Glutamic Acid

Many other amino acids are made from glutamic acid such as arginine, GABA, glutamine, glutathione, ornithine, and proline. There is a mechanism for moving, modifying, and recycling amino acids that depend on glutamic acid. Glutamic Acid is found in most protein-rich foods such as beef, poultry, fish, and dairy. It is also found in protein rich plants such as wheat.

Glutamine

This is the primary fuel for the enterocytes, the cells that line the gut. It's the energy source also for kidney cells and one of the energy sources for brain cells. It promotes memory enhancement and ability to concentrate on a subject. Lastly, it helps build the immune system. Animal-based sources include beef, chicken, lamb, saltwater fish, cow's milk, and eggs. Plant-based sources include almonds, peanuts, hazelnuts, cabbage, whey protein, kidney beans and soybeans.

Glycine

Glycine helps mobilize glycogen into sugar, and as such, curbs sugar cravings. It also helps build other amino acids. It's made naturally in the body, but is also found in the connective tissues, tendons, ligaments, skin, cartilage, bones, collogen, and gelatin of meats.

Histidine

Histidine is useful in the treatment of allergic diseases, rheumatoid arthritis, and digestive ulcers. It's involved in the manufacture of white and red blood cells. Our skin is designed to absorb ultraviolet light for the manufacture of vitamin D. Histidine is involved in the ultraviolet absorbing molecules. Animal-based sources include pork chops, skirt steak, chicken breast, tuna, tuna, milk, and eggs. Plant-based sources include navy beans, pumpkin seeds, squash seeds, almonds, sunflower seeds, whole wheat, teff, and quinoa.

Isoleucine

Our red blood cells carry oxygen because of the iron attached to hemoglobin, which is built from isoleucine. It also is used for the treatment of muscle wasting in the elderly and AIDS patients and is used for a quick muscle energy source. Animal-based sources include pork, beef, veal, lamb, chicken, turkey, fish, and cheese. Plant-based sources include wheat germ, legumes, seeds, and baker's yeast.

Leucine

Leucine promotes the healing of broken bones and skin lacerations. Like isoleucine, it protects against muscle breakdown and is a muscle fuel source. Animal-based sources include lean portions of meats, and poultry, most fish including tuna, salmon, haddock, whitefish, tilefish, and trout, and dairy products including milk, yogurt, parmesan, colby, cheddar, and bleu cheese. Plant-based sources include raw and fermented soy, white and kidney beans, lentils, tempeh, dried spirulina, and peanuts.

Lysine

Lysine has long been used for viral cold sores and other viruses. It's easily destroyed by heat, i.e., normal cooking. Corn, which is in everything we eat, is lysine deficient. So it's common these days to be deficient in lysine. When taken with adequate doses of vitamin C, it forms L-carnitine, one of the critical components of our mitochondrial energy cycles. Lysine deficiency also affects protein synthesis and muscle and connective tissue repair mechanisms. So when we are deficient in lysine, we fall apart, breakdown, get easily fatigued, and get frequent viral illnesses. Plant-based sources include avocados, dried apricots and mangoes, beets, leeks, tomatoes, pears, green and red peppers, potatoes, tempeh, tofu, soybeans, soy milk, kidney beans, navy beans, black beans, chickpeas and hummus, lentils, edamame, pumpkin seeds, pistachios, cashews, and macadamia nuts. Animal-based sources include yogurt, cheese, butter, milk, oysters, shrimp, snails, beef, pork, and chicken.

Methionine

Methionine is critical for the formation of glutathione, our primary antioxidant and liver detoxifier. It helps regenerate liver and kidney tissue, reduces blood cholesterol levels, and is a precursor to the formation of cystine and creatine mentioned above. Animal-based sources are the richest and include beef, chicken breast, crab, lobster, cod, salmon, ham, turkey, shrimp, milk, yogurt, eggs, and cheeses. Plant-based sources include coconut milk, wheat, quinoa, wild rice, white and brown rice, buckwheat, millet, teff, hominy, lentils, mung beans, refried beans, chickpeas, tofu, almonds, chestnuts, hazelnuts, bananas, kiwi, blueberries, apples, apricots, grapefruit, melon, oranges, peaches, pineapple, plums, squash, brussels sprouts, pumpkin, peppers, tomatoes, onions, okra, mustard greens, cabbages, collards, beets, and asparagus.

Ornithine

Ornithine is important in growth hormone secretion, for the immune system, and liver function. It can be found in most protein sources including freshwater clams, fish, dairy, cheeses, and eggs.

Phenylalanine

Phenylalanine suppresses appetite, helping with weight loss. Most importantly, it's the major ingredient in the manufacture of tyrosine which as seen above forms our feel-good neurotransmitters. It can be found in beef, chicken, pork, tofu, fish, beans, milk, nuts, seeds, pasta, whole grains, and vegetables like sweet potatoes.

Proline

Proline is an important building block in the formation of connective tissue and heart muscle. It's also used for muscle energy. Animal-based sources include beef, chicken, pork, monkfish, cod, and shark cartilage. Plant-based sources include asparagus, mushrooms, and cabbage, soy, buckwheat, and watercress.

Serine

Serine helps memory and improves nervous system functions. It can decrease production of harmful levels of stress hormones by switching off the stress center in the hypothalamus. Stress hormones decrease sleep quality, trash memory ability, and raise blood sugar and blood pressure. So optimal levels of serine are important for health and memory. It's also used to build up the immune system and help the energy systems in the cells. Serine is made by the body. Animal-based sources include meats, fish, shellfish, and eggs. Plant-based sources include soybeans, peanuts, almonds, walnuts, chickpeas, and lentils.

Taurine

Fat absorption and elimination is influenced by taurine. It helps like a neurotransmitter in the retina and brain. It's found mostly in animal proteins and is made in the human body.

Threonine

Threonine builds collagen, helps detoxify the body, prevents fatty liver degeneration, and is found mostly in animal proteins.

Tryptophan

Tryptophan is converted to 5 HTP, then to serotonin, the feel-good hormone, then to oxytocin, and lastly to our good sleep hormone melatonin. Sources include chicken, eggs, cheese, fish, peanuts, pumpkin and sesame seeds, milk, turkey, tofu, and soy.

Tyrosine

Tyrosine is probably one of the more important amino acids for forming our critical neurotransmitters in our brains such as dopamine, norepinephrine, and epinephrine, thereby improving our mood. It's also critically important in the formation of thyroid hormone and growth hormone. It's made by the body. Animal-based sources include pork chops, salmon, tuna, turkey, chicken, roast beef, and parmesan cheese. Plant-based sources include roasted soybeans, large white beans, lentils, split peas, wild rice, and oatmeal.

Valine

As one of the branched chain amino acids, it helps muscle function. In order for the brain to make feel-good neurotransmitters, it has to import their amino acid precursors. Valine helps them get into the brain. Exercise helps tryptophan get into the brain. Valine can be found in chicken, pork, beef, salmon, halibut, sardines, mackerel, peas, beans, chickpeas, lentils, fenugreek, soy, cheeses, peanuts, mushrooms, whole grains, and vegetables.

So getting a healthy and diverse balance of the amino acids keeps many of the body's systems functioning at optimum levels. However, when the balance of these nutrients becomes tipped to excess, either by fake proteins or excessive proteins, the balance of health shifts to the negative side. For instance, NutraSweet, or aspartame, has phenyl-alanine as 45% of the weight. Overconsumption of foods and drinks containing this artificial sweetener cause the phenylalanine levels to sky-rocket. Unfortunately, some people have phenylketonuria deficiency (PKU) which is an enzyme needed to utilize and breakdown phenyl-alanine. Consequently, there is a black box warning on chewing gum for those who have this deficiency to not to consume those products. About 1 in 10,000 have the full genetic disease. However, 1 in 50 have the trait, which means they are not as robust as others at getting rid of phenylalanine. Recent lab rat studies show that the overconsumption of phenylalanine depletes the levels of multiple essential amino acids causing numerous diseases. The aspartame depleted amino acids are threonine, valine, methionine, isoleucine, leucine, histidine, trypto-phan, and tyrosine. The branched chain amino acids were most affected with drops intracranially of 38% to 64%. Tyrosine excess also depleted the essential amino acids but not as drastically. Tyrosine is often added to energy drinks along with aspartame.

Everyone is bombarded by advertisements for gym membership. They all know exercise is good for them. However, some people get sick when they exercise. Exercise like other strenuous physical, emotional, and mental activities can cause metabolic stress. So if their immune systems and repair systems are compromised already, they injure them-selves and get sick. Whey protein studies are robust in showing the pro-tection against metabolic stress with exercise. Whey protein promotes muscle synthesis, aids in weight loss, and has immunologic stimulating properties that protect against illnesses. Whey protein supplementation does the opposite of NutraSweet by increasing the levels of essential amino acids, especially the branched chain amino acids. Studies in athletes show increased antioxidant glutathione production. Calcium absorption and subsequent weight loss that was caused by increasing intracellular calcium was demonstrated with whey protein supplemen-tation. Whey promotes the growth of friendly bacteria in the gut. Whey is rich in glutamine, which is a fuel source for enterocytes, the cells that line the gut and keep bad things out of our bodies. So in general, eating high quality unadulterated protein such as whey, or products that contain only essential amino acids has been proven scientifically in numerous studies to produce significant health benefits. Eating damaged amino acids, toxic amino acids, and foods with missing essential amino acids has been shown to destroy our health.

Lysine helps the energy cycle in our mitochondria in a very important way. Some weightlifters supplement with L-carnitine to boost their energy and burn fat. It turns out that lysine is the precursor to L-carnitine. Without enough good L-lysine, you don't make enough L-carnitine. Without L-carnitine, the fatty acid shuttle of fats into the mitochondria to be burned as fuel does not take place. So fatigue and weight gain ensue.

Not only do we need more L-carnitine, we also need more than just a supplement called L-lysine, its precursor. Many people take L-lysine for cold sores. It works for that. But nature is picky in what it wants for making L-carnitine. It needs a special form of L-lysine called trimethyllysine found only in certain proteins most of which are in vegetables.[12] The free form amino acid L-lysine will not suffice. Once again, the numerous health problems caused by eating nothing but poor food cannot not be alleviated by taking supplements. Nature cannot be fooled. Whole health needs whole foods in their most natural and least processed state. What many food manufacturers do to increase the supposed quality of health food store snack bars is to add hydrolyzed soy protein. Normally corn, wheat, and rice flour that are often used in these bars are all lysine deficient. So to make a complete protein for better health, soy flour is added. Only raw soy flour causes gas and digestive issues. The Chinese got around this gas problem by fermenting the soy. But in America it's hydrolyzed into separate amino acids and added to food. But now it has at least two toxic aminos in their free form, glutamate and aspartic acid, and the wrong form of lysine in its free form that will not be available to make L-carnitine. So that health food bar is looking less healthy by the minute. The proteins that have trimethyllysine have used S-adenosyl-L-methionine (SAMe) to methylate lysine so that it can become L-carnitine.[13] So we have to rob our precious SAMe stores to make L-carnitine. So not only do we lose SAMe and become poor methylators because of its loss (more heart disease and cancer) but have fatigue and weight gain because of the lack of trimethyllysine and its final product L-carnitine.

For natural health people also need an unadulterated supply of essential vitamins. Only the body prefers vitamins to be piggybacked with other nutrients. In order to get the blood levels of certain vitamins high enough to do some good, massive doses are required. Since this alters physiology and liver function, and often people do not know enough about vitamins to balance high doses of them, people can actually get sick on them. The blood levels go up, but they do not have the health benefit. To get around this conundrum, some vitamin companies mix natural foods with their vitamins to make them more absorbable at lower doses. But after this additional processing, the consumer is paying extra for what nature does so harmoniously with the vitamins already packaged with the proper nutrients for their absorption in fruits and vegetables. One world class athlete eats several pounds of juiced vegetables daily. He set the world record for any age for the amount of weight lifted in one hour, 50,000 pounds, at age fifty-five beating out all the younger competition by a wide margin.[14] I tried eating two pounds of vegetables daily without a juicer for four months when I lived in Afghanistan and found that I doubled my weightlifting ability during that time when I had just turned sixty-two years old.

Part 6: Real Flavors

The flavors in natural foods are so savorful and intense that many people, on consuming whole foods for the first time in years, are shocked at how good they taste. Fresh spices without MSG or lead and pesticide contamination round out the culinary surprise. Raw food cooking at low temperatures and raw food restaurants are gaining in popularity. Food can then be eaten slowly like our digestive system wants because the more we chew these healthy delights, the better they taste. Try eating a fast-food hamburger slowly. You will quickly find the fake flavor gone and a gagging taste to replace it. Flavors from the real world of nature cannot be faked. We have forgotten how wonderful they are because we rarely if ever experience them anymore. They each have their own role in our health.

For example, freshly crushed raw garlic has a potent antibiotic in it called allicin. Garlic powder or flakes from the seasoning rack does not. Not only is the flavor better, but we are actually healing ourselves when we use the raw food as a flavor. Garlic is also used for arterial inflammation, lowering blood pressure, digestive aid, and for asthma.[15]

Cinnamon bark flavors sticky buns, chocolate, hot apple cider, and coffee cake to name a few. It has been used for centuries as a stimulant, astringent, and as a stomach and bowel tonic.[16] But lately, research has shown that it's quite useful for lowering blood sugar and preventing, along with a proper diet, blood sugar highs and lows.[17]

Curry, a member of the ginger family of plants, is used worldwide as a spice. Its health benefits have been studied for many years in the 20th century. Lately, a group showed that whole turmeric spice was better absorbed than the curcumin extract from it that has been studied so much. Not only that, but they were also able to demonstrate that the inflammatory cytokine levels went down with the whole root and not with the curcumin extract of the root. So nature trumps our efforts to find the one ingredient in the herb that can cure cancer as injectable curcumin can. Oral curcumin is not only poorly absorbed, but also does not lower inflammatory cytokines. Whether oral curcumin or curry spice could have the same effect on upper gastrointestinal cancers than the injectable curcumin form remains to be established.[18]

Horseradish or wasabi has potent antibacterial properties in addition to its role as a spice.[19] Perhaps that makes sushi covered with wasabi less likely to cause food poisoning. Nutmeg has been shown to kill the oral pathogens that cause caries.[20] Anas Muchtaridi extols nutmeg's medicinal qualities, "Nutmeg has aromatic, stimulant, narcotic, carminative, astringent, aphrodisiac, hypolipidemic, antithrombotic, antiplatelet aggregation, antifungal, antidysenteric, and anti-inflammatory activities." Although consuming it in large quantities would be ill advised since it has effects on the fetus in pregnant mothers even though historically it was used for the nausea of pregnancy.[21]

Cardamom also has wide ranging medicinal uses. It has been used successfully to treat "constipation, colic, diarrhea, dyspepsia, vomiting, headache, epilepsy, and cardiovascular diseases." Cardamom has been used to treat spasms, hypertension, anxiety, and even as a preventive for colon cancer.[22]

In the age of MRSA and VRE and other flesh-eating bacteria, one would want protection from the zombie plagues. Recent studies show that clove oil was one of the top three in killing these pathogens.[23] It also kills dental cavity pain and is useful in dental emergencies as a topical treatment relieving pain in a matter of minutes. Studies also show it was just as effective as topical benzocaine gel in providing dentists with a topical pretreatment to reduce needle pain.[24]

There are many more spices than these that we use daily that not only taste better in their organic forms, but also provide numerous health benefits. So natural organic spices have many useful medicinal properties in addition to making our food tastier and safer. Real flavor heals us while fake flavor trips our health.

In order to prevent Salmonella and other food poisoning, commercial spices are treated with approved techniques such as irradiation, propylene oxide, ethylene oxide, steam heat, and dry heat.[25] For food purists, this process would ruin the taste and medicinal value of the spice. Growing your own for your own use in flowerpots on a window sill is far healthier than these sanitized versions.

The reward of old age used to be respect, honor in the community, being sought out for advice and sage wisdom. Now we have become a nation that ruins the health of our elderly with toxic food that makes them so sick they can't take care of themselves. Then they are placed a nursing home that feeds them even more toxic processed food that quickly makes them invalids. We should reward them with good food from mother earth. Then their last days would be far more peaceful and disease free than presently. If we start this process now, it might become the norm by the time we are at the end of life too.

13

Make Meals Last

Imagine that the body snatchers have invaded your body. Now you have the munchies and can't stop eating. You just ate thirty minutes ago and are back in the refrigerator for more. The munchies control your eating habits. You may not realize it, but you're living in a snackaholic nation. People get all hyped up about hundred calorie snack bags that make you think you aren't eating a lot of extra calories per day. If we multiply 365 by 100, we get 36,500 extra calories per year. This is about ten pounds of fat per year in weight gain. I exercise a lot on treadmills, gliders, rowers, stair steppers, and exercise bicycles. The calorie counter doesn't lie on these machines. It's so disappointing to see that I only burn a hundred extra calories by an intense thirty-minute workout on three different machines. That hundred calorie snack bag doesn't look so good after one trip to the gym to get rid of the unnecessary calories. So the important question is: Why do we get the munchies and how do we control them?

The only way to control the cravings is to make each meal last as long as possible. There are, for starters, at least twelve ways to do this:

1. A good one to try is the *Zone Diet* by Barry Spears. In this model, each meal and snack follow the One-Third Rule: One-third carbohydrates, one-third vegetable, and one-third protein.[1] Lately, a similar diet called the Paleo Diet is all the rage and there

are numerous books out that are all good on how to make it work for you.[2] The body builders have gotten into it in order to have less body fat and a more ripped look.[3]

2. We need fat to burn and L-carnitine to help move the fat to the mitochondria where it is burned and keeps us full for hours. But we need the right kind of fats for this to happen. Trans-fat will not do the trick. Until recently almost all the snack foods were made of hydrogenated soybean oil which is 50% or more trans-fat. Since the package labeling of trans-fat was mandated by the FDA in January 2006, there has been a 42% to 45% decline in the amount of trans fat in chips and cookies.[4]

3. Whenever we snack, we should balance insulin with glucagon. The first lowers blood sugar and the second raises blood sugar causing a feeling of wellbeing and fullness. We can do this by eating protein with each snack. The protein increase causes glucagon release which raises blood sugar while at the same time suppressing insulin release which lowers blood sugar.[5] Often insulin over-secretes, blood sugar goes too low, and we get anxiety, panic attacks, and tremendous food cravings designed to rescue the brain which needs glucose to survive. If we do not get glucose, we go into an insulin induced mini-shock called hypoglycemia with numerous symptoms such as palpitations, anxiety, hunger, trembling, numbness and tingling in hands and feet, sweating, a sensation of warmth, confusion, weakness, and fatigue. In severe cases, one passes out and goes into coma. I have personally seen quite a few cases of hypoglycemic people passed out on the floor who were revived when sugar was put into their mouths.[6]

4. To prevent high and low blood sugars caused by rapid sugar absorption and subsequent insulin release, we need to eat more complex carbohydrates like whole grains cooked at home or in locally owned bakeries rather than in commercial bakeries. Wholegrain foods take a while to digest and they slow down the release of glucose into the blood minimizing the insulin release.

Animals without any insulin at all live longer in an environment with constant food supply than animals that have insulin. It appears that insulin's role is to preserve us in times of famine.[7] Crash dieting and poor eating activates insulin's role in preventing starvation by storing nearly every calorie as fat and burning muscle for fuel instead. An important study was done with cafeteria breakfasts that contained regular oatmeal cooked from scratch compared to instant oatmeal of the same caloric density. All other foods in the experimental cafeteria were the same. At the end of the month, the regular oatmeal subjects weighed one and a half pounds less than the instant oatmeal subjects. The difference was the rapid rise in blood sugar caused by the instant oatmeal that triggered higher insulin releases and more storage of the calories as fat.[8] When insulin is overactive, you feel tired, irritable, hungry, and exhausted. Eating more quick calories for temporary energy causes the problem to repeat itself every half hour with rapid weight gain and more fatigue. One diet plan that counteracts this effect suggests that snacks should be cheese sticks. Cheese is high in proteins and fat which do not trigger insulin release.[9] This makes more sense than the low-fat snacks that made the whole nation gain weight in the last decade.

5. If you have reactive hypoglycemia with sudden surges of insulin while getting tired and shaky two to four hours after a meal, you can split up an ideal calorie count for ideal body weight among six meals eaten every two to three hours. For a 2,400-calorie diet, this would be 400 calorie meals eaten six times a day. For an 1,800-calorie diet, you would eat 300 calorie meals.[10] Evening out the blood sugars prevents the surges in sugar that cause insulin release and fat storage.

6. Eating more soy and vegetables has also been shown to even out blood sugars and make meals last. Barry Sears, PhD, says that replacing some meat and wheat with soy evens out blood sugar levels within two weeks.[11] It's easier to fill up a stomach on

non-starchy vegetables than grains. If you give a horse unlimited grain to eat, the horse will eat till it founders and its stomach explodes from the gas caused by the excess grain. On a day of donuts, Coke, pizza, and cake, people will often feel like the horse foundering with exploding gas. They will get sugar cravings and want more rapid rises in blood sugar as a result.

7. Corn is not a vegetable and causes all kinds of weight problems. In its worst form, high fructose corn syrup, it can only be stored as fat.[12] It's in almost all processed foods because it tastes sweeter than sugar and, due to corn subsidies given to farmers by the government, it's cheaper to buy than sugar. Regular table sugar needs sucrase, an enzyme, to be digested properly. Sucrase works much slower than amylase which breaks down white flour starch and corn starch. An equal calorie amount of white flour or corn starch will cause a more rapid rise in blood sugar than sugar itself. In addition, this will cause more insulin to be released and more storage as fat. This does not mean we should eat most processed white sugars which are poisons in of themselves. They are devoid of the nutrients they have to rob from our cells to be processed and stored as fat.[13] Raw cane sugar has many nutrients that aid in its proper digestion. A few healthier types of unrefined sugars include Sucanat, Rapunzel Organic Whole Cane Sugar, and Jaggery from India. They have significant levels of antioxidants, polyphenols, calcium, phosphorus, chromium, magnesium, copper, iron, zinc, manganese, vitamin A, vitamin B1, vitamin B2, vitamin B6, niacin, and pantothenic acid.[14] One of my hypoglycemic patients who spent the day chasing one tiny carb snack after another in order to feel good for just a few minutes tried the Sucanat that I suggested. When she made cookies for her children with organic whole grain flour, organic butter, and Sucanat, she snacked on them. She didn't get the horrible hypoglycemic symptoms that she had with regular brown evaporated cane sugar cookies made with the identical ingredients. Some experts say that the medical

75-gram glucola drink we use in our three hour glucose tolerance test is mostly sucrose, so it's released more slowly and triggers less blood sugar rises than the regular breakfast. So to mimic home eating, it's recommended that the glucola drink be replaced with a medium size bagel covered with two tablespoons of grape jelly. Since white starch causes more rapid blood sugar rises than straight sucrose, it's more reliable to match the problems at home during the test. However, all simple carbohydrates consumed in excess have been found to be stored as fat in liver and muscles whether they be glucose, fructose, or sucrose. Fat in excess is preferentially stored as fat more than the simple carbs.[15]

8. There are many books and websites devoted to people with hypo-glycemia and the sugar cravings it causes. They talk of eating low glycemic index (GI) foods. These are foods that slowly release their sugars in order to prevent insulin over-secretion and sub-sequent low blood sugar and food cravings. The new science also takes into account low glycemic load (GL) or total carbohydrate calories in the fully absorbed foods. So now it's important not only to know which foods release their carbohydrates slowly, but also which foods have low total carbohydrate load. The website that best lists the foods that meet both criteria is Medosa.com.[16] The website has an Excel spreadsheet with over 1,500 foods color coded green, yellow, and red. Another book you should check out that has both low GI and low GL diet advice is entitled *New Glucose Revolution Guide to Living Well with PCOS* by Dr. Jennie Brand-Miller and Nadir Farid.[17] So if your blood sugars and moods are like a yo-yo, research the best carbohydrates to eat in addition to the best proteins and fats to balance them with.

9. Cinnamon bark has been shown to lower blood sugar and insu-lin.[18] I had a patient on two oral medicines for lowering blood sugar who also had hypertension. He walked three miles a day and did not seem to eat much of anything. His blood sugars were very high at 140 mg/dL to 150 mg/dL in the morning before eating.

When his daughter bought an eight-dollar bottle of cinnamon bark and he took one pill twice a day, his blood sugars lowered in two months to 110 mg/dL fasting and his blood pressure normalized also. There were no other changes in his high-pressure executive lifestyle to account for the sudden changes other than the cinnamon bark.

10. Chromium and zinc are also deficient in overly stressed people and are important for steady blood sugar levels.[19]

11. After all this exploration into sugar cravings, it would seem wise to avoid sugar altogether. The sugar substitutes most commonly used, aspartame and acetylsulfame K, not only act as brain and thyroid poisons, but they also trick the brain causing problems. The brain knows it did not get the sugar it was promised by the sweetness on the tongue and food cravings actually go up. Drinking a diet Coke while eating causes experimental subjects to eat more calories than they would when just drinking water.[20] The brain rewards this deception by causing food cravings for the very calories that are missing. The cravings persist till the calories are eaten. This is one reason why American food portions are 30% larger than they are in France.[21] We supersize everything because of the aspartame drinks and the aspartame gum we chew.

12. When we get rid of sugar and wheat, we have intense food craving for them for about two weeks until the yeast in the gut that feed on them die off. It appears that the yeast secretes hormones that make us hungry and take over our metabolism tricking us into eating the very foods they want. Yeasts do more than cause us to eat the wrong foods, they also release poisons called mycotoxins that poison our livers and ruin our health. They also kill off the friendly bacteria our mothers may have given us in breast feeding. The friendly bacteria make all our B vitamins that support many functions in our body including the brain's sense of wellbeing. Without B vitamins, we get anxious and cannot sit still. Our detoxification pathways shut down and we fill up with poisons we

cannot get rid of. The yeast overgrowth from all the simple sugars and carbohydrates in our diets causes the intestinal permeability to increase which causes food allergies, arthritis, and many other diseases.[22]

If we want to get rid of sugar cravings and the sweet tooth the tooth fairy loves so much, we need to start a program involving one or two of the points mentioned earlier. Perhaps radical diet changes are too much to start out with. If this is the case, you can start with small changes like reaching for a piece of cheese after that cookie you just ate. Plan a healthy snack, like celery and almond butter, just once a day during a high temptation time. At the beginning keep it simple and enjoy small successes. Over time, more change will come naturally as you feel better and have fewer mood swings. When you cannot adhere to the diet every day and go into long relapses off the diet, consider staying on the diet just during the weekdays, with weekends off, until it becomes a natural part of your healthy lifestyle.

14

Feasting on Fermentation

We are not cows. We do not have four stomachs to digest the wide variety of foods we eat. Yet the modern food industry, Big Agra, and the modern food crop industry assume we are. We are fed the same foodstuffs that are fed to cattle and hogs to fatten them up. Corn, high fructose corn syrup, and grains of every kind are in virtually everything we eat. A recent mass spectrometry test of all the edible products in a grocery store revealed corn's presence in 95% of the foods sold there. It's found in nearly all the meat and boxed food.[1] How can we not imagine that eating this modern food will not make us fat in the same way that it does the cattle and hogs we consume?

But more and more I see another health disaster that is a direct consequence of the consumption of these foods. Gastric distress, acid reflux, irritable bowel syndrome, and Crohn's disease of the intestine are natural consequences of putting four-stomach-foods into a single, overwhelmed gastrointestinal tract. For these reasons, it is important to understand how a cow digests grain in order to understand how foreign these foods are to the human body.

The first stomach uses fermentation by lactobacillus as the main pretreatment for grains. If the grains bypass this important first step, the cows would probably develop many of the same problems humans have. Whole grains and milled processed grains have many proteins and chemicals that are toxic to the human digestive system. In order to prevent germination until enough moisture is present, grains have enzyme inhibitors. When beans, seeds, or grains are soaked in water for twelve to forty-eight hours, depending on the grain, the enzyme inhibitors are turned off.[2] The cow's first stomach mimics this process by fermenting these grains.[3]

The grains also have very compact proteins like gluten that are extremely difficult for a single stomach to digest properly. If gluten is not properly digested and the lining to the intestine is compromised by high levels of chronic stress, then the entire gluten protein is absorbed into the blood where it creates allergies, arthritis, fatigue, mental fog, and depression. If a person becomes allergic to wheat gluten, which is the case of 12% of the population, then he or she will have an allergic reaction taking place in the intestines and colon that destroys the delicate lining needed to absorb important vitamins and nutrients.[4]

A cow does not have this problem because the first stomach prepares the food for the rest of the digestive track. The cow's first stomach uses lactobacillus to predigest the proteins and make them more digestible for the other stomachs. There are other lectins, glycoprotein complexes, in grains, beans, nuts, and seeds that cause gut and health problems. These are likewise destroyed or predigested by fermentation in a cow's first stomach.[5]

Our ancestral genes are designed for the hunter-gatherer lifestyle of the people of the African savanna. The cultivation of grains by our ancestors is very recent. Our ancestors knew much more about how to make food healthy than we do. They created an artificial first stomach in a bowl, in a hole in the ground, or in a hollow tree. There they fermented whatever grain they wanted to eat before they cooked or ate it. The discovery of fermentation of grains allowed our migratory ancestors to settle down and build cities and civilization.[6] The recent discovery of mass milling of grains for profit and convenience threw out thousands of years of the refinement of the fermentation process by our ancestors. Not only have the wheat germ and vitamins been stripped off and the flour bleached white with chlorine before it's brominated, but the messy, gluten destroying fermentation process has been thrown out as well.[7]

Please refer to the below to learn more about the beneficial effects of fermentation:

1. It preserves food.
2. It prevents scurvy.
3. It preserves nutrients in food.
4. It makes nutrients in food more digestible and absorbable.
5. It improves bioavailability of minerals in food.
6. It doubles starch digestibility.
7. It scavenges free radicals like an antioxidant.
8. It generates copious amounts of nutraceuticals: superoxide dismutase, GTF chromium, glutathione, phospholipids, digestive enzymes, and beta 1.3 glucans.
9. It removes toxins like cyanide from foods.
10. It removes phytic acid from foods which blocks the absorption of zinc, calcium, iron, magnesium, and other essential minerals.
11. It removes toxic chemicals such as nitrites, prussic acid, oxalic acid, nitrosamines, and glucosides.[8]
12. It floods intestines with probiotics and helps heal damaged intestines.
13. It helps digest other foods that are not fermented.
14. It provides less indigestion and more rapid clearing of food from stomach.
15. It drives out bad bacteria.
16. It improves function of immune system.
17. It reduces allergies and asthma.
18. Fermented milk (Kefir) curbs unhealthy food cravings, increases levels of B vitamins, and has a calming effect.[9]

With all of these benefits, it's hard to argue that fermentation doesn't belong in the modern human diet. Our ancestors were free from the digestive assault of the US food industry, free to eat legacy foods, free to listen to the wisdom of the ages. By balancing our diet with fermented foods, we can destroy the phytic acid and gluten and enzyme inhibitors in the rest of the non-fermented foods eaten at the very same meal. A little bit of fermentation goes a long way.

15

Your Quality of Life Is the Quality of Food You Eat

I see people with migraines at work all the time. People with allergies and sinus infections are more prone to migraines. After seeing multiple doctors for many years, these patients were finally referred to me to treat their allergies and sinus problems. Often, they did not know that certain foods trigger migraines in susceptible people. A common culprit would be beer nuts or aged peanuts cooked in rancid oil. Another is overly ripe bananas (green bananas are good for you).[1] So the quality of food affects the overall health of the individual.

In the US, people tend to go with dollar meals at a fast-food place. Nothing could be worse for their health. I had a friend at college who ran out of money part way through school. He bought a fifty-pound bag of pancake mix and began eating pancakes three meals a day while bumming meals off of anyone who would feel sorry for him. Pancakes made with brominated bleached white flour are perhaps the worst food we have. This is especially true when covered with fake foods like trans-fat margarine and fake syrup which is made from the poisonous high fructose corn syrup, trans-fat, and sawdust in the form of cellulose. The fast-food dollar meal has replaced quality nutrients with Frankenstein-ian modified proteins, fats, and bleached bromated white flour.

When we substitute margarine and canola oil for butter in order to save money, we really put on weight and develop many health problems from the trans-fat and toxic seed oils including obesity, heart disease, and Alzheimer's. So cheaper, supersized foods are not really a bargain after all. The cheaper foods not only contain lots of altered food-stuffs, but also lots of high glycemic foods. Dr. Cara Ebbeling of the Children's Hospital Boston says, "Consumption of meals composed predominately of high glycemic index foods induces a sequence of hormonal events that stimulate hunger and cause overeating in adolescents."[2] She goes on further to summarize research that shows when children eat out they eat more calories than when eating at home.[3] Fast-food meals are so bad for children that they change their hormones and make them fat. Lots of cheap, low quality fast food is not anywhere near as good as a more filling lesser amount of high-quality food cooked at home. Modern-day eating patterns will cause so much disease that it will be more expensive for the family, the obese child, and society in the long run while seeming to be cheaper in the short run.[4]

This quality issue with our food is more than tragic. Old people who make unwise food choices have enough information to know better. But children are naïve and unaware of the consequences of the food choices forced on them by lazy adults. The following is a list of diseases and health problems caused by fast food obesity in children:

Psychosocial

Poor Self-Esteem
Depression
Eating Disorders

Neurological

Pseudotumor Cerebri

Pulmonary

Sleep Apnea
Asthma
Exercise Intolerance

Cardiovascular

Dyslipidemia
Hypertension
Coagulopathy
Chronic Inflammation
Endothelial Dysfunction

Musculoskeletal

Slipped Capital Femoral Epiphysis
Blount's Disease
Forearm Fracture
Flat Feet

Endocrine

Type 2 Diabetes
Precocious Puberty
Polycystic Ovary Syndrome (Girls)
Hypogonadism (Boys)[5]

As you can see from the list, these are not inexpensive diseases to treat. This tragedy is spreading worldwide because the fast food franchises are spreading worldwide. The high cost of natural traditional foods and the cheap cost of fast-food is changing the eating habits of the entire world for the worse.[6] According to the World Health Organization, worldwide obesity rates in adults have tripled since 1975 while 39% of the world population is overweight. In most of the world's countries, obesity causes more deaths than starvation. Another troubling statistic is that many poorer global youth populations are simultaneously battling obesity and malnutrition at higher rates than ever.[7] In the US, those on food stamps were more obese than those eligible but not on food stamps as well as higher income groups. Shelley Hearne, DrPH, director of Trust for America's Health said, "We have reached a state of policy paralysis in regards to obesity."[8] No one knows what to do, but many states are starting with educating elementary students in proper nutrition and trying to give them more nutritious choices in the school lunch program. Michelle Obama started a healthy food choices curriculum for school lunches in the US. It was not favorably received by the public in part by a misinformation campaign started by the tobacco companies that own most of the food corporations.[9] In Japan, students spend the first part of their school day preparing their own delicious and natural lunch to eat later. They learn how to eat, how to prepare, and how to enjoy the whole process. Adults and children can't always eat at home, but they need to be educated about the dangers of food that is consumed in places where nutritional quality and processing information is not available. As Americans, we need to ask that our food standards are kept high and that our kids are given healthy choices when they are away from home.

16

Life Begets Life While Anti-Life Destroys All Life

Imagine a meadow of beautiful Kentucky bluegrass the size of two football fields. The ground is soft and velvety. There are no gouges, cracks, or dead areas. There are no weeds to sticker your feet and legs. There are no gopher holes and snakes. Life would be so wonderful. You could roll over and over again across the downy grass with no discomfort.

Our intestines have two football fields of surface area and recruit one-third the output of our hearts every minute even when at rest.[1] The intestinal grass carpet is made of delicate cilia that are completely covered with one hundred trillion friendly bacteria that keep away all the bad bacteria, parasites, and disease. The lining is intact in perfect conditions. It's a barrier against bad bacteria entering our bodies and causing extraordinary destruction. It produces 90% of the neurotransmitter serotonin in our bodies that makes us feel good. The friendly bacteria also produce most of the B vitamins we need to be healthy, to think, and feel well. Even the dreaded candida albicans that causes so much human disease cannot grow when the carpet of trillions of friendly bacteria is flourishing.[2]

So how do you go from healthy to sick intestines? Why are some people born to have sick intestines their whole life? The answer is simple. We are not human without trillions of friendly bacteria to support us. Vast armies of defenders and helpers reside in the gut. In utero, as fetuses, babies have a sterile gut. When they are born naturally, they traverse the birth canal where they become colonized with lacto-bacillus, one of the friendly bacteria. When they begin to nurse soon after birth, their alimentary tract is also colonized with bifidobacterium from their mother's breast milk. So what about the one-third of babies born in America by cesarean section[3] or the many babies who are bottle fed? Some babies are missing one essential friendly bacterium necessary for lush green garden-like intestines and some are missing another. But what happens to the 15% who are both C-section and bottle-fed babies?[4] They are missing all of the friendly bacteria necessary for health. What if they are further cleansed with antibacterial soap containing triclosan? This will kill friendly bacteria and often lets in the nasty bacteria that can be resistant to antibacterial chemicals and antibiotics.[5]

It turns out that the immune system is tolerant to bacteria for about two years. During this time, the friendly bacteria get a pass to live forever protected by the immune system while the foreign infectious bacteria can never escape the power of a healthy immune system and gut lining. If a person has no friendly bacteria and gets sugar water and sterile formula with substances that promote unfriendly bacteria, the wrong bacteria get the pass. This person then has a lifetime of gut problems not curable by simple means. This person's normal status is to have unfriendly bacteria with the tendency to return to this state at every turn. While others who had a better start with vaginal birth and breast feeding have a normal status of friendly bacteria and tend to go back to this default position after invasion and illness pass.[6]

Research shows that it takes at least six weeks for friendly bacteria to recover from one course of antibiotics. Sometimes the infection with the nasty Clostridium difficile that follows antibiotic use lingers for years.[7] A simple test can determine if this is causing your gut problems.[8]

Can a bad start in life be reversed? Can the gut be healed after a prolonged course of antibiotics? Numerous studies show that different treatments help. Certain conditions have to be administered with life-long treatments. Recently, people awaiting surgery for Crohn's disease of the colon had their disease reversed so well with probiotic treatment that they did not need surgery. For months, they were treated daily with literally trillions of friendly bacteria. The protocol was developed by an Italian researcher.[9] Helicobacter pylori can cause not only ulcers, heartburn, and atrophic gastritis, but also coronary artery plaques. It can be reduced 70% by just adding the pro bacterium Lactobacillus rhamnosus. If a person develops insulin resistance, diabetes, and toxic fat inflammation, bifidobacteria can improve that person's health. Rheumatoid arthritis is helped by healing intestinal permeability with probiotics. Protection against salmonella food poisoning is provided by probiotics. Probiotics that contain Saccharomyces boulardii heal the leaky gut by neutralizing the Clostridium difficile toxin that burns holes in the velvet bluegrass intestinal lining. Colon cancer is also prevented by the probiotic healing of the gut.[10]

So how do people heal their guts and prevent these diseases? They should avoid the four apocalyptic horsemen of death: trans-fat, high fructose corn syrup, white death (white flour and white sugar), and soda drinks. Eat a well-balanced diet with lots of vegetables and some fruits. Balance meat with carbohydrates and fat. Avoid meats with anti-biotics and in their place eat organic meat raised without antibiotics. The antibiotics fed to the animals and injected into the meat cause the friendly bacteria to die off. When friendly bacteria are wiped out in animals by the antibiotics in their feed, they gain weight more rapidly and put on the extra fat that makes the meat taste better. If people eat meat laced with antibiotics and take too many for themselves, they can gain weight too for the same reasons.[11] Avoid antibacterial soaps and kitchen cleaning compounds. Whatever is put on the skin goes right into the body. Eat lots of fermented foods that have not been pasteur-ized like yogurt, miso, natto, real sauerkraut, natural pickles made the old-fashioned way, and fermented beans. If you cannot eat fermented foods, take lots of high-quality prebiotics, sporebiotics, or probiotics before meals or between meals.[12] Sporebiotics have become somewhat popular lately in treating gut issues. They are the fungal elements clinging to organic fruits and vegetables. Avoid antibiotics for the common cold and cough. Reduce the stress in your life by reframing events in a more global perspective, avoid unnecessary stress, get enough quality sleep, and pray or meditate long enough to find peace in your heart.

During the flu season, I see lots of people with obvious flu prodrome. After they are infected with the virus, they go through stages of infection that last six weeks. The actual flu is nausea, vomiting, or diarrhea. Before that, they usually have a stuffy and runny nose. After the intestinal part of the flu, they usually get a sinus infection or bronchitis. Many people come to me either before or after the flu and want antibiotics for their runny nose or, later, their sinus headache. The antibiotics are usually totally unnecessary during these six weeks of one type of misery after another.[13] If no antibiotics are given, the patient will get better faster. Sinus rinsing with salt and soda solutions, of which NeilMed kits are a great option, helps more and can cause less harm than antibiotics. It will hurt the flu ravaged intestines even more to use antibiotics.[14] People get over the respiratory tract symptoms in practically the same length of time whether they use antibiotics or not. Since the illness is mostly viral with occasional bacterial superinfection, the antibiotics will not do much.[15] But they will certainly destroy the friendly bacteria for at least six weeks causing people to feel tired and not their usual selves. If someone is dying from pneumonia, gall bladder infections, bladder and kidney infections, appendicitis, or meningitis, then they will need antibiotics and certainly will need them to work. If they have had too many unnecessary antibiotics for viral illnesses, then they could develop resistant bacteria along with the life-threatening illness. That person may die when the first round of regular strong antibiotics doesn't work. This is what happened to Jim Henson, the muppeteer and movie producer, when he died of highly drug resistant Streptococcus pneumonia. This illness is not usually resistant to any antibiotic treatments.[16]

When I was an intern in Aurora, Colorado, the neurosurgeon I worked with told me of a soldier in Germany who had gotten a sinus infection and was treated many times with different antibiotics. The doctors did not know till after he died from multi-drug resistant meningitis that he had never finished taking any of the antibiotics he was prescribed. He only took them for three days until the symptoms went down. Within a week, he went back for more antibiotics.

If we follow the guidelines of the CDC and the infectious disease specialists, we need to avoid antibiotics and stop demanding them from doctors who would rather not prescribe them. Remember, if you do nothing, you will get better in a week or two from most flus and colds just like you would if you had taken the antibiotics. Twenty-five years ago, a study on sinus infections found that the average sinus infection lasted ten to fourteen days without treatment. With antibiotics, it lasted seven to ten days.[17] The vitamin C study done in Canada more than thirty years ago showed that vitamin C, taken 500 mg daily, shortened colds by 30% fewer days and the subjects had 30% fewer colds than the placebo group. So it was just as effective as antibiotics in shortening the illness. More recent studies have been equivocal. Meta-analysis of pooled double blind and placebo-controlled studies show vitamin C was ineffective as a prophylactic against the common cold. However, studies in arctic weather military training, skiers, and marathon runners taking 250 mg to 1000 mg a day showed a 50% reduction in risk of catching a cold.[18] An even more recent five-year randomized controlled trial from Japan showed three times less colds in the high dose (500 mg) vitamin C group compared to the low dose (50 mg).[19]

So the maintenance of the digestive system is tied to more than just weight loss and the gratifying feeling of being full. It is the point where we are directly taking the elements of the earth into our bodies. We cannot be separated from these outside forces that control the integral roots of our health. When people say, "you are what you eat," it's true! Your body could not function without the assistance of foreign bacteria and your health would deteriorate without the regular maintenance of these good bacteria.

Flow states are marked by the simple elegance of synchronicity. Maintaining this balance and harmony within the digestive system is crucial for our longevity and healthspan in this increasingly polluted world. Our bodies are more important than our homes. We can't move out of them after years of bad choices and neglect. Our bodies are our defense against the elements that would disrupt our flow and take us out of equilibrium.

Guiding Flow Away From Toxins and Excess

17

Returning to Paradise

We find ourselves in this weary world with great, almost super-human, powers to return it to Eden paradise. And yet we can't muster our collective will to do it. Utopian dreams have historically been with us. This utopian Eden has been a dream from time immemorial in every culture. Many schemes have been tried with great failures. Force has always been a failure. Extermination of enemies supposedly disturbing the peace has never worked. Toxic governments create toxic waste. Anarchy creates civil war and great pollution. There seems to be no middle ground. The melting pot way of bridging the cultural divide has worked on some levels, but the war of opposing wills is ever with us.

As Americans, we have encouraged the slow ruin of the planet and our health as a result of our greedy behavior. Unless we change, we will self-destruct through wars, toxic chemicals, and famines that will come when our genetically modified and chemicalized crops fail to adapt to the new toxic planet. There are limited resources on this planet, and we are going to use them up. However, like T.S. Eliot said in 1925 in "The Hollow Men,"

> Between the idea
> And the reality
> Between the motion
> And the act

Falls the Shadow[1]

The problem with the shadowy world we live in is that it's increasingly more toxic and poisonous than people realize. Fertility rates are dropping so fast world-wide that some say there will be very few children born fifty years from now due to environmental poisons.[2] We can't live under this shadow anymore. We have to act and create our own reality, our own utopia, and return to paradise.

There is a better way. Why not teach people how to be self-reliant, how to grow their own food and medicinal herbs, and take their energy production and wise consumption off the grid. We have lost this rugged frontier independence. In Mexico, many peasant farmers who were formerly living a subsistence lifestyle providing for their own have moved to the most polluted city on the planet to live on government welfare and have forgotten how to take care of themselves.[3] In New Jersey, 95% of the food was grown locally fifty years ago. Now 95% of their food is imported and the farms were replaced by financed money-making and man-made structures.[4] Nothing would make the oil barons happier than to use oil to move food vast distances across the world and then to move it by truck vast distances within a country. For this monetary reason nations are taught to be dependent on others and not be self-reliant.

Self-reliance would bankrupt the money-makers. They fear the old adage of make do, do without, fix it up, don't throw it out. It would be a huge loss for them to go back to the days when appliances would last forever like my grandmother's washing machine. Several years ago, I worked in a town where the city water works decided to replace the main submersible pump that provided the water for the sprinklers in the city park. It was still working but no one knew how long it had been running and they were afraid it would break down. When they pulled it out, it turned out to be seventy-five years old. Nothing being made today could last that long. We would be lucky to get three years out of an appliance because failure is built into them.[5]

Eating food grown within twenty-five miles of your home is healthier. Our immune systems don't like to be overwhelmed by foreign toxic molds that come from multiple soils across the planet. Our bodies like to grow up with predictable bugs that they can figure out how to handle and keep in their place. So what is good for globalist money bags is not good for the gut. There are restaurants in the Southwest that specialize in serving only locally grown foods. Detroit has made a move to turn vast acres of abandoned homes back into farms. So we build megacities, destroy the natural beauty, make it an eyesore, abandon it, and then return it to paradise all in five generations. The circle of life is not what we imagined fifty years ago with our futuristic vision of a megacity world.

Paradise, Kentucky is the ancestral home of my wife's family. They had emigrated from Germany to Pennsylvania, to North Carolina, and then followed the Shenandoah Trail through the Cumberland Gap into southern Kentucky. Paradise lies on a big bend in the Green River. The county history records the tale of old grandmother Barbara Hamm getting up in the Conestoga wagon, stepping off and putting her cane down saying, "This is it, I'm going no farther. Build us a home right here."

John Prine, a second cousin of my wife, wrote a song called "Paradise" about my wife's ancestral home. It goes like this:

> And daddy won't you take me back to Muhlenberg County
> Down by the Green River where Paradise lay
> Well, I'm sorry my son, but you're too late in asking
> Mister Peabody's coal train has hauled it away
>
> Then the coal company came with the world's largest shovel
> And they tortured the timber and stripped all the land
> Well, they dug for their coal till the land was forsaken
> Then they wrote it all down as the progress of man.[6]

Our family went back to Paradise to try to find the ancestral home, the one riddled with bullet holes left over from the Cherokee Wars. Two Cherokees were invited to live with the family after the war and were later buried in the Hamm family cemetery nearby, the original Cherokee writing engraved on their tombstones. When we arrived at the homestead site, all we found were broken shards of burnt glass and pieces of wood. The coal company had torn it down to construct a tower and pulley assembly in order to move loads around the hill. The entire landscape looked like a child's drawing. Nothing seemed right. The hills looked artificial and the grassy fields boringly uniform. The angles of the land jutted out unnaturally. The coal company was contracted to return the land back into all its paradisiacal glory. But all they accomplished was to make it appear alien and uninviting.

When the Americas were discovered by Christopher Columbus and others, many came looking for gold, or their own imagined paradise. Ponce de Leon spent years in his quest of finding the fountain of youth. This is not dissimilar to the modern dream of discovering disease-free health or even living in perfect health forever. Jonathan Swift, known for his satires, made a joke of living forever. He wrote in *Gulliver's Travels* a piece on the Struldbrugs of Luggnagg who had figured out the magic of living forever. The only trick was that they had not figured out how to prevent the ravages of disease and aging. They were all blind, deaf, crippled, diseased, and senile living forever in a misery worse than hell.[7]

Modern medical science has succeeded in fulfilling this nightmare satire that has proven to be prophetical. We can now keep people alive for twenty or thirty years beyond their normal death age by poisonous chemicals that make them sick in numerous other ways. I routinely see people in my medical practice that are in a partially petrified state maintained by drug-chemicals that they can't live without. Some are so sick from the side effects of these properly prescribed drugs that they beg me to take them off the drugs. I can't do it without making them sicker. So many medicines have such disastrous drug withdrawal symptoms that

I refer them back to their doctors for proper drug maintenance plans, a safe withdrawal from the offending drug, and replacement with a less toxic one that does the same beneficial thing.

We don't need an increased lifespan. We need increased healthspan. We need to be healthy every day we live till the last few years when we decline rapidly into a sweet and peaceful death. Jack LaLanne, founder of the first exercise gym in America, lifted weights every day of his life from age fifteen to the day before he died at ninety-six from pneumonia. He had written another book the year before. He was only sick one week before he died suddenly.[8] He had maximized his healthspan. Paul Bragg, an early nutritional guru, once told the then fifteen-year-old pimply and sickly Jack, "You're a walking garbage can." At the time when Jack heard that, his daily diet was basically comprised of "cakes, pies, and ice cream."[9] After Bragg opened Jack's eyes to the truth, he changed his life and the world forever. Later, a fifty-four-year-old Jack LaLanne would beat twenty-one-year-old Arnold Schwarzenegger, the newest Mr. Universe, in a fitness match so badly that Arnold exclaimed, "That Jack LaLanne's an animal!"[10]

Fortunately, wisdom, both ancient and modern, has shown us the way back to paradise. This path can be discovered by beginning to consume healthy vegetables and herbs grown naturally. In fact, we are beginning to know more and more about these medicinal herbs as research funding has increased over the years. The book *Herbal Medicine: Biomolecular and Clinical Aspects* states that, "In 1989, the US Congress established the Office of Alternative Medicine within the National Institutes of Health to encourage scientific research in the field of traditional medicine, . . . This led to an increase in investment in the evaluation of herbal medicines. In the United States, the National Center for Complementary and Alternative Medicine at the National Institutes of Health spent approximately $33 million on herbal medicine research in the fiscal year 2005."[11] Each herb and vegetable has thousands of natural phytochemicals in their natural form and ratios between them that have medicinal properties. The properties of these phytochemicals, plant chemicals, have been extensively studied for their effects on our health and the eradication of disease for many years. One third of all prescription drugs originated from these natural plant substances.[12]

But nature is more complicated than our simple one drug for one disease paradigm or the narrow viewpoint that accompanies it. In nature, groups of phytochemicals work together to produce healthy plants and then in turn increase the health of the beings that consume them. Returning to paradise means returning to whole organic herbs and foods, finding the tree of life, the healthy lifespan, the happy life meant for us from time immemorial. Fortunately, we have a guide in Traditional Chinese Medicine and in Ayurvedic medicine. These preventive, food, and plant-based medicinal approaches have been in practice for thousands of years and have kept populations of people balanced and healthy. Western Medicine would be blindsiding itself to not consider and include these tried-and-true health paradigms.

18

The Chaos Theory and
Homeostasis

On the sloping side of Mount Rainier, there is a high mountain meadow that in June is covered in tiny blue and yellow wildflowers. As a youth while I was hiking there with my Boy Scout troop, we saw a bear amble by about a hundred yards away. We waited till he passed. Then we hiked along the stream that meandered through the meadow. Despite the cool air at that height, the stream was soaking up the sun and was warm. Trickling over the edge of a chasm, it fell in a granite pool ten feet across and three feet deep. We hopped down and jumped in. It would have been serene except for the cacophony of the glacier fed icy river just five feet away, cold and wild. Dropping steeply down the mountain, the glacier river was full of swirls and eddies that were always changing. Watching for several hours, we could see patterns of whirlpools coming and going. They repeated themselves in the same place, yet were slightly different and the intervals were not predictable. It was a memorable yet contradictory exposure to chaos theory. I was at peace with the serene mountain stream and the chaotic mountain rapids. I was warm in the natural mountain Jacuzzi, but a cold mist hung in the air.

Explaining the mathematical and chaotic return of patterns in cascading water had not yet been invented. Later, it became to be known as chaos theory after James Gleick published the first popular book on the subject.[1] Among scientists it's better known as non-linear dynamics. Slight changes in initial conditions that create vastly different outcomes is one of the predictions and demonstrations of the theory. The lungs breathe and the heart beats with the irregularity predicted by the chaos theory. If they beat with cuckoo clock precision, like patients with pacemakers on mechanical ventilation in the intensive care unit, they can develop congestive heart failure and pulmonary edema. Apparently, our heart and lungs march to the beat of a different drummer, the chaos theory. This allows for the impossible to happen, good blood flow and breathing without the heart and lungs fighting each other.

The Chinese were aware of this thousands of years ago, calling it yin yang. For them, nothing was black or white with scientifically sharp edges. It was all a chaotic swirl, like the yin yang symbol. Even the yin had a little yang dot in the swirl, and the yang contained a little yin. They appreciated nature's chaotic balance millennia before modern scientists had the computers to show how it worked its magic.

For example, all vitamins need to be balanced with each other. We need a given amount of each one so that they average out within a month. Any given day we may need more of one than another. The balance is hard to predict, and the pattern might be obvious in retrospect, but there is a chaotic equilibrium between the vitamins.

There are many equilibriums within our bodies. The first are barrier equilibriums which keep some things out and other things in. They allow either passive diffusion or active transport of nutrients and excretion of waste. The blood brain barrier is critical for health and many diseases are the result of it breaking down. Worse yet, it breaks down during certain disease states making us more susceptible to life-threatening toxins. The kidney has a barrier in the loops of the nephron or kidney cell. The blood and waste are pushed through, and the good things are brought back through it into the blood. The intestines have a barrier that is one cell layer thick. It allows for absorption of nutrients and keeps bacterial endotoxins and food particles out of the bloodstream. When it breaks down, and it does with IBS, Crohn's, and acute and chronic diseases, people get sick from bacteria moving through the holes and into the blood. Endotoxemia is the name of the illness. When people get it they feel like they have the flu. The endothelial layer is one cell layer thick and it has many important functions for vascular and heart health. It is also one of the most diseased areas for older Americans who have hardening of the arteries, plaques, and inflammation. Basically, when it's healthy, we are healthy.

All these membrane boundaries create balance in the body so that when they are healthy, the whole body is healthy. They create, essentially, a yin yang balance between two different areas. This yin yang goes throughout the entire body. Humans have a balance between bone building and bone resorption called constant bone remodeling. We need both for healthy bone maintenance. Many American women have osteoporosis which means this process has been out of balance for years.

There is a balance between oxidation and antioxidation called reduction. The balance is called redox. When people fast, or go without eating for a while, they are actually causing oxidation. The body's response to this is to make more natural antioxidants like glutathione which helps clean out the poisons in the body while it gets a rest from further poisoning by more toxic food. Fasting too much is harmful, because too much oxidation occurs. Too many antioxidant pills are harmful if there is not enough oxidation through fasting and exercise. This balance is critical for health, yet all you hear in the media is about breakthroughs in this or that antioxidant pill that will make someone rich. Plants have the right balance between starches that oxidize us and antioxidants that put out the fires of burning starches for fuel in our bodies. So plants in their more natural states help give us this balance.[2]

Hormones build muscle and repair damage to the body. They are called anabolic hormones and they include in part growth hormone, testosterone, estrogen, DHEA, pregnenolone, and progesterone. Other hormones are catabolic such as the stress hormones, cortisol, and its metabolites. You would think that only the anabolic hormones are necessary. But when people get the flu, their bodies have to make the main defense against it, glutathione. It can't be made in the body without eating. They also need to make armies of white blood cells and immunoglobulins to fight the virus. Where does all the protein come from to fight the flu? The body pours out stress hormones to quell the inflammation and also break down or catabolize muscle proteins so the body will have the raw material to mount a proper defense against the flu. The flu kills 20,000 to 40,000 elderly a year in the US. The reason is simple, they have lost so much muscle from disuse, loss of anabolic hormones with aging, and poor eating that they don't have enough reserve muscle and fat to breakdown to fight the virus. They are more susceptible, so they often lose the battle. Hormone balance is critical for aging. Women take estrogen for hot flashes while men take Cialis instead of testosterone for impotence. But all anabolic hormones go up with exercise and the need to supplement them goes away in most cases. Exercise keeps muscle mass high enough to withstand the flu, keeps bones stronger, prevents falls that cause hip fractures, and improves mental health. So balancing hormones between catabolic and anabolic is critical,[3] especially as you grow older, and exercise with proper nutrition are the best ways to find your health flow.

There is also a balance between estrogen and testosterone as they are both able to be converted to the other in both men and women. Polycystic ovary syndrome (PCOS) causes increased aromatase enzyme activity which increases testosterone in women giving them acne, oily skin, and facial hair. Older men have increased aromatase activity which converts their testosterone to estrogen. They get fatter in the hips and belly, get prostrate hypertrophy, and have problems urinating. So if the balance is out of whack in females or men, they will get disease. While hormonal balance is important in the human race, we are also connected to and are balanced by the incredible diversity of the plant life on the planet.

There is an interesting mirror between our bodies and the plant world. We make porphyrin in our red blood cells. Porphyrin keeps iron in the middle of the molecule in order to carry oxygen.[4] Plants make the identical porphyrin which has magnesium in the center for its energy production. Humans have a balance between different types of teeth with large molars for chewing plants and grains and a significant number of incisors for tearing and chewing meat into pieces. So from meat we get iron, from plants we get magnesium. This style of flow and symmetry runs all through nature.

We have a balance between right brain and left brain, between artistic tendencies and analytical math ability, between abstract thought and concrete deductive reasoning. There is a beautiful balance between each. There has to be balance in our lives between focused attention and relaxation. If there isn't, we secrete stress hormones and develop the numerous diseases caused by stress. This balance is further mirrored in the two main nervous systems of the body. On one hand, we have the power system, full of get up and go, energy to spare, and intense focus and action called the sympathetic system. On the other hand, we have the house-keeping nervous system that kicks in when we relax and sleep properly. It fixes things that wear or break, rebalances all the acids, and restocks the used-up supplies of hormones, neurotransmitters, and nutrients. It helps us digest our food properly so we can extract the nutrition that we need from it. These two systems are opposed with miles of nerves carrying each system's different neurotransmitter to each muscle, organ, and even skin area.

Sympathetic tone is set by norepinephrine, the fight or flight hormone. Parasympathetic tone is set by acetylcholine, the relaxation hormone. Stressed people have high sympathetic and low parasympathetic tone causing the mouth to dry up, the bowels to stop moving food through and digesting it, and anxiety or anger set in. The balance is found in reasonable work hours, relaxing after work, not taking work home, avoiding workaholic vacations, and practicing meditation and prayer. Where there is balance and flow, there is happiness.

There are nutrient balances in the body that are critical for health. There is roughly a two to one balance between calcium and magnesium.[5] Too many Americans do not eat enough vegetables, get no magnesium, and have numerous health problems from subclinical hypomagnesaemia. So the calcium which is needed is too high relative to the low magnesium. For one thing, calcium helps contract our muscles and magnesium helps relax them. Magnesium deficiency causes nocturnal leg cramping. Low sodium from excessive sweating at work and water replacement without electrolytes causes Stoker's cramps, a different cramp needing a different salt. There is a balance between sodium and potassium. When people eat too much salt (sodium) and eat too few vegetables (which have high potassium), they get hypertension. Low potassium is a problem for diabetics and needs to be corrected. There is a balance between copper and zinc. Supplementation of one without the other causes illnesses. Zinc deficiency is common in stress situations because zinc is needed as a cofactor in so many stress adaptive responses in our bodies. So it gets depleted. Copper excess or deficiency causes many different disease symptoms that are often missed.

Considering all the above, you might come to the conclusion that supplementing willy-nilly with minerals can cause problems. As I explained earlier in this book, a lot of research has gone into some supplements to make them balanced properly in this regard. In most supplements, there are obviously bad ratios and the wrong form of the mineral. Pondering this chaos of minerals in our bodies and the diseases various imbalances cause might make you wonder if any vitamin or mineral supplement will help. The ancient wisdom of "let food be thy medicine," Traditional Chinese Medicine, or Ayurveda goes far beyond the modern hawking and hype of vitamins and minerals. The minerals in a vegetable-based diet are already properly balanced if the diet includes a large variety of vegetables, colors, and some fruit. The minerals are more easily absorbed from these than from a supplement.

As mentioned earlier, there also has to be a balance between omega-3 (fish oil and flax oil) supplements and the omega-6 oils (plant oils used in cooking) or we get sick. Omega-3 makes PGE2 series of prostaglandins in our bodies. These are anti-inflammatory. Omega-6 makes PGE3 series of prostaglandins that are inflammatory. So we need inflammation to protect us from influenza and shark bites. Other than that, it's a disease in its own right. The PG2 series can not only cause inflammation but also cause mitogenesis of fibroblasts which is a precancerous condition.[6] Studies have also found that many are consuming too much omega-6 seed oils. These include canola, sunflower seed, sesame seed, corn, peanut, and cottonseed oils. These oils are used extensively in fried foods, crackers, cookies, and cakes. On the surface, they have all the markers of being healthy for us, but they oxidize easily in our bodies causing numerous diseases.[7] Conversely, omega-3 supplementation, or just eating flax like the ancient Israelites in Egypt did, suppresses the aches and pains of everyday work.

To understand balance, we need to go beyond culture and habit and understand how we work on the inside and fit into the larger world without. In harmony and balance, there is flow. There is no us or them. There is no body part or function that exists in complete isolation. By breaking down these barriers and the excessive compartmentalization of western thought, we can become healthier and more balanced people operating for a greater good within our communities.

19

Who Wants to Eat Like a Caveman?

Who wants to eat like a caveman? Or more currently, who wants to spend most of the time gathering and preparing food like the nearly one billion subsistence and small farmers worldwide do in order to survive?[1] In their circumstances, there are no grocery stores or fast-food restaurants. Their reality is what they grow, harvest in the wild, capture, or share. Americans like the luxury of spending very little time obtaining or preparing their food. We like it fast, and we like it hot. We want it on the doorstep in thirty minutes or we get it free. Since most of the food is old and rancid anyway, we've grown accustomed to it being loaded with artificial flavors, salt, and sugar to make it taste better. We also like to eat lots of it. We weren't always this way though. The old TV advertisement, "Where's the beef?" introduced super sizing with a bang. Fortunately for the food producer's wallet, the same flavor enhancing chemicals also made the food addictive. It was by no coincidence that the tobacco companies created research labs to study addictive chemicals that could be added to cigarettes in the 1960s and 1970s.[2]

The food industry got involved and mimicked the dirty games played by the tobacco industry. "You can't eat just one" from the potato chip commercials was not a psychological ploy to get us to eat more chips, it was a fact based on the research of the addictive nature of the MSG that was added to the potato chip.[3] The super sizing was based on additives that were known to make people crave more food after the food that should have filled them up had just been eaten. According to the studies, soft drinks with artificial sweeteners made people eat more food in the same sitting than if they had drunk a regular sugary soft drink. No matter what you eat, if it came from a food company, it had flavor enhancers that made you eat more.[4]

The science behind this is troubling. Too much phenylalanine in the form of the aspartame found in diet sodas interferes with tryptophan absorption. Tryptophan is necessary for formation of serotonin, the feel-good hormone. People get depressed if they have a diet drink with a meal. They don't get the tryptophan surge after the meal which would have made them feel happy, satisfied, or satiated. The body thinks it didn't get enough tryptophan which is critical for wellbeing. So they end up craving even more food, start gulping more of their super-sized diet drink, and cave in to keep eating. So the diet sweetener causes ravenous eating and even more weight gain.

The Standard American Diet (SAD) created a whole new diet and exercise industry that created wealth for many companies. Exercise could burn calories if someone had the healthy body and motivation to do several hours a day. But after following this routine for a while, the exercise would stop working as well. When the weight was lost and the person resumed the SAD diet, the weight would come back with a vengeance. After a while the body's famine protection systems prevented further weight loss by dieting and the weight loss programs stopped working. Then a whole new industry making billions in weight loss surgery grew to fill the need for something that worked quickly. But even such drastic measures failed half of the people, and the average weight loss was only around twenty pounds. The effects of this along with yo-yo dieting induced famine protection genes in the unborn fetuses of that era.[5] Now we have whole new generations of Americans that can't lose weight on 500 calorie-a-day diets. Their genes are so efficient at extracting calories from food that they can gain weight on empty salads with no salad dressing added.

Most people are familiar with the Mediterranean Diet that helps people stay healthy and lose weight. It's also commonly understood that Japanese cuisine helps keep people skinny. But what is it about North American food that causes people to gain weight? Fresh foods have none of the added chemicals that make people eat more and gain weight—right? The answer is no! Our food is loaded with altered, unearthly genes (GMO), pesticides, herbicides, and toxic metals. It is also irradiated before shipping and later nuked in microwave ovens. It's far from fresh by the time you eat it. So it's not the same food grown organically in the volcanically rich soil of Japan or on the hillsides of Italy. It is Frankenstein food far removed from the food of our ancestors.

So how do pesticides in food cause weight gain? That question has been answered through research completed at the National Institute of Health (NIH). One researcher performed liposuction on obese people and sent the fat in for analysis to see what environmental pollutants could be found in the fat. He found that the more obese the person, the more pesticides and herbicides were found in the fat. In fact, the fat globules had formed around the pesticides with more pesticides concentrated on the inside of the fat globules than the outside. This suggested to him that the body was storing the poisons in fat in order to keep them away from critical organs.[6] So weight loss would release the poisons and make people feel ill causing them to quit their diet and exercise programs.

People also get discouraged about starting weight loss programs due to their bodies naturally changing as they age. When we are young, we have a number of fat-burning hormones that help us burn fat. These include thyroid hormone, testosterone, pregnenolone, DHEA, and progesterone which burn fat into heat and energy. The fat storage hormones are insulin, the estrogens, leptin, and adiponectin. Our own fat makes additional fat storage hormones that are released into the blood in addition to the ones that we make in our endocrine organs.

Some young people have more fat-burning hormones than fat storage hormones. But as they get older, they run up against the hormone poisons that cause these fat-burning hormones to decline and even they start gaining weight. The plastic world we live in has plasticizers that mimic the fat storage hormone estrogen.[7] Our first exposure to this is in the womb and our second is in the plastic IV bag hung on our mother's arm during labor.

Cord blood now contains high levels of phthalates, the ingredient that makes plastics soft, which can cause estrogenic effects in newborns.[8] Later, the baby is exposed to plastic bottles, pacifiers, plastic wrapped fast food, and microwave food. It's nearly impossible for a child to avoid this poison in their life. As adults, we are constantly exposed to plastics. You can find it in so many products used in daily life. Even the new car smell that is sprayed in used cars to trick customers is phthalate—an estrogen mimicker.

In addition to estrogen stimulating poisons, the otherwise skinny child is continuously exposed to thyroid poisons that reduce the fat burning thyroid hormone levels. These are common additives in soft drinks, water purification, Teflon pans, hot tub sanitizers, etc. They are so widespread in our environment that no one can escape them. The plasticizers are causing testosterone levels to drop in men at earlier and earlier ages, causing infertility, and early erectile dysfunction.[9] Without testosterone, a fat burning hormone, men in America are gaining weight and growing large prostates, something that not even Cialis can fix.

Pesticides and herbicides also mimic estrogen and our food is loaded with ever more increasing amounts of them.[10] The big agriculture giants are taking one staple crop after another and making them GMO in order to make them resistant to the damage from herbicides that are sprayed directly on the crops. This allows them to spray more herbicides more frequently in order to improve yields and make more money. This means that foods in our stores have more of these chemicals than ever before. Apples are often sprayed up to sixteen times.[11] The poison is not just on the surface where it can be washed or peeled off, it's found all the way through the fruit or vegetable. Increased levels of these chemicals are found in our blood and fat every year, matching the rise of obesity.

These chemicals enter our lives from other sources as well. Our water is no longer pure. An example of this is found in the fact that fish swimming downstream from Denver are mostly female while fish swimming upstream from Denver are equally male and female. Estrogens in the water produce this effect.[12] These forever chemicals are so prevalent, they are now falling out of the sky in rainwater.

The estrogens do not all originate from herbicides and pesticides. They are also real human and horse estrogens, and they are at high levels in the water. Tap water all over our country is being tested for the presence of these hormones and increasingly they are being found everywhere. Where does tap water get its estrogen? The answer is that people flush birth control hormone laced urine down the toilet, and it ends up downstream where it's taken in by a water purification plant and pumped into the city water there.[13]

Water purification can remove toxic metals and bacteria, but it cannot remove hormones. Even Premarin, a pill made from horse urine estrogen, is found in drinking water. Chemotherapy agents and heart medications are also found but they are at levels that supposedly do not cause health problems. The trouble with estrogen-like compounds is that they cause severe effects in our bodies at the smallest levels imaginable. The estrogen concentration in our blood is like one drop of estrogen in a railroad tank car holding 44,000 gallons of water. Often, the concentrations of these environmental estrogens are much higher than that.[14] If they are at higher levels than our own hormones, they can hijack our hormone system, override its built-in protections and natural feedback mechanisms, and cause huge estrogenic effects in our bodies such as weight gain, mood swings, infertility, low sperm counts, large prostates, male breast enlargement, and depression.[15]

So in addition to feeling out of whack from an imbalance of artificial hormones, the Standard American Diet throws the internal balance off even further. When we eat the SAD foods, we often feel immediately tired and want to take a nap. This helps our bodies store the food we just ate as fat. The fatigue, mental fog, and desire to sleep come from the action of insulin in our bodies. Insulin takes the high starch, white flour, corn, or sugary meal we just ate and turns it straight into fat. This causes us to overproduce insulin. The high insulin takes all our blood sugar from the meal and turns it into fat, but leaves us with low blood sugar, fatigue, irritability, and mental stupor, or brain fog.

The low-fat diet craze of a few decades ago led the nation on a true carbohydrate binge. We replaced fat calories with carbohydrate calories which resulted in a surge of obesity and diabetes. Even our children developed diabetes. I will never forget the first time I saw a skinny aerobics instructor on TV in the early nineties with a blond buzz haircut frolicking around saying fat makes you fat. I had never heard that before and it didn't make any sense to me at the time. After the popularity of her show and videos exploded, the food industry was quick to answer this low-fat food fad. We had been told for years prior to this that saturated fat caused heart disease. When the original studies on heart disease and fat were done in the fifties, most people were consuming trans-fat margarine and trans-fat Crisco in the form of hydrogenated soybean oil. The studies didn't differentiate between these fake fats and natural saturated fats, so all fats were presumed to be toxic to the heart and brain.

By the time the eighties rolled around, it wasn't hard to sell the American people on a scientifically groundless fad of eliminating fat altogether. It was conveniently forgotten for monetary reasons that many cultures throughout the world ate a large amount of fat without any heart disease. Many of these cultures also have no obesity. It turns out that carbohydrates, especially white flour, cause nutritional deficiencies that lead to heart disease too.[16] So now the trans-fat heart disease epidemic was magnified by the refined carbohydrate heart disease epidemic. The wheat flour used in these low-fat foods was bromated which also caused thyroid hormone problems which led to more obesity.[17] Apparently, we do not have precise enough genetic control over the wildly fluctuating blood sugar levels we get from eating SAD foods. Our brains are made from saturated fat and omega-3 fatty acids so, in addition to all the other cons, low-fat diets are also harmful for our brains. The only solution to this is to eat like our ancestors did before the rise of the corporate takeover of our food supply.

The fun foods, the snack foods, the addictive foods, the fast foods, and the mood foods can never be a regular part of our lives again if we want to be healthy. Some people would rather die than give up these foods. When I was a teenager, I had a neighbor who died from diabetes. I played with his children all the time. His wife started cooking a specialized diabetic diet when she found out he had diabetes. He did not like it, so he snuck out each morning and ate a big stack of pancakes with maple syrup poured all over them. The doctors couldn't control his blood sugar and he died happy, but early, leaving a widow and children.

Balance is very important in maintaining a changing diet. It's very easy to go too far in one direction. Some fad diets encourage imbalance. People want to see immediate results, but if these diets aren't followed very carefully, health problems can ensue. Many fad diets advise in reducing fat intake dramatically. While it's true that too much fat and cholesterol clog arteries, too little fat and cholesterol trashes the good feel hormones, energy hormones, and sex hormones. A diet that contains too little meat results in the loss of the B12 vitamin which causes a mental decline in the elderly that is irreversible at the later stages. This meat deficit also causes inadequate taurine: an amino acid neurotransmitter, membrane stabilizer, and protector from neurotoxicity of glutamate. People also tend to develop abnormal insulin/glucagon ratios and their blood sugars become unstable going too high or too low.

Too much meat causes increased acidity in the blood, acidosis, which causes osteoporosis.[18] It causes inflammatory polyarthritis[19] and benign prostatic hypertrophy.[20] Grilled red meat and barbecue are associated with increased risk of pancreatic cancer that is independent of alcohol, tobacco, and vegetable intake.[21] It also causes delayed gastric emptying where the stomach can't clear the food out quickly. This can overwhelm the digestive enzymes in the elderly. This causes gastric distension which dilates the lower esophageal sphincter and causes heartburn.[22] The US has an explosion of esophageal cancer because of it. Americans double up on the antacids which cause atrophy of the stomach lining. This causes the wrong bacteria to grow in the stomach where it rots the food by fermentation. The next stage is even more delayed gastric emptying, irritable bowel syndrome from rancid food entering the intestines, and poor nutrient absorption.[23] They get constipation from too much meat which causes increased bacterial glucuronidase activity in the gut. This is associated with colon cancer.[24]

The FDA suggests a minimum amount of protein in our diets in order to be healthy. This recommendation is based on old research. The level might be too high. However, even with this higher level, Americans consume meat at about twice the global average.[25] I am not recommending that everyone be vegetarians here. I am only pointing out that excesses lead to disease. Too much sugar, too much fat, too many carbohydrates, too much trans-fat, too much alcohol, too much water, and too much salt all lead to various disease states. Our bodies like variety.

There are some problems with the purely vegetarian diet as well, especially the vegan diet. These problems are not as severe as the carbo-hydrate excess diet or the protein excess diet. If a vegetarian supplements his or her diet with nutraceuticals and eats a wide variety of vegetarian foods that are not over processed, he or she can have excellent health. Vegans tend to get amino acid deficiencies and B12 deficiency which leads to anemia.[26] If our cholesterol gets too low, then we have trouble manufacturing our hormones as well. Two essential amino acids found only in meat are taurine and carnitine. One helps make neurotrans-mitters and the other helps build muscles among other things. I don't want to castigate the vegan diet too much here because it has helped a lot of people get rid of modern diseases and it's good for the planet. It's not an easy diet to follow and requires a lot of work. It's easy to become malnourished on it and end up in the doctor's office with nutritional deficiency diseases. I only want to point out that we should have a balanced diet. The one most recommended is the whole food Mediterranean Diet. It appears to be best at preventing most of the modern diseases while being varied and enjoyable to eat.[27]

The Mediterranean Diet promoted in this book has been researched by the scientific community more than many of the other diets out there. One reason for this is because there has been a record of very few sudden deaths from heart attack by the Italians who were reported to have followed this style of eating. However, when purchased in the United States, these same types of foods are more toxic than those sold in Italy. The wheat crops in Italy, for example, don't have toxic glyphosate sprayed on them prior to harvesting. This is a common practice with large corporate farms in the US so they can dry the wheat crop out in preparation for rapid harvesting and milling. Another drawback of an American trying to follow the Mediterranean Diet is that it doesn't prevent diabetes and hypertension. But overall, this diet is a good model to start with, it can be modified, and it's sustainable for a lifetime of healthy eating.

Fad diets are many and they come and go. The Genotypic Diet is one of them. Some people have had success with it. More currently, the Keto Diet is all the rage, but it has its drawbacks. It causes alterations in the liver's metabolism after six months, followers tend to develop "keto breath," and it's hard to sustain in a family or social setting where everyone else is eating differently. Lectin-Free Diets have become popular lately because a significant portion of the US population has irritable bowel syndrome (IBS), Chron's disease, or ulcerative colitis and those people can benefit from this diet. Lately, the modified Keto Diet with 10% healthy carbs added to it has been gaining popularity. It's too early to tell if it's beneficial scientifically because we don't have long-term studies completed as of yet. Other promising methods are the Anti-Cancer Diet which has been well-researched and used at many cancer centers, and there's the Anti-Inflammatory Diet which has been popular for years.

In Functional Medicine, there are many diets that have stood the test of time, are simple to learn, and have proven benefits for each category of illness they target. If you need to discover what aspects of your diet are making you sick, the Elimination Diet is a great place to start. If you need more testing to discover food allergies, the Allergen-Free Diet uses blood testing to find which food allergens need to be eliminated. Heart and diabetes patients have found healing with the Cardiometabolic Diet. If you are chronically fatigued, the Mito Food Plan for boosting mitochondrial energy could be helpful. The Detox Diet can be used to eliminate toxins. The Anti-Candida Diet can be used to fight yeast infections and restore gut health. The Phytonutrient Spectrum Diet, also known as the Rainbow Diet, is full of multi-colored fruits and vegetables that add variety and nutrients to an otherwise dull diet of processed foods. The Low FODMAP Diet (Fermentable Oligo-saccharides, Disaccharides, Monosaccharides, and Polyols) recommends avoiding simple chain-link sugars that irritate the small intestine and cause gastrointestinal distress and diarrhea. All of these methods require testing and careful examination to discover which diet or diets would be best suited for a specific ailment. So visiting a Functional Medicine doctor would be the first step. Many people find it difficult to start a specialized diet without a nutritional coach or counselor. Checking in with your physician periodically is a great way to keep you on track and ensure progress.

Diet alone can't fix everything and balancing any food program with regular exercise is a must. However, similar strategies of leaning toward extremes can turn what is normally a health benefit into a disease or injury when done in excess. Our bodies are not meant for extreme exercise. Overtraining syndrome can result in those addicted to exercise or to those who are pushed too hard as athletes.[28] The large animals that run do so intermittently. They eat vast quantities of natural foods to get the necessary resources for such intense activity. Americans eat vast quantities of carbohydrates with little nutritional value. So when they exercise too much every day, they burn through all their vitamins, minerals, and hormones.[29] Humans make a fixed amount of hormones every day. When the hormones run out, they feel exhausted beyond belief. But like the horse ridden till exhaustion and then beaten to go some more, they force themselves to keep going. Many athletes who reach this wall of exhaustion resort to elephant size hormone supplements to keep training. They become temporarily as strong as an ox, but their bodies are not meant for that level of exercise. The human joints, heart, and support systems are smaller. Built-in human feedback loops respond to gargantuan doses of hormones by adapting to the overload and making people very ill in the long run. Many of these athletes never recover from steroid abuse and live in hormone hell the rest of their shortened lives. Over exercise produces a lot of free radical oxygen which tears up the mitochondrial DNA that power the energy cycles in cells. When enough of the mitochondria fail, the person falls ill or gets cancer.[30]

Running and exercise are also hard on our joints. We have a native joint repair mechanism. It has so much damage it can repair in a given day. If we exercise beyond that point, the joint wears out prematurely and needs to be replaced. One jogger I knew ran every day. When she wore out both hips doing that in her fifties, she had both hips replaced. She immediately started walking an equal amount and I began to wonder how long her hip replacements would last.

So where is the happy medium between couch potato lethargy and jogger collapse? People need to exercise at least three times a week, maybe five at most. If they exercise every day, they don't have enough time to repair the damage and replace the nutrients that the exercise depleted. If this happens, the nutritional deficiencies multiply, the oxidative damage is not repaired, the cartilage damage accumulates, rapid aging occurs, and people get into trouble sooner.[31] A balanced program includes getting the heart rate up to the safe range for a person's age for thirty minutes three times a week. Preferably, the exercise should not tear up joints. Stair steppers or glider steppers are good for preventing this. Weight training is also recommended with low repetitions of heavy weight for thirty minutes three times weekly, enough to break out a sweat. The weight training should exercise all of the muscle groups.

Our bodies, and similarly the environment around us, like variety, balance, and moderation. So should we if we want to be simply healthy for the remainder of our lives. The diet of various indigenous or ancient cultures is extremely varied. Depending on the season and location, they can eat over a hundred different foods every week.[32] They often won't have the same breakfast twice in a week. I teach this to my allergy patients who on average, like most Americans, eat only twenty different foods every week. It's not unusual for them to become highly allergic to the foods they eat on a daily basis. They will often eat the same thing for breakfast every day. It's not long before their revved-up allergy system becomes allergic to the milk and wheat cereal they have every morning. So they switch to soy milk and become allergic to it. Indigenous peoples who haven't lost their connection with their original lands listen to their bodies and eat a wide variety of foods. Their bodies tell them when they need this or that nutrient and they listen to the promptings of their interconnected souls.

This inner wisdom is also evident in the nutrition studies done in babies and toddlers. It was originally opinioned that they would not get the right nutrition if left to themselves. We are always trying to get them to eat peas every day thinking that nutritious peas are good for the baby's health. Soon they become allergic to them, like I did. During one experiment conducted in the last part of the 20th century, a wide variety of foods were placed before infants in highchairs. Large plastic mats were used under the chairs to catch the food falling from the highchair tray. After each meal, the food was gathered up and weighed to see how much had disappeared. Some days the babies would eat only several food items. Other days they would eat multiple foods. Some foods were eaten once or twice a month. Other foods were eaten regularly. At the end of the experiment, each baby had eaten the perfect RDA for all the nutrients and vitamins. But they had consumed a balanced diet over time and not in a single meal or day.

Older Americans could learn from these infants. So how do we start to change permanently from one way of eating to another that is so unfamiliar? At the beginning, it's best to start slowly. Limit fast food meals to twice a week at first. Then cut the sugar out and replace it with Stevia, honey, or agave. Don't use the appetite stimulators such as NutraSweet. Sucralose is a thyroid poison but is perhaps better than NutraSweet. Then replace the white flour items one at a time with stone-ground whole-wheat foods. Then reduce the carbohydrates and increase the non-starchy vegetables. If it seems too much, go slower on the transition. Eat good food all week and have your favorite desserts on the weekends. If you do this, you will soon see that they make you feel ill on the weekends. Before long, you will have dropped them as well in favor of better snack foods. Some people need help from doctors, medical food diets, personal trainers, and gym and club memberships. Changing one's lifestyle can be fun and rewarding even though it seems hard at first. Take one baby step at a time and you will get there.[33]

If you need additional guidelines or a set diet to follow, look into the diets from the American Heart Association,[34] the American Diabetes Association,[35] and the American Cancer Society.[36] These diets all tout balance and natural foods that are free of toxins. Interestingly enough, some of them also mention following the Mediterranean Diet. One thing to remember when following a "Mediterranean" style diet is that many people don't fully understand what that entails. "Mediterranean" isn't referring to an Americanized-style Italian diet heavy in processed white flour pastas, canned tomato paste sauces, and bottled, dusty "parmesan" cheese. It is comprised of freshly caught fish and freshly chopped vegetables with steamed, minimal, or no cooking. These vegetables are often produced in an organic, or near organic manner causing them to be mostly toxin free. They also use fresh and properly cured flavorings or spices such as freshly chopped and crushed garlic, fresh ginger, dried spices in their whole form and ground right before cooking, and fresh greens. They freshly grate parmesan or Romano cheeses from blocks of fresh cheese. These hard cheeses keep forever in the fridge. They don't use salad dressing that you would buy in the grocery store. They sprinkle their salads with freshly produced and bottled Italian olive oil and then they dash the salad with some type of balsamic or wine vinegar. If you get these two ingredients in a bottle already combined, it might be too heavy on the oils. Europeans use a salad dressing serving tray as part of a table setting. This includes a serving bottle of olive oil and one matching serving bottle of a type of vinegar. You can monitor how much oil is going into your salad and manually reduce the caloric intake.

Don't bother with canned vegetables or at least use them sparingly. Try making your own broths. You can simmer up a large batch of homemade chicken or vegetable broth once a month and freeze it into single servings for use throughout the month. They won't have the heavy and artificial sodium of the store-bought cans, they will be fresh, and you don't have to thaw them in a microwave. Just place the frozen bit in a pan and melt it into the other ingredients. Freezing food in meal containers prevents histamine reactions. If you want to make a large meal to cover a few weeks of quick meals, freezing is by far the best way to store them. In the fridge, leftovers begin degrading immediately and the degraded elements of the food can cause symptoms of an allergic reaction. Silicon baggies and covers can be boiled, are dishwasher safe, are biocompatible, and contain no plastic hormones. Glass containers with freezer safe lids are a great option for this type of storage as well. If you can't live without breads, make large batches once a month, let the dough rise once, and then freeze it. When you want a loaf, put the dough in the fridge the night before, then take it out and let it rise one more time before baking. You will have fresh bread whenever you want without the toxic preservatives. Just make sure you are using a healthy recipe and eat it in moderation.

Eating healthy isn't a death sentence for your taste buds and cravings. Eating healthy is actually the key to a rich and fulfilled life. Build a library of cookbooks that call for all natural ingredients. Find an authentic foreign cookbook and slowly learn how to use whole spices. Visit your local Asian or Indian grocery stores for new flavors. In the same amount of time it takes to drive to the fast food restaurant or order a pizza, you can whip up a healthy, tasty, and fresh meal that will leave you and your family satiated, satisfied, and with enough energy leftover for homework, play, or relaxed socializing. The slow food restaurants and trends are another way to introduce yourself to the never dull world of fresh cooking. Farmers markets or co-ops are another place to find intriguing ideas and locally grown foods. Get excited about your lifestyle changes, learn to love new flavors and foods slowly, gradually redirect the energy you formerly put into bad habits towards habits that are fulfilling, long lasting, and rewarding. Whatever you do, don't belly flop into the new lifestyle. It will hurt and make you want to quit. Cultivate an educated flow attitude of balance, elegance, and positivity surrounding everything you do. Every moment is precious. Live them to their fullest.

20

The Monte Carlo Diet

But the House Always Wins

Overeating and indulging are encouraged and manipulated by restaurants and grocery stores. It's not unlike driving along the dusty roads into Las Vegas where inhibitions are thrown to the wind. The experience is all smoke and mirrors, a great illusionist act, but there is nothing substantial to take away. The appearance of the good life and good eating betrays the empty reality. The glitz, the glamour, the fabulous hotel suites, the entertainment, the thrill of gambling, and the elaborate food are all forgotten on the deflated trip home from Vegas. The soul is left unfulfilled, yet hungry for more emptiness.

We are taking crap shots with our health when we eat out, eat fast food, eat comfort foods, or eat with the hope that this last morsel will bring contentment. Odds are that we will feel lousy but still go back for more. The science of addiction teaches that intermittent rewards are highly addictive.[1] Eating that chocolate mousse once felt so good. Like winning the jackpot once and trying vainly to win it again, the treat becomes an addiction. It's consumed over and over again in an attempt at finding that original feeling. Every once in a while, the taste buds hit the jackpot and feel good again.[2] Sometimes that first mouthful of melting chocolate mouse or truffle is heavenly. The natural desire is to duplicate the sensation with the next bite and the next. But with each bite the enjoyment lessens or becomes bloated and hours after the over-consumption, feelings of lousiness and depression set in.[3] The modern American portion sizes are slowly killing us.

I visited Paris in 1971. The Parisians eat very differently than we do. When I ordered a meal at a local restaurant, all the portions were in small sizes. I was still hungry after the meal because I wolfed it down like a typical naïve American. The other French patrons were eating slowly and were full at the end of pleasant conversation and slow eating that lasted at least forty-five minutes. Their blood sugars had time to rise from chewing the food properly and slowly. This creates satiety. So before my blood sugars told me to stop eating, I ordered desert which was expensive but still a quarter of the size I was used to eating. I ate it so fast I hardly tasted it. I was still hungry, but couldn't afford any more food.

When Big Tobacco started buying up all the major food companies,[4] I began to notice more advertisements saying, "You can't eat just one." They had already discovered the chemistry of addiction and added numerous addictive chemicals to the cigarettes in the 60s and 70s. Now they wanted to play with the big boys and get into the huge arena of food addiction. It was a gamble that paid them royally and at our expense. When we eat their food, we are throwing the dice. We are only as good as our last meal or snack, and that could have been filled with toxins that not only cause addiction, but damage to our bodies.

Pulling into the drive thru is like cruising the Vegas Strip. Which glitzy place or piece of food is going to be the jackpot? But how are we going to feel tomorrow? It's pure roulette, and the odds are against us. The little guy can't win in the long run. The house always wins. Health is gambled away for a fleeting pleasure. The vast majority of commercial food is basically a Molotov cocktail of toxic chemicals. The ingredient lists have become so complex that they have a hard time fitting the numerous lines of small print on a package anymore.[5] The chemicals make it taste good, make it addictive, and create toxic effects in the mind, body, and soul later.[6]

On the other hand, home cooking is a win-win situation. Here, the house always wins. We get all the profit, and we share it with our families. The word "companion" comes from the Latin language and means "to eat bread with" someone. Those we eat with become our lifelong companions. A family that eats together, stays together. When we cook at home, we can add our favorite mouth-watering raw ingredients, smell them cook, and look forward to eating and enjoying them with our family. How different this traditional American home life is from the new reality that has replaced it. The modern meal consists of a family ordering pizza which often doesn't show up despite four phone calls and over a two hour wait. The family gets bored, hungry, losing their minds before it finally shows up. And then, surprise, it's cold upon arrival. Fortunately, most Americans still have a Thanksgiving meal with numerous guests cooking their favorite dishes. These meals are prepared for several hours and a happy meal results, although overeating tends to be the goal.[7]

I often tell my patients that if a food has more than five ingredients on the label, it's bad for their health, and it's a gamble to eat it. Most of the undecipherable additives are addictive substances and stabilizers that keep the food fresh tasting and looking good for months on a grocery shelf. In Europe, they would never consider eating such food. When I was in Norway several times over the years, I noticed that they have much less selection in grocery stores. But the bread was made fresh every day. The leftovers were thrown out at the end of each day. They have a taste for fresh food. We have a taste for rancid food that is chemicalized to make it seem like it tastes good. The Europeans will not eat our wheat. Our wheat has been genetically modified to contain fifty times the gluten than was there originally. Gluten is a glue-like protein in un-sprouted wheat that keeps it from germinating when there is no moisture around. It causes numerous health problems in the majority of people because of how hard it is to digest. The American gluten content in wheat exceeds the health standard for Europe, so they won't buy wheat or wheat products from the US. One of the reasons for putting more gluten in wheat, also called enriched flour, is an effort to make it rise higher and fluffier. In other words, appearances are more important than health. It's just like the Monte Carlo casino where the glitz and glamour distract you from the cold reality that you are losing your hard-earned money and that the house is always winning.

The only way to win is to build your own resort. Cook at home and you'll change the odds to your favor. Recent studies show that more than three fast food meals a week damage children's health causing a 27% increase in allergies, asthma, and eczema.[8] Eating beef, pork, and lamb daily doubles the risk of Non-Hodgkin's lymphoma compared to those who eat them less than once a week.[9] Food colorings and additives have been shown to cause hyperactivity in children.[10] A county in California banned fast food kiddie meals with toys that have too many fat calories.[11] The movie *Super Size Me* showed how quickly a 100% fast food diet can destroy one's health.[12] It was like gambling every day for a month, hoping for a win, and then going bankrupt.

There is no question that Americans are addicted to food as childhood obesity rises higher every year with no end in sight.[13] Albert Einstein is often misquoted as saying, "Insanity is doing the same thing over and over again but expecting different results." But the quote really comes from *Sudden Death* by Rita Mae Brown.[14] But before her, a similar quote was found in the *Basic Text of Narcotics Anonymous*.[15] The way we gamble our health away by eating in these culinary casinos is very similar to a narcotic addiction that for some will cause a painful, early death later in life.

The health benefits of eating right have been known since antiquity. Hippocrates said in 450 BC on the Greek island of Kos, "Let food be thy medicine and medicine be thy food."[16] When people would get sick in the polluted eighteenth century European and American cities, they moved out to the countryside with their relatives to eat wholesome food, drink fresh water, and breathe in some fresh air. It wasn't long before they were better and could resume their city life and work. We no longer have such privileges or country folk. Instead, we turn to quick fixes sponsored by toxic Big Pharma for instant symptom relief with no cure. We borrow from our health bank account to gamble on toxic food and toxic drugs. But sooner or later we have nothing left to gamble and, like the prodigal son, we return home empty handed hoping for some decent food on the table. Eating at home is a royal flush nearly every time. Most of the time we can predict what will happen with the food we make and eat. Eating out is a true gamble. We have no idea what we are going to feel like later because we have no idea what they put in the food. Let's ditch the sham and build our homes and diets around the foundation set by our ancestors. The positive energy we grow in our gardens and homes from conscientious buying of local and healthy foods will have a ripple effect into the broader market. It is the only way to truly lessen the power of these megalithic companies.

21

The Milky Whey

As we fine tune the approach to nutritional flow, we narrow the focus even more by honing in on a diet staple rooted deeply in American culture and traditions. Namely milk and its byproducts. Many modern health critics are decrying this diet standard as being unhealthy overall, but there is a reason our ancestors have been consuming it for so many generations. And the answer why isn't always that simple. There are multiple components in milk. Some are good and some are really bad.

Calcium is good for our bones, if we can absorb it. There is a problem with pasteurized milk in that it coagulates proteins, and it binds calcium thereby preventing absorption. Lactose is a milk sugar that is good for energy unless a person is lactose intolerant. A significant portion of the world's population suffers from lactose intolerance.[1] Babies make lactase in the lining of their intestines. Lactase breaks down lactose into glucose and galactose which are types of simple sugars. Genetically we are wired to stop making this enzyme, lactase, when we are weaned at age two. This is the average age of weaning in aboriginal cultures unaffected by the pressures and stress of modern urban life. Without lactase, the sugar runs through the gut without being absorbed. It attracts water that is not absorbed either and causes osmotic diarrhea in lactase deficient or lactose intolerant children and adults.

Northern Europeans and most white Americans have a genetic malformation or adaption that allows them to continue making this enzyme their whole lives. But even they will have problems if they get influenza, rhinovirus, Norwalk virus, or other viruses such as measles that attack the lining of the gut. The attack destroys the villi in the stomach lining where lactase is made. This causes diarrhea if milk is consumed in the recovery period from these viruses. With a severe gastrointestinal viral infection, this temporary lactase deficiency can last up to six weeks.[2]

Conversely, milk has been used for treating gastric ulcers. High stomach acid during a stressful period causes the lining to the stomach to break down and secrete less mucous to protect itself causing gastritis and even ulcers. Over the centuries, grandmothers have advised their families to drink milk with the intent that it would absorb stomach acid and reduce stomach pain.[3] This actually works in some people. I have seen many patients who consume a gallon or more of milk a day. Some because they become addicted to the morphine effects of milk, and others who need another glass of milk every half hour to hour or so for stamping out stomach pain. Unfortunately, the pain returns because milk fat causes an increase in stomach acid within thirty to sixty minutes. So what seemed to work so well in the beginning ends up being an ulcer treatment with serious side effects. The modern antiulcer drugs also have side effects such as long-term calcium loss from bones or even osteoporosis after seven years or more of continuous use.[4]

Whey is one of the best proteins known to man.[5] For decades the biological value of different plant and animal proteins were compared. The following table lists the biological value of each by how much nitrogen was absorbed from the protein into the body:

Protein Type[6]	Biological Value (BV)	Protein Efficiency Ratio (PER)	Net Protein Utilization (NPU)	Protein Digestibility Score Corrected for Amino Acids PDCAAS	Decline in BV with Overconsumption[7]
Whey Protein	104	3.2	92	1.0	70
Egg	100	3.9	94	1.0	70
Milk	91	2.5	82	1.0	
Casein	77	2.5	76	1.0	
Beef	80	2.9	73	0.92	
Soy	74	2.2	61	1.0	
Gluten	64	0.8	67	0.25	25
Peanuts		1.8		0.52	
Black Beans		0.0		0.75	

Whey protein improves HDL levels and stabilizes blood sugars better than casein.[8] Whey protein supplementation of an otherwise unchanged diet has been associated with a dramatic weight loss over three months in several scientific studies.[9] Twenty grams three times a day was the optimum dose. Weightlifters use whey protein to build muscle rapidly because it's so effective. More muscle helps burn more fat which enhances that ripped look that is so desirable. All our neurotransmitters are made from amino acids. If the toxic or incomplete proteins people consume do not have all the amino acids found in whey, they become depressed, lack energy, and become anxious. Whey supplementation can correct amino acid deficiencies behind many emotional, social, and learning disorders.[10] Since whey is so good for overall health, why not drink more milk to get more of it? Unfortunately, whey protein is completely destroyed by the temperatures of pasteurization which are between 62° C and 71° C.[11] There are many products that have been studied to boost the immune system such as colostrum, which is the milk produced in the first several days after a cow delivers her calf. The calf's own immune system is activated by the colostrum which is full of immunoglobulins. Immunoglobulins are also considered to be one of the whey proteins. The whey proteins are: alpha lactalbumin 2%, beta lactalbumin 10%, serum albumin 1%, immunoglobulins 2%, and other proteins 2%. So the benefits of colostrum are a more concentrated fraction of a portion of whey protein immunoglobulins.[12] In other words, whey is just a weaker form of colostrum.

On the other hand, casein is not a good protein source for humans. It is heat stable and is not destroyed by pasteurization. Not only does it cause numerous health problems, but it is also toxic in many ways to humans. Casein is meant for animals with four stomachs. It literally takes four stomachs to digest this compact protein. That is why most cultures consume fermented milk such as buttermilk, kefir, and yogurt. This fermentation acts like another stomach to predigest casein.[13] Because casein enters the intestines intact or as casomorphin, it causes many health problems. Casomorphin is a morphine-like molecule. It puts us asleep. That is why warm milk has been used as a nighttime treatment for insomnia. However, morphine also causes histamine release. This causes flushing of skin and engorgement of mucous membranes. The nose becomes congested and fills up with mucous. So do the lungs.[14] This is a typical allergy response without even being allergic to milk. It's even worse if one is allergic to milk. So if the nose plugs up, the beneficial sedative effect of milk is destroyed by a stuffy, mucous nose that degrades the quality of sleep and causes disrupted sleep rhythms, less deep refreshing sleep, and more awakenings.

However, casein can be ingested without the negative side effects so long as it is processed correctly. Casein is found in unusual places like Greek yogurt which is spiked with extra casein. Original yogurt has predigested casein in it and is not as bad as regular milk. But real Greek yogurt from Greece is naturally high in casein which is digested by the probiotics in the yogurt. However, in the US, profits, not preventive health, dominate FDA thinking and actual practice. So instead of getting more predigested protein, we get more casein as an additive in fake Greek yogurt.[15] Why not spike it with whey protein which is healthier? Casein is also a natural part of butter. Ghee is clarified butter without the casein.

Another serious problem with undigested casein is that it activates macrophages in the intestines. Seventy percent of the entire immune system is in the lining to the gut or intestines in the form of Peyer's patches. The white blood cells kill viruses, pathogenic bacteria, parasites, and harmful foreign particles. They also gobble up toxic food proteins like casein. If they don't, the casein ends up in breast milk causing food allergies in breastfed babies. The casein also ends up in inflamed joint fluids, bursitis effusions, and can be the direct cause of a painful joint.[16] So if the white blood cells are allowed to do their job, the joint pain will be prevented. However, once the casein is taken up by the white blood cells, they become activated and secrete numerous hormones, cytokines, and other inflammatory chemicals, and attract more white cell warriors to the area causing inflammation in the gut. These activated white blood cells are the culprits behind excessive food and environmental allergies, excessive mucous in the nose and lungs, foggy thinking, and mental and behavioral problems in children and adults.[17]

Casein has components that act as antioxidants. Alpha s1-casein has a peptide fragment that is a powerful antioxidant. Alpha s2 fragments have been shown to have antimicrobial properties. Beta casein has fragments that activate macrophage phagocytosis and cause them to release peroxide.[18] Many scientists, doctors, and allergists believe this to be one of the main initiating and promoting factors in food and environmental allergies. Behaving like a light switch, the beta-casein flips on genes that have been initially turned off and promotes their expression. Then, the epigenetically switched-on macrophages digest food particles and swallowed environmental pollens and create antibodies to them and present them to antibody producing B cells. These cells become memory cells devoted to the production of antibodies to that particular food or pollen. These memory cells persist and replace themselves and this process can go on for decades if not one's entire life.[19]

Raw milk is a major source of diseases spread worldwide. Raw milk can go bad, but there are many factors that prevent putrefaction in raw milk. A pathogen, Streptococcus pyogenes, can only grow in heated milk, not raw milk. The heating destroys the antimicrobial properties of raw milk.[20] Raw milk preservation has many steps including immediate cooling, straining, centrifuging, and Lactoperoxidase System (LP-s). In Cuba and many Central American, South American, and African countries, over half of the milk would spoil because of lack of refrigeration if it weren't for this processing. So the LP-s preserves the safety of the milk. Cuba preserves over half of its milk production this way.[21]

So there are other options that would protect the US food supply of milk products without sacrificing the quality of the nutrients and food. Unless they are all chemists, most food labeling is Greek to the average American. Without a detailed knowledge of what, how, and why the US food supply is so corrupt, the answer about fixing it becomes unclear and even a little scary when considering the monolithic companies that are behind it.

The body likes order and balance along with comfort and safety. Consuming foods randomly from the supermarket is like opening all the doors and windows of your home in the middle of a thunderstorm. Luck might get you through the night, but wouldn't you rather warm up by the stove over a simmering saucepan while the rain beats relentlessly against the windows?

22

Shangri-La Versus Sugar Shack

As we are beginning to understand, natural foods are not always healthy for us. Natural foods that are processed heavily or incorrectly become harmful creating blockages in our energy and overall health. One such food is refined sugar which is sourced from sugar cane and sugar beets. The refining process is so intense, that all nutrients from these plants are destroyed leaving only a very concentrated simple sugar. The body likes to have balance, but these sugars are not attached to a nutrient-rich food that can be eaten slowly and in healthy quantities. Eating refined sugars in homemade or commercially-processed foods gives us unhealthy doses of simple sugar that throw body systems out of balance and into disorder.

The symptoms appear like a Jekyll and Hyde personality switch. At first, sugar makes us feel good with a transient rise in serotonin.[1] Refined sugar enters the bloodstream quickly acting not unlike a drug in the body. For people with a sensitivity to sugar, it can be as addictive as heroin. Refined sugar creates a biochemical reaction in the mind causing more beta-endorphin release. The resulting euphoria increases the potential for addiction.[2] Addiction leads to increased consumption which in turn amplifies the negative effects of sugar in the body.

This isn't the only hormone that is surging after an overdose of re-fined sugars. The other hormone people with diabetes are all too aware of is insulin. This hormone is released to regulate the sugar, or glucose, so that it doesn't stay heavily concentrated in the blood. Insulin takes the sugar out of the blood and places it in fat storage. Messing with this hormone by overdosing on sugar causes irregularities in its production causing the body to end up with too much or too little of the essential hormone.[3]

These effects can destroy our health and at the same time distort our behavior and feelings of wellbeing. After a sugar high, the withdrawal-like sugar lows kick in. This is the body's attempt at creating balance after extreme imbalance. At this point, cortisol is released into the bloodstream in order to alert the liver to send stored sugars back into the blood. Through this process, the sugar is actually depleting the body of the essential hormone cortisol.[4] Essential as it is, this rush of cortisol, a hormone mostly needed for emergency situations, contributes to paranoid, fearful, blaming, and I-have-the-worst-life thinking.

Another drawback to the sugar highs and lows is that it affects adrenalin levels. When the body is thrown off balance from the disturbance caused by sugar consumption, the adrenal gland compensates with adrenalin.[5] This influx of adrenaline zaps the adrenal glands of their production power creating another low after the sugar is gone. This type of back-and-forth pivoting can cause mood swings and anger outbursts, irritability, jitteriness, and trembling hands.[6]

This crisis obviously affects the brain. Chemically, the brain needs blood sugar to function properly. Without blood sugar balance in the brain, we are likely to feel confusion, forgetfulness, mental fog, and fatigue.[7] Low blood sugar also affects tissues and organs. Low blood sugar triggers the liver enzymes that create inflammation.[8]

Conversely, when sugar levels are spiking with each new high carb food, the continual outpouring of insulin will eventually lead to insulin resistance.[9] This insulin resistance leads to higher insulin levels in the body.[10] High insulin levels make people feel lousy and are also associated with inflammation. The inflammation affects the brain, heart, coronary arteries and carotids, gut, and joints.[11] In worst case scenarios, this insulin overproduction wears out the pancreas and leads to pancreatic failure.[12] Pancreatic failure leads to high blood sugar diabetes where not enough insulin is produced in the body.[13]

High blood sugars also poison nerves and harden arteries.[14] This petrifaction occurs naturally on earth in many other processes. There is a river in northern England that petrifies objects placed in it. It takes a few weeks to months, but eventually, the object turns to stone. The river has a high mineral content. The local people of Yorkshire put their objects at the top of a small waterfall. The calcium rich water flows over them, and soon, they are hard as rock.[15]

When people eat sugar, they are doing the same thing to the insides of their bodies. Sugar hardens arteries with calcium plaques. First, it's turned into fatty acids, then the fatty acids get into the space under the lining of the arteries, then the body puts calcium in the fatty plaques, and the artery gets stiffer. The inflammation in the underlying muscle caused by the rancid fat accumulating on top of it causes the muscle to get stiff as well.

Advanced glycation end products (AGEs) worsen this inflammation and oxidant stress and are present in increased amounts in people suffering from diabetes and cardiovascular disease.AGEs cause the nerve damage that leads to foot ulceration and eventually amputation in diabetic patients. AGEs are formed when proteins are cooked with sugar and without water. The browning of the food forms the AGEs. This process can also occur inside the body due to the overconsumption of simple sugars and the chronically elevated blood sugar levels of diabetics. Eating foods that are low in processed sugars and eating proteins that are cooked with minimal browning or in liquids can prevent the formation of the AGEs that cause increased aging symptoms and damage to the body.[16]

Another browning action of cooking is called caramelization. Caramelization is the process of attaching sugar to protein. The color changes from white to orange brown. When we eat sugar, we are caramelizing our proteins. Hemoglobin A1c is a sugarized blood protein in red blood cells that carries oxygen when not full of carbon monoxide from smoking. The level of hemoglobin A1c goes up the higher the average blood sugars go. It's kind of like caramelizing ourselves from the inside. The level of it represents the average sugar level in our blood for the last several months.[17]

High levels of sugar intake can also cause intestinal problems, especially for people with a tendency for fructose intolerance. In these cases, sugar can cause constipation and bloating symptoms.[18] Another intestinal problem from elevated processed sugar intake includes a leaky gut.[19] This causes toxins, partially undigested foods, and larger chain proteins to seep out of the intestinal lining and into the bloodstream. These toxins end up in the liver and overtax it. Leaky gut is also a cause of runaway inflammation in the body.[20]

Even if someone doesn't have diabetes or an intolerance to refined sugar or fructose, the negative effects extend beyond digestion, weight, or mood problems. Flu season is an especially important time to reduce sugar intake. In the intestinal tract, where most of the body's immune system operates, sugar actually feeds pathogenic bacteria. This depletes the immune system when the body needs it most to fight off viruses.[21] Avoiding sugary cough drops is also a good idea when the flu strikes.

All this being said, if we want to live a somewhat balanced and satisfied life, we will want to have, on occasion, that slice of wedding cake or a cookie from the neighborhood bake sale. There are ways to counterbalance occasional treats. For example, sugar competes with vitamin C for entry into every cell.[22] Consuming more vitamin C before a sugary snack or dessert will reduce some of the side effects of sugar. Vitamin C has also been found to reduce blood sugar levels in diabetics.[23]

Sometimes a shift in the direction of eating habits will also help the sugar detox have a lasting effect. A sustainable and balanced way to heal from a sugary diet is to slowly switch into eating more foods from the Paleo Diet.[24] It takes about thirty days to detox and get the metabolism back on track. It's not a drastic diet and won't cause rapid weight loss without intense exercise and portion limiting. Overtime it will prevent, possibly even slow or reverse, modern diseases from sugary diets including obesity, cardiovascular disease, type 2 diabetes, cancer, autoimmune diseases, osteoporosis, acne, myopia (nearsightedness), macular degeneration, glaucoma, varicose veins, hemorrhoids, diverticulosis, and gastric reflux.[25]

It begins with the elimination or gradual reduction of dairy products, cereal grains, legumes, refined sugars, and processed foods. These foods are replaced with an increase of fresh foods including fresh meats from grass-fed or free-ranging animals, beef, pork, lamb, poultry, and game meat, fish, seafood, fresh fruits, vegetables, seeds, nuts, and a variety of healthy oils including olive, coconut, avocado, macadamia, walnut, and flaxseed oil.[26]

This diet is just one way of reducing refined sugar intake and eating for the long run rather than for short term satisfaction. Eating whole, fresh, and minimally processed foods will reduce excessive cravings of unhealthy and sugar-laden foods. It will also train the palate to crave freshness and loathe anything pretending to be real food. It will create a harmonious state of wellness in the body that will extend into the mental state and outward toward relations with others creating effortless flow on many levels.

23

Foodborne Illnesses

Revenge of the Superbugs

Invariably though, no garden exists without its snake. Even when you are making healthy decisions, you still have to have your guard up. Eating whole and minimally processed foods can expose you to some very unhealthy pathogens. Superbugs salmonella, Shigella, E. coli, and Staph aureus are not only common throughout our food supply, but are increasingly becoming antibiotic resistant. So educating ourselves about the signs and risks is the best way to eat healthy foods safely.

Salmonella is found in nearly all chicken ovaries in the USA and thus is in nearly all chicken eggs.[1] If an egg is infected severely, it will float in water because these gas forming organisms provide gas buoyancy. Less severe infections are detected by the odor of the egg at room temperature. Other sources of Salmonella infection are milk, meats, fresh fruits and vegetables, farm animals, turtles, iguanas, and petting zoos. Outbreaks in 2008 were found in cantaloupe melons (March 2008),[2] Malt-O-Meal cereal (April 2008),[3] peppers (June and July 2008), and frozen chicken dinners (October 2008).[4] In the past, there have been outbreaks associated with pancake mixes, frozen pot pies, and peanut butter. When food production is contaminated with human and animal feces at any stage, then salmonella infection is likely.

Symptoms are variable but fever is almost always present. Other symptoms are nausea, occasional vomiting, dehydration in children and elderly, diarrhea, abdominal pain and cramping, and headache. The symptoms usually last four to seven days and usually common oral antibiotics suffice for the simple cases. In 1963, we had 18,000 cases per year documented, but recently it has climbed to 40,000 cases per year with 600 deaths reported yearly. The *Centers for Disease Control and Prevention* estimates there were 1,412,498 unreported and reported incidences in the United States between the years of 1983 to 1992.[5] Although these numbers are astounding, prevention is still simple. Cook all meats till pink is gone, wash hands, use separate utensils and cutting boards for cutting uncooked meats, cooked meats, and fresh vegetables. In fact, keeping a separate cutting board for raw meats only is a good way to keep track.

Shigellosis, another bacterial pathogen from feces, can cause some of the most severe cases of gastroenteritis. High fever and massive diarrhea with blood is the hallmark of the worst infections. Mild infections can cause stomach upset and last four to eight days. Severe infections last three to six weeks untreated. Shigella is resistant to a number of antibiotics. It's diagnosed with a stool sample. Antidiarrheals can make it worse. Produce is commonly infected with Shigella so it can be picked up from raw vegetables in addition to dairy products and meats. Often it is found in potato, tuna, or chicken salads. Reported cases number 22,412 with actual incidence twenty times higher.[6]

E. coli is commonly found in the gut. What is not so common is the kind that causes bloody diarrhea. It's called E. coli O157:H7 which produces a toxin that hurts the delicate lining of the intestines. Because of the way cows are slaughtered, E coli contaminates the meat. E. coli is not normally in the meat but in the intestines of cows. Our efficient slaughterhouses reduce costs to the producer but do not reduce contamination. Fortunately, not many cows carry E. Coli O157:H7. But in 2007 alone, there were twenty-one recalls involving thirty-three million pounds of beef. Lately, retailers are not recalling all of the beef sold in their stores when there is an outbreak of bloody diarrhea traced to their meat.[7]

So how do we avoid E. coli contamination concerns? The following is some of the best advice I've found which was largely borrowed from FamilyDoctor.org:

- Wash your hands carefully with soap before you start cooking.
- Cook ground beef until you see no pink anywhere.
- Don't taste small bites of raw ground beef while you're cooking.
- Don't put cooked hamburgers on a plate that had raw ground beef on it before.
- Cook all hamburgers to at least 160 °F. A meat thermometer is helpful.
- Defrost meats in the refrigerator or the microwave. Don't let meat sit on the counter to defrost.
- Keep raw meat and poultry separate from other foods. Use hot water and soap to wash cutting boards and dishes if raw meat and poultry have touched them.
- Don't drink raw milk unless you really trust the producer.
- Stay away from unpasteurized dairy products if pregnant.
- Keep food refrigerated or frozen.
- Keep hot food hot and cold food cold.
- Refrigerate or freeze leftovers right away or throw them away.
- People with diarrhea should wash their hands carefully and often, using hot water and soap, and washing for at least 30 seconds. People who work in childcare centers and homes for the elderly should wash their hands often too.
- In restaurants, always order hamburgers that are cooked well done so that no pink shows.[8]

Like E. coli, Staph aureus has a toxin that can make us sick. Staphylococcus aureus is one of the most common foodborne illnesses.[9] It can produce symptoms with a very small dose of less than .1 microgram.[10]

The symptoms are not always the same for different people. Most common are nausea, vomiting, retching, abdominal cramping, and prostration. In severe cases, someone might experience headache, muscle cramping, and fluctuations in blood pressure and pulse. Usually, the infection is over in two to three days depending on the severity.[11]

The FDA Center for Food Safety Applied Nutrition has sobering statistics on Staph aureus. Foodborne diseases are suspected to cause 76 million illnesses, 325,000 hospitalizations, and 5,200 deaths each year with 20% of these numbers being clearly documented pathogens.[12] It is suspected that one in six outbreaks of foodborne illnesses is caused by Staph aureus. In 1983, 7,082 cases of food poisoning were investigated and 1,257 were found to be Staph aureus.[13]

Staph aureus can be killed by pasteurization, but the toxin secreted by some strains of Staph aureus survives the high temperature pasteurization process. The only way to prevent toxin exposure in the purchased food is to prevent Staph aureus contamination during the food making process. Most countries allow low levels of contamination in purchased foods like unpasteurized European cheeses made from raw milk. Fermentation drives down levels of all Staph aureus including the toxin producing strains. Salt concentrations above 12% and acetic acid (vinegar) inhibit release of the toxin from the bacteria.[14]

The most common foods infected with Staph aureus involve human processing by hand and include "meat, meat products; poultry and egg products; salads such as egg, tuna, chicken, potato, and macaroni; bakery products such as cream-filled pastries, cream pies, and chocolate éclairs; sandwich fillings; and milk and dairy products."[15] Common sense ways to prevent starting your own Staph aureus with your infected hands is to wash hands carefully before and after all food preparation, avoid preparing food when you have skin infections or wear gloves, don't prepare foods while you are sick with Staph-like symptoms, and keep hot foods over 140°F and cold foods under 40°F.[16]

So by following these guidelines and being aware of the types of infections that can be transmitted through foods, we can keep ourselves and loved-ones safe while we prepare them healthy and satisfying meals. These infections aren't always preventable, but if we know the signs, we can get people the right treatment as soon as possible. This is especially important for the immune compromised and elderly. While a healthy and younger person may be able to bounce back after treatment for such illnesses, they can be life threatening for others.

24

The Yin Yang of Moldy Mycotoxins

In many traditional and culturally distinct African villages, a chieftain or shaman would watch over their villagers with a wisdom beyond modern science. Their tribal rituals had been passed down through the ages. Depending on the tribe and their location, villagers typically lived in grass roofed huts made with curved sticks. In this type of setting, their lives would be nearly devoid of our Greco-Roman rectangles and right angles. After growing up in such surroundings, they wouldn't see the optical illusions dependent on the visual cortex computing of straight lines.[1] The cultural limits of our observations are even more apparent when compared to that of the South African bushman. It is said that the bushman could see like eagles with far vision so acute that they have described the moons of Jupiter.[2]

One such observation occurs when the people of a village would all get sick around the same time. The tribal chieftain would often move the village five miles down the road. He would make the villagers build new grass huts and their health would be magically restored. This wisdom also extends to burial practices. A practice of the Kalahari people is to burn the hut of a deceased person after they are buried.[3] What is this ancient wisdom that restores or preserves the health of an entire village?

Grass huts are vulnerable to mold infestations. Ridding mold of an environment, village, or home has been happening for centuries. Methods for eliminating mold have been documented in ancient texts spanning from the Bible to the Roman "de Architectura." In the book of Leviticus, removal of moldy housing materials and the replastering of walls was used to combat molds. According to Marcus Vitruvius Pollio in "de Architectura," the alignment of the home with the four directions and the sun is very important. A room facing to the East with morning sun exposure is preferable for libraries and bed chambers. This would reduce the influence of heavy afternoon sun and southern moisture-laden winds that might produce mold in books, shelving, and bedding.[4] This is very similar to the directional positioning taught in feng shui architectural design. The proper energies, flow of water, sun, and wind, all determine where certain rooms and activities are favorably situated within a home or building.

Native Americans would often burn the land alongside streams and rivers.[5] The purpose of this could have been for constructing settlements along the water source or to clear it of occasional toxic fungi that poison fish and plant populations.[6] Early American settlers also found ways to reduce mold toxicity. Settlers used to sleep on straw ticks and lived in houses composed of straw roofs and clay dirt floors. Every spring, the cotton bags holding the straw were emptied and fresh straw was used. The grass was taken off the roof and new grass replaced it.

People are very sensitive to certain molds. Some common soil fungi are good for intestinal health such as Streptomyces badius. Eating shitake and reishi mushrooms for their phytonutrients is good for you. Mushrooms, fungi, and molds are all the same organisms. On the other hand, there are many molds which are not good for you. In fact, some are lethal. Certain toadstool mushrooms look very much like the edible ones, but numerous deaths are caused worldwide when people mistakenly eat them. The poisons they contain are called mycotoxins. When they dry out, the toadstools release toxins from their spores to kill off competitor bacteria during drought times. When the moisture comes back, they will be the only ones living to eat all the new food. That way they can grow like crazy and take over their local environment. Some of these toxins are harvested to make antibiotics like penicillin that kill off nasty bacterial infections.

Our lives are full of molds and their toxins. We have poorly constructed homes where the plumbing leaks, the bathroom tile cracks, and water moisture seeps into the paper on the drywall. In the 1970s, drywall replaced plaster in the construction of new homes and buildings. The paper on the gypsum drywall board gets moldy when wet. Stachybotrys chartarum is the kind of mold that grows on the surface of drywall. It has more mycotoxins than other indoor molds and causes allergies and respiratory inflammation. Most buildings that have flooding or other water damage need to replace these walls or the people who work or live in them will get sick or have increased allergies.[7] Everywhere there is moisture and a place that harbors it, mold grows and releases its spores and mycotoxins into our sickened lives.

If you catch them early enough, there are ways you can combat these household molds that don't require major repairs such as replacing tiles, floors, or drywall. For smaller jobs, I suggest cleaning molds with food grade hydrogen peroxide rather than chlorine bleach. Hydrogen peroxide is a naturally occurring element in the environment. We drink hydrogen peroxide laced water all the time because it is a part of rain water. When sunlight breaks down oxygen high in the sky, it forms ozone which interacts with water vapor and becomes hydrogen peroxide. This rains down on oceans, lakes, rivers, and streams and acts as a natural disinfectant in them. Using this natural and cheap water treatment for city water is a common practice in Europe.

The healing waters of Lourdes, France are high in hydrogen peroxide containing about 0.25% H2O2. David Farr, MD PhD, was a leading proponent of H2O2 therapy and worked at the Geneses Medical Research Institute in Oklahoma City. He believed that using medicinal, food grade, H2O2 helps tissue repair, cellular energy, growth of normal cells, immune function, the mitochondrial energy system, and hormone regulation. He treated many conditions with H2O2 therapy including candidiasis, chronic fatigue, depression, arthritis, AIDS, and cancer. These therapies are not based on word of mouth testimonials like the old patent medicines, but on basic science, numerous scientific research articles, and animal and human research studies.[8]

Many people use it for simple cuts and wounds. When 3% hydrogen peroxide is placed on a wound infected with bacteria, the H2O2 bubbles as the oxygen is being released. This release kills the bacteria in the same way that our own immune cells release hydrogen peroxide in order to kill microbes.[9] Many also use it in toothpaste with baking soda and salt.[10] It's an important component to have in your daily life because it kills off the things that are harmful to you, while not increasing the chances of lung or cancer problems like chlorine bleach can. It's extremely important to note that drinking either bleach or concentrated hydrogen peroxide will likely kill you. So using it does come with risks. Keeping it away from kids and animals is an absolute must. But I still recommend using food grade hydrogen peroxide in place of chlorine bleach as a household cleaner and disinfectant to combat mold problems as a great way to keep the non-toxic flow of your home in good order and balance.

Keeping our homes and environments mold free is a must, but molds are also prone to creeping into our food supply where they continue wreaking havoc on human health. There is a long history of this being observed. Bedlam was the house for the insane in Renaissance England. During this time, mental illness was a favorite theme of the playwright Shakespeare. Whether we read King Lear and his lunatic yelling in the pouring rain, the Macbeths' decent into evil and bloodshed, or Othello who is slowly driven into madness by Iago, the lives of the insane fascinate us, scare us, and create an unsettling paranoia in our lives. One of Shakespeare's plays stands out as the most fascinating glimpse into the minds of the insane ever written. The play *Hamlet* revels in the Machiavellian twists and turns of the royalty in Denmark during the 1200s.[11]

What some readers of Shakespeare do not know is that the intrigues, suicides, and deranged thinking that make the play so famous actually existed to some extent in Denmark at the time. Denmark has no mountains. It's flat and surrounded by water. Until wheat prices collapsed in the 1880s, wheat was the main crop of Denmark. Because of the constant rain and high humidity from sea winds, the common wheat fungus or rust made the bread moldy.[12] Some speculate that this moldy bread was a culprit in causing insanity in the play Hamlet.

The molds produced toxins that had both a beneficial effect and a negative effect on the Danes. The Danes were considered to be the hardiest of the Europeans and had fewer physical illnesses than the rest of Europe. This might be theorized that they received some health effects from moldy breads and grains, the precursors to penicillin, as it was used in ancient healing methods around the world in earlier eras.[13]

Citrinin is a mold that is also found in wheat, rice, corn, barley, oats, rye, and food colored with Monascus pigment. Citrinin has been proven to have a natural antibacterial and penicillin effect on pathogens.[14] However, this mycotoxin has both a light and a dark side. On one hand, it's used to produce many foods that have nutrition and great flavor including cheeses, sake, miso, and soy sauce. On the other, is has been blamed for yellow rice disease in Japan and can be toxic to the kidneys if consumed in large quantities from improperly cultivated grains.[15]

Mycotoxins from molds, fungus, and yeast also cause widespread hormonal and neurotransmitter changes. About 2000 years ago in Denmark, a man was brutally murdered and dumped in a boggy swamp. His body was preserved in the mud of the swamp, and he was named the "Tolland Man" by his discovers. The mycotoxin that produces ergot was found in his stomach during the autopsy. The hallucinations caused by ergot poisoning may have led to his violent death.[16]

Ergot is a common fungus found on the rye grown in Denmark, France, and other European countries. The blisters it caused were called St. Anthony's fire. But the mental effects were even more painful. The Salem witchcraft trials were thought to be the result of ergot poisoning causing mental illness in the supposed witches.[17] It's similar to LSD in chemical structure and caused widespread hallucinations. It caused seizures, spasms, itching, headaches, nausea, and vomiting. The mental symptoms were dramatic: mania, melancholia, psychosis, and delirium.[18] So Shakespeare's Hamlet set in Elsinore, Denmark in the early 1200s captures the full spectrum of ergotism which was not discovered to be connected to moldy grains until 1676.[19]

Another mold found in the wheat and corn that plagues humans and animals is called Fusarium.[20] This mold is highly toxic affecting the nervous system of horses and having lethal effects in humans and animals. It's not a common mold found in our food supply, but has been known to crop up in the hay or feed given to horses. This mold can be passed on from horse to human, so horse feed needs to be inspected for molds as well.[21]

Can we get ergotism from eating moldy grains today? Can a high white food (starchy diet) and sugar diet cause similar mental problems so common in the Denmark in Shakespeare's play? The short answer is that although mold is usually not on our grains today, over-consumption of white foods and sugar can cause the molds to grow in our intestines. When they grow there, they usually make mycotoxins which then cause the same problems the Danes experienced so long ago.[22]

I recently had a patient who came to me with both his ear drums eaten away by a mold that had filled his ear canals as well. He had been getting the mold cleaned out of his ear canals and off of his ear drums weekly for quite some time. The other doctors who took care of him prescribed all the commonly used ear drops and pills for treating this disorder, but nothing had worked. He came to me in desperation willing to try anything. I found that he also had bad jock rot and the steroid creams were not working very well either. He also had fungal toenails and was very obese. I could then see the whole picture. He had a disseminated fungal infection. It was most likely originating in his intestines from the white food and sugary diet he was on. I gave him my special anti-candida diet which is a stricter version of the William Crook anti-candida diet. I cleaned his ears every week and soon the mold dis-appeared, and the ear drum perforations healed quickly. He lost twenty pounds and the mold disappeared completely from his body.

To prevent molds from entering the body from already moldy foods, it is also important to know the shelf life of foods and condiments. Sometimes a person will assume his or her allergies are acting up, but upon inspection of the fridge, it's full of outdated food and condi-ments. Sometimes the mold can be present in processed cottonseed oil, peanuts, spices, pistachios, and maize. The molds that most commonly grow on these goods are called aflatoxins.[23] These molds are actually very carcinogenic and cancer causing. So that peanut butter that's been sitting in the fridge for months (or more!) could have had carcinogenic molds growing on the actual peanuts before it was made into peanut butter or has had these molds growing in it during its stay in the fridge. Ways to avoid this are to choose different ground nuts, like cashew or almond butter, because peanuts are loaded with other health problems like inflammation and allergies too. You can also run the nuts through a grinder so you see whether or not they are contaminated before buying them. This would be one of the safer ways to eat peanut butter if it's really difficult to give up.

Another mycotoxin that throws health off balance is called an ochra-toxin.[24] This mold is found in cereals, coffee, dried fruit, and red wine. The best way to avoid this and other mycotoxins is to stop buying mass marketed processed foods and only buy fresh foods or good quality processed foods from trusted sources. Seeing foods in their natural form is a great way to avoid molds. Buying coffee beans and grinding them on clean equipment, making homemade cereals of nuts and whole grains, drying fruit at home or eating fresh fruit, and buying only quality wines from respectable growers are ways to avoid this type of mold.

When possible, buy whole and organic fruits and vegetables to avoid the mold Patulin. This mold is found in all store-bought concentrated fruit juices.[25] This is a case for looking at each fruit and vegetable to inspect for mold before buying it at the grocery store. Home juicers are a great investment and are worth your child's health. For the adults, fermentation kills the mold in the juice used for ciders.

This is a helpful list from the USDA for foods and their approximate storage life in the fridge for the prevention of ingesting molds:

Food Spoilage Safety Guide from USDA[26]

FOOD	REFRIGERATION TIME
Bacon	7 days
Commercial brand vacuum-packed dinners with USDA seal, unopened	2 weeks
Cooked egg dishes	3-4 days
Cooked meat, poultry and fish leftovers/pieces, casseroles	3-4 days
Corned beef in pouch with pickling juices	5-7 days
Eggs fresh, in shell	3-5 weeks
Fresh chicken or turkey, parts	1-2 days
Fresh chicken or turkey, whole	1-2 days
Fresh fish and shellfish	1-2 days
Fresh giblets	1-2 days
Fresh meat (beef, veal, lamb, pork) steaks, chops, and roasts	3-5 days
Gravy and broth, patties and nuggets	3-4 days

Ground beef, turkey, veal, pork, lamb	1-2 days
Ham, canned, labeled "Keep Refrigerated"	Unopened 6-9 months, Opened 3-5 days
Ham, fully cooked, half	3-5 days
Ham, fully cooked, slices	3-4 days
Ham, fully cooked, whole	7 days
Hard sausage, pepperoni, jerky sticks	2-3 weeks
Hard-cooked eggs	1 week
Hot dogs	Unopened package 2 weeks, Opened package 1 week
Liquid pasteurized eggs, egg substitutes	Unopened 10 days, Opened 3 days
Luncheon meat	Unopened package 2 weeks, Opened package 3-5 days
Mayonnaise, commercial	2 months
Pre-stuffed pork and lamb chops and chicken breasts	1 day
Raw yolks, whites	2-4 days
Sausage, raw from meat or poultry	1-2 days
Smoked breakfast links, patties	7 days
Soups and stews	3-4 days
Stew meats	1-2 days

Store-cooked dinners and entrees	3-4 days
Store-prepared (or homemade) egg, chicken, tuna, ham, and macaroni salads	3-5 days
Summer sausage labeled "Keep Refrigerated"	Unopened 3 months, Opened 3 weeks
Variety meats (tongue, kidneys, liver, heart, chitterlings)	1-2 days

So we have moldy mycotoxins that permeate foods, buildings, the air, and our bodies. If we do not clean our homes, refrigerators, and bathrooms of the mold that eats into drywall and other surfaces, the healthy energy of our homes will be compromised. If replastering after mold damage is not an option, remodeling with mold resistant drywall can heal an infested home as will cleaning it with hydrogen peroxide rather than bleach. If we do not watch our diets, we can end up with the same infestations living within and without our bodies. Grinding wheat using a hand grinder and making homemade bread is another way to avoid wheat molds and it is also more delicious and nutritious than store-bought and preservative-laden breads. If you can't see what the food was like in its natural form before processing, there is no way to know that it was mold free and you run the risk of poisoning yourself. We need to avoid mold exposure and make sure our bodies are not the prime spot for molds to grow to maintain optimal health.

25

Microwave Madness or Nuke 'Em Puke 'Em

There are, in the food industry, several schools of thought that are a great source of pride to many Americans. One is that we have the safest food supply in the world. The other is that we have the widest variety of convenience foods in the world. Another is that food is just an assemblage of parts small and large that can be added, subtracted, or changed to produce another model or flavorful designer food. This food is then marketed for its color, flavor, tastiness, or for some scientifically promoted fad. Commercially manufactured foods were conceived with but one purpose, to generate more revenue with the least amount of investment possible.

Our ancestors would be quite confused by the vast army of foods present today because they ate to live. They would not understand the gluttonous desire to live to eat. They ate living food that satisfied them for hours. Modern Americans eat dead food that brings on reactive hypoglycemia and glutamate (MSG) induced food cravings within an hour or two. Because of this, they think of food all day long and what they are going to eat next. In a land of plenty, people spend vast quantities of time and polluting gasoline driving around to get "convenience" fast foods.

The same amount of time and effort driving and shopping would have produced a good meal at home that would be filling giving enough energy to last for hours. Instead, after quickly running out of the fake energy in fast food, the impulse is to resort to heavily marketed caffeinated beverages to get a quick fix of empty energy. This energy comes at the expense of draining the last dregs of precious hormones needed for feeling good, immune system support, and inflammation control. The end result is another run to the doctor for antibiotics and anti-inflammatory drugs.

Recently we have had outbreaks of foodborne illnesses. Very few people die from these although some 76 million contract some type of foodborne illness per year.[1] There is an awareness of this, but most people take risks despite the fear. Like most fears, people end up suffering the very thing they fear the most despite all their gargantuan efforts to avoid getting it. Foods that are the "safest on the planet" are making people sick in numerous other ways. However, these other illnesses take time to develop. They end up being explained away by other causes like working too hard, bad genes, or a poor night's sleep. Americans are seeing doctors more than their ancestors and for more diseases than those people experienced precisely because of modern food processing. Modern food processing designed to prevent infectious diseases is causing more illness and deaths over time than the acute diarrhea from unprocessed food has ever done.[2]

There has been a long history of fascination with nuclear power ever since the days of Madam Curie, Rutherford, and Niels Bohr. As a child I participated in the 1950s duck and cover drills for possible nuclear war with Russia. The only time we ever used it was during a violent 7.5 earthquake that cracked our school walls, shattered windows, and flung stuff off the walls. We literally bounced up and down three feet with each wave. The anti-nuclear activism of the late 1960s shut down the nuclear anti-missile sites surrounding the coasts of America. Six years later, as fire direction control officer in South Korea, I would take care of those same missiles now retrofitted with conventional explosives during the Vietnam War. As Reagan negotiated the first ever nuclear missile reduction treaty (START I), the fear of nuclear radiation was put on the back burner of the American psyche. It wasn't until recently that the ongoing calamity of the Fukushima Daiichi nuclear meltdown in Japan brought nuclear radiation to the forefront yet again. However, unbeknownst the general public, another nuclear threat has crept its way back into our lives with very little news coverage or alarm.

As the population has grown and food production become a global and national industry, new methods of preventing spoilage and bacteria have become commonplace over the years. One of which is the irradiation of foods. What does radiation do to the quality of the food that has already been depleted of so many vital nutrients? Quite literally, it destroys vitamins, proteins, and fats.[3] When I worked in the Veteran's hospital in Louisville, Kentucky, we had a name for the governmentally "safe" hamburgers.[4] We called them "leather burgers." They had been previously cooked according to government standards of safety to high temperatures, and then were frozen. Later they were thawed out and re-cooked again. It sounds like fast food with a government twist. The twist was the half hour of chewing it required to eat the tough beasts. Later, as a head and neck surgeon, I would literally see fifty patients in clinic every Tuesday. Most of them had been radiated after their radical neck surgery. Their necks were just as tough and hard as the "leather burgers," and for the same reason. Irradiated food will have similar but not so extensive alterations in the proteins. But along with the goal of eliminating the bad bacteria or aging agents acting upon foods, the life of the nutrients is cut short even though the food is edible for quite some time longer.

Radiation levels in produce and meats have gone down from their originally higher levels over the years, and while many people acknowledge irradiation destroys nutrients, they describe it as being minimal or compare it to other forms of food preservation like canning.[5] The problem with this comparison is how many of us really prefer canned chicken over buying it fresh from the grocery meat section? Some of the major vitamins that are highly sensitive to irradiation are vitamins B1, C, A, and E. It's theorized that freezing foods before irradiating them can help prevent nutrient loss,[6] but freezing also adds another level of nutrient loss.

Anyone with even the least developed sense of smell and taste can tell you that fresh green beans and peas from the garden are exquisitely different from the canned or even frozen variety. The closer these foods can get to being fresh without undue processing, the better. The depletion of nutrients from these preservation processes could be compared to the depletion of nutrients that occurs during the cooking process.[7] Both processes truly reduce the nutrient value of foods. When you combine both the irradiation nutrient loss with cooking nutrient loss to the foods that have already suffered nutrient loss from excessive fertilizers, poor growing soil, or early (green) harvesting,[8] the food is rendered practically lifeless by the time it reaches the dinner table.

While living food produces life, dead food causes disease and death. The government, which is increasingly catering to the wishes of corporations over the needs of the people, requires that whole foods be labeled with the irradiation symbol, processed foods with irradiated ingredients aren't required to carry the label, and restaurants are not required to disclose that they use irradiated foods.[9] Many national and international groups are pushing for increased percentages of the food supply to be irradiated.[10] So in the near future, possibly 25% of the US food supply will be irradiated. Will we ever be able to move beyond last century's nuclear fascinations? Haven't we played doomsday so long and hard that we are tired of it? Irradiating food seems unnecessary and excessive when we haven't controlled all the foodborne diseases that are preventable with available technology.[11] Better procedures at processing plants would not only benefit the consumer with foods that are safer but would also create better work environments for the poor people who are subjected to unsafe conditions for minimal pay. The laws that protect these workers and our food supply are under constant threat from lobbying groups in congress and the paid off politicians that are whittling away our public health.

The "nuking" that occurs during food irradiation does not make the food radioactive and generally the X-rays, electrons, or gamma rays pass through the foods are only being absorbed where they kill off some bacteria or part of the food. The facilities where irradiation occurs are not nuclear reactors, but they are built with underground pools used to absorb the radiation of the radioactive material, usually cobalt 60 or sometimes cesium 137. Concrete walls two meters thick encase these buildings to prevent radiation leaks and these buildings are regularly inspected by the Nuclear Regulatory Commission.[12] So while these buildings sound like they are safe, they don't sound very appetizing, and indeed, radioactive materials are the burden of future generations that will have to dispose of the radioactive water, concrete, and nuclear waste at some point.

Speaking of units designed to contain radiation and alter foods only leads to a discussion of microwave ovens which are a standard in nearly every American household. Before microwave ovens there were pressure cookers and convection ovens that also cooked foods quickly, but in safer ways. When long range microwave radars were first invented to detect Russian nuclear missiles coming into the US through Alaska and Canada, microwave radiation was experienced by humans in large numbers for the first time.[13] The soldiers asked to guard these large microwave radars preferred to be in front of them rather than behind. In front, they found that they did not need their coats. It felt like a warm summer day in front of the radars even though the outside air temperature was way below zero. Microwaves would heat up their bodies in slow cook fashion by exciting their water molecules to vibrate more rapidly. Before that, there was an isolated report of a GE engineer who put himself in a large microwave oven to see how long it took his body temperature to rise. These early experiments with human microwave radiation, remind us of our nation's experiments with nuclear radiation where the soldiers were asked to march across ground zero shortly after atomic bomb blasts in Nevada to see what the health effects would be. I once took care of a patient who worked in the atomic weapons laboratory. He looked through leaded glass to watch the nuclear material. Only one day, the leaded glass failed to come down between him and the radiation. Ten years, later he developed brain cancer behind the eye that took the radiation. All radiation is bad, just like sunburns teach us. We have enormous antioxidant systems to handle the poisoning from just the sun. The sun's gamma rays are filtered out by the earth's thick atmosphere. Space travel significantly shortens astronaut lives. So now we are on the verge of shortening our lives with radiated food.

Unlike thermal heat from regular cooking, microwaves heat food unevenly. So there is the need to rotate the food or mix it mid-microwaving to more evenly distribute the radiation. Even with that there are cold spots, so there is the suggestion that the food be stirred or let sit until the heat distributes more evenly. These cold spots lead to heating times that are excessive in order to get the temperature higher in order to kill bacteria in meats or mixed foods likes casseroles or stir fries. This leads to overall nutritional loss.[14] The other trick is to precook the food (back to the "leather burgers") so that the bacteria are supposedly killed already.

Microwaves destroy the quality of proteins by ripping them into unnatural amino acid segments. Certain essential amino acids are destroyed by microwaves and excessive cooking leading to nutritional deficiencies for the consumer.[15] It's important to cook meats to the point that bacteria are killed. Different meats require different internal temperatures to be safe. When checked with an internal thermometer, the safe temperature is at its lowest 165 °F for chicken, 160 °F for eggs and ground meat, and 145 °F for steaks and pork chops.[16] When overcooked, the loss of essential amino acids leads to nutritional diseases which will push people towards doctors who do not correct the underlying nutritional deficiency. Then the vicious cycle begins where symptom relief medical treatments are given, their side effects ensue, and this leads increased risk of other diseases. And even if this worst-case scenario doesn't occur, the patient still ends up with a handful of pills and a nutritional deficiency that is worsened by the very medications they are taking. Almost all prescription medication causes depletion of critical vitamins and nutrients.[17] The depletion of these vitamins causes more disease.

Tryptophan is an essential amino acid found in foods that contain protein. The body uses it to make serotonin and melatonin. These hormones make people feel happy and increase their quality of sleep. Without them depression and insomnia occur. Tryptophan is very sensitive to heat. So microwave heat destroys it and makes the food less helpful in keeping body levels up. Precooked microwave meals already have lower tryptophan levels because of the precooking. Microwaves just add to the tryptophan destruction already present. The result of this is that people will get depressed and go to the doctor who diagnoses depression and gives a drug that boosts serotonin in the brain through some gimmick that does not always work with low serotonin levels. People can't sleep without melatonin, so they take sleeping pills to get to sleep only to find themselves drugged during the day, getting in car wrecks, and forgetting important things. These things happen because they eat food that is deficient in tryptophan.

Other nutritional issues combined with microwave cooking have nothing to do with the microwave itself. People are more likely to eat frozen dinners or frozen lunches at the office because of the quick preparation time. These frozen meals are often highly processed, but in addition to that, may have spent too much time in the freezer. Another cause of bacterial contamination of microwave foods is due to their frozen status. Modern frost-free freezers have frequent daily defrost cycles that melt the ice and partially thaw the frozen microwave food. Some bacteria and fungi can grow at near freezing temperatures like Listeria. So the longer a frozen dinner sits in the frost-free freezer, the more chances it has had increased bacterial contamination. The constant cycle of freezing and then thawing ruins the nutritional value of the proteins and vitamins in the food. The answer to this potential problem is to radiate the food with gamma rays which takes us back down the line of nutritional loss added upon nutritional loss from the seedling to the dinner table. Deep freezers that grow frost always stay cold, but many people will leave food there for many months where it slowly loses nutritional value.

Other concerns with microwave ovens include safety issues. There are warnings on microwave ovens that people with pacemakers should not stand too close to them. I was curious as to how far away from my microwave oven I would get a safe reading on my microwave meter instrument of less than two milliwatts per square meter. It was nearly ten feet. The way we cook microwave popcorn and other microwave meals in the kitchen is to put the stuff in the microwave and then continue preparing other foods on the stove two feet away where the reading was twenty times higher than the safe level. Worse yet, people stand in front of it wanting for the thirty seconds to be over. These levels are even more harmful than cellphone radiation which is bad enough.[18]

So what should we do to be safe here? We should, for starters, not stand next to the microwave when operating. We should be at least six feet away or move it to the laundry room. We should not cook fresh meat in it unless we overcook it. It's hard to tell if the fresh meat is done since fresh meat does not brown in the microwave. So temperature probes help determine if the meat has reached the optimum 165 °F needed to kill bacteria. We should keep meats and frozen dinners in a real deep freezer without an automatic defrost cycle. These are the ones where you have to unplug them every six months and open the door till all the frost melts and water runs out.

If this seems too complicated, maybe we should get rid of the microwave and replace it with a far cheaper convection toaster oven. These can cook foods almost as fast and are ten times cheaper than a microwave to buy ($70 will buy a good one). They require a little reading to figure out cook times for different foods. They even have defrost cycles and can cook microwave dinners. But microwave dinners are not the most nutritious foods to eat in the first place because they are already precooked. Another option for defrosting meats is to leave them in their packaging and put them in water or defrost them overnight in the refrigerator. This works great for fish or thin pieces of meat that can be monitored so they aren't left out too long after they are thawed. These suggestions are made so that we can simply adapt our present practices immediately in order to be healthier. Over time, we can gradually progress on to real food cooking which keeps the Italians far healthier than we are when it comes to heart disease.

We already live in a world where the ozone is being depleted and more radiation is coming through. The nuclear fallout from Chernobyl in the Sahara Desert was picked up by strong winds and dumped on Greece where the radioactive cesium levels went sky high. The nuclear fallout from Chinese atomic bomb testing has dumped radioactive dust all over the USA. Now we are radiating our food like never before and sun tanning our bodies like never before. It seems we have a love affair with radiation. We have successfully reduced nuclear missiles on the planet but increased our exposure to radiation and radiated products. The key to keeping the kitchen a life harboring place is to root out the foods and cooking methods that deaden the nutrient life of the foods. A happy kitchen is a place where fresh and dried vegetables or herbs are hanging from well ventilated bowls or baskets. There is a flow of aroma, flow in the cooking of natural foods, and flow in eating for a healthy life. It's not only aesthetically appealing, but nutritionally appealing as well.

26

Infuriating Inflammation

Inflammation is peculiar to living things. Inanimate objects don't swell when injured. Hitting a rock with a hammer doesn't cause inflammation of the rock. A sheet of paper in flames is burning into ashes, not suffering from swelling. But if you smash or burn your thumb, it swells. For living beings, inflammation is an inevitable part of the healing response. And while it certainly has the power to heal, it can do some damage along the way.

The body's natural reaction to stress, injury, disease, and infection is to send more blood and resources to the distressed body part. For minor issues, or for people who naturally inflame less than others, the inflammation does its job and is a bump in the road on the way to healing. For some people, and for more serious health issues, inflammation can explode into a serious threat like a thousand-degree flame spreading through the body burning everything in its path. So how do we know when inflammation, specifically pain and swelling, is potentially lethal or not? Most of the time, inflammation can be healed with simple remedies. But when it turns into an out-of-control fire, it must be doused strategically, thoroughly, and swiftly before it turns chronic or, in worst case scenario, deadly.

When inflammation rears its ugly head, we run to the medicine cabinet for aspirin or Motrin to take away the pain. Sometimes it works and all is well. But sometimes it doesn't work so well, and we go to doctors who are trained exquisitely in the use of drugs to relieve the symptoms of disease. In allopathic medicine, the symptom is considered to be the disease itself and all kinds of anti-inflammatory drugs are thrown at it. Drug companies want us to believe that for every symptom there is an appropriate drug that quickly cures the symptom. With such powerful sledgehammer medicines, is it any wonder that we begin, as doctors and patients, to think of the pain and inflammation as the disease itself? Fortunately, many doctors are now getting smarter about finding the disease behind the pain. They are getting better at finding the ultimate causes of inflammation and treating them.

At the onset of an illness or injury, inflammation might be the obvious culprit and manifest as an acute response. This is a one time or initial cause for inflammation. It could be in the form of an allergic reaction, chemical irritant exposure, an infection, trauma or injury, a burn, lacerations or cuts, frostbite, animal bites, or even breathing in smog or particulate air. If we follow the pathway of an acute illness, we see that it could begin with a pathogen, such as a virus, entering the body. The immune response would be to send white blood cells to where the virus is located. These white blood cells, or leukocytes, will then release cytokines which are basically protein messengers that rally and stimulate the immune system. These cytokines alert the hypo-thalamus to release prostaglandins. These prostaglandins are lipids that behave like hormones. They are the cause of fever or inflammation at the site of infection or injury. In many cases, the body heals itself and everything returns to normal. But ironically, this very immune response that could save you, often times is the very thing that will make you perilously worse.

For years, I have seen the ravages of infection inflammation. I have seen literally thousands of patients caught in the vicious cycle of infection causing inflammation and the inflammation causing more infection. I have done a large number of tonsillectomies on adults who still get four to five strep throat infections a year. Many of them are women who feel tired all the time and gain weight because they are too exhausted to exercise. As soon as I take the infected tonsils out, they experience a dramatic change in their lives. They lose fifteen pounds on average from the postoperative sore throat and get newfound energy that they never had before. For the first time in their lives, they can exercise without becoming exhausted. It turns out that infection does not stay put in the place where the pain is felt. The tonsils have five arteries and veins each. The pus gets into the blood and makes it thick with inflammation. The bacteria get into the heart, the joints, and numerous other locations. The net result is feeling like you have the flu all the time. The sinuses and ears cause bacteremia in the same way. If the source of the problem isn't found, the acute infection becomes chronic and can lead to generalized malaise and fatigue.

Over the last thirty years as an Ear, Nose, and Throat doctor and allergist, most of the diseases I see are related to inflammation in one way or another. Someone may come in with sudden hearing loss. It could be caused by swelling of the eustachian tube from a virus, sinusitis, allergies, or swelling of the adenoids which lie in front of the eustachian tube. It could also be caused by swelling of the hearing nerve in a tight bony canal due to a viral infection. The treatments are usually centered on removing, shrinking, or bypassing the blockage. We put PE tubes in and do balloon eustachian tuboplasty to bypass the blockage of the eustachian tube. We also take out the adenoids to remove the blockage of the eustachian tube. We give steroids to take the swelling out of the hearing nerve to restore blood flow to the hearing organ. Blocked sinuses from inflammation of the sinus outflow tracts cause a backup of the mucous. It then stagnates and grows bacteria and fungi which cause more inflammation and more symptoms. It's a multibillion-dollar industry to medicate the inflammation that blocks the sinuses and causes people to be miserable for months at a time. This is very common with 14% to 16% of people in the US having chronic sinus infections.[1] If the medications and allergy treatments don't work, then surgery may be needed to open the sinus so that it can drain properly. The inflammation goes away, and with it, the patient's symptoms.

There are numerous other obstructions that cause chronic infection and inflammation and I've detailed them in the following chart:

Obstructive Inflammatory Disease	Causes of Obstruction
Otitis Media	Eustachian tube obstruction from viruses, pathogenic bacteria, thick mucus, adenoids
Sinusitis	Blockage of sinus openings, deviated septum, large turbinates, nasal fractures, viral, thick mucus, fungal, pathogenic bacteria, dental problems
Tonsillitis	Viral damage to tonsils, strep carrier, sinusitis
Cholecystitis	Gallstones
Kidney Infection	Kidney stones caused by oxalates
Prostatitis	Milk, estrogen excess, aging male, infection caused by a weakened immune system
Mastitis	Iodine deficiency
Bladder Infection	Prostate swelling
Diverticulitis	Chronic constipation, food allergies
Dacryocystitis	Tear duct obstruction from sinusitis
Periodontitis, Periapical Abscess, Endodontitis	Bad gums and teeth from dental neglect

So as a surgeon, I strongly recommend that anyone with a chronic infection get rid of it as soon as possible. You aren't saving money by not going to the dentist regularly and letting a toothache get worse. Living with infection anywhere in the body is asking for more secondary diseases than you can imagine. When the fire of inflammation is low, people get away with ignoring it most of the time. But sometimes there are other factors at play that prolong the illness or injury. The inflammation can then mushroom into a bigger problem as the inflammation itself can injure and reinjure the body if it never goes away. And there are quite a few serious diseases, cancers, and debilitating health issues that can develop with runaway chronic inflammation.

I made the following list to give you just a brief overview of the scope of chronic inflammation and how it manifests with various diseases:

Chronic Inflammation Diseases	Sub-Categories of Diseases
Cancer	Well over a hundred cancers result from chronic inflammation.[2]
Neurological Diseases	Alzheimer's Disease, Parkinson's Disease, Multiple Sclerosis, Lou Gehrig's Disease, Guillain-Barre Syndrome
Pulmonary	Chronic Asthma, Chronic Obstructive, Pulmonary Disease, Hay Fever, Chronic Bronchitis
Bone and Joint Disease	Osteoarthritis, Osteopenia, Osteoporosis, Rheumatoid Arthritis
Metabolic Diseases	Type 2 Diabetes Mellitus, Renal Failure, Fatty Liver Disease

Cardiovascular Diseases	Atherosclerosis, Hypertension, Congestive Heart Failure, Stroke
Auto-Immune Diseases	Irritable Bowel Disease, Crohn's Colitis, Multiple Sclerosis, Type 1 Diabetes, Mellitus, Lupus, Auto-Immune Thyroid Disease, Sjogren's Disease (and nearly a hundred more)
Miscellaneous	Depression, Autism, Pediatric Acute Neuropsychiatric Syndrome, Fibromyalgia, Chronic Fatigue Syndrome, Chronic Inflammatory Response Syndrome, Post-COVID-19 Syndrome, Systemic Inflammatory Response Syndrome, Lyme Disease

All of these late stage and chronic health issues started small, started with genetics, or started with prolonged unhealthy lifestyles. Many people, especially Americans who are afraid of exorbitantly expensive and ineffective medical treatments, will ignore the beginning signs or just live with prolonged discomfort. If they do seek treatment, they'll often trip into the rabbit hole of Western Medicine's symptom-based treatment schemes. For example, the success of varying treatments of lower back pain shows how finding the right cause of inflammation is paramount to curing it. Many pain-free people have stenosis and lesions identical to the patients who went into surgery to have them removed. Perhaps there are more causes for the pain than meets the eye of the physician. They are likely only trained in one specialty and can't see how the body flows and communicates between organs.

We have pain clinics where doctors directly attack the pain itself with pharmaceuticals and surgeries. But the cause of the pain, and the source of the fire of inflammation, will often be hidden from their view. Many doctors and patients are finally beginning to see how all this pain starts. Around half of all back surgeries actually relieve the pain for which the surgery was intended.[3] Other causes are intermittent claudication of the arteries going to the muscles in the lower back. When bad food choices along with inflammation in the arteries from low testosterone in men and low estradiol in women cause a blockage, the muscle gets starved for oxygen and begins to cramp with severe pain. If this sounds like a heart attack process within the coronary arteries, that's because it is. Aspirin and Motrin can get the blood flowing again and relieve the cramp, but it's not treating the cause.

The anti-inflammatory drug industry has become a maniacal expert at creating misinformation in their marketing to trick you into treating the symptom and not the disease. The true disease cures are never mentioned because you'd be using a more natural remedy in place of these drugs. Since the drug companies represent one third of the stock market's Dow Jones Industrial Average, the Dow would collapse if people favored natural remedies over their drugs. The World Health Organization (WHO) recommends natural remedies for worldwide use for some illnesses because herbs don't pollute the planet in contrast to massive drug industry pollution.[4]

By being one of the few nations that allows drug manufacturers to advertise to the public, we have created a monster of misinformation. Through advertising, the public is made aware of the many treatments for symptoms but never informed about the cures for the underlying diseases. This creates a nation with an ever-increasing number of people who have chronic diseases, and each sick patient collects more chronic diseases as he or she ages. Each of the inflammatory processes requires their own group of drugs for treatment. This leads to polypharmacy where one patient is taking forty pills. Every day I see patients who are taking more than twelve medications. Each of the prescriptions has side effects. So many of the patients I see every day have, as their only reason for seeing me, one or several of the side effects of the medications they are consuming. So I get out the *Physicians' Desk Reference* and show them where their side effect is common. The drug companies would be all too happy if I just gave them another drug to treat the side effect of the first drug. In fact, the whole industry is built around this approach. After all this behind-the-scenes manipulation, it's no wonder people often live in fear, disempowerment, and at a disconnect from themselves.

While the foreign invaders of virus, bacterium, and fungi will stoke the inflammation fires, the culprit is often more homegrown. As people age, they lose growth hormone and testosterone. As a result, their muscles get weaker and smaller and can no longer hold up their beer bellies caused by more inflammation of a different sort. Then the posture sags and they develop mechanical low back pain. Their shoulders also slump over their upper back and the neck begins to hurt for the same reason. Recently, it has been noted that with bottled water lacking bad tasting magnesium, Americans have become magnesium deficient.[5] Over half of the liquids in the US come from bottles that contain very little magnesium. Magnesium relaxes muscles and causes cramping and pain to go away quickly. Many drugs are prescribed for treatment of midnight leg cramps. Magnesium glycinate works the best and quickest at preventing leg cramps with none of the dangerous side effects.

When the bowels become inflamed from poor food choices, outright poisons, and overgrowth of bad bacteria and yeasts like candida, people get constipation or diarrhea. So they will often run to the corner grocery store and buy poisons for relief. Little thought is given to the cause of the constipation or diarrhea. The fire continues on inside and for some, it consumes their entire colon, and they lose it through a surgery that sticks them with an ileostomy bag. There are many natural cures for this inflammation, but the simplest one is eating lots of vegetables and some fruits in order to get the required 45 grams of fiber daily. When people get full on these naturally cleansing fiber-rich foods, there is little room for that triple decker fudge cake that plugs the piping and requires a lot of medical Drano to unplug the clog.

The acid reflux pandemic that has swept the nation is another example where the inflammation caused by stomach acid actually blocks
the esophageal plumbing. I see three to five patients a week who can't
swallow very well. An excess of too much stomach acid has been blamed
as the ultimate cause of acid reflux which causes upper esophageal
swelling and difficulty swallowing. The drug companies that make acid
blockers blame acid as the cause. Nothing could be further from the
truth. We actually make too little stomach acid, and this relaxes the
sphincters allowing acid to go up.[6] There are a large number of other
diseases that are also rooted in the inflammation that arises from acid
reflux. There is Barrett's esophagus, esophageal cancer, reflux laryngitis
(chronic non-productive cough), and some cases of asthma caused by
aspiration of the acid that gushes past loose sphincters up to the voice
box. Even some cases of ear disease and sinusitis can be caused by nighttime acid reflux reaching all the way into the nose. Once the acid gets
into places it shouldn't be, it causes more inflammation and more disease. The most common symptom of too much stomach acid is upper
stomach pain with inability to belch caused by acid tightening up the
lower esophageal sphincter too strictly.

If problems such as these are caused internally or are a result of diet
choices, people have more agency in healing themselves than the pharmaceutical companies would have them believe. Why is our immune
system so fragile in the first place? What can be done to enhance its
effectiveness? The answer lies in the gut where over 50% of our immune
system lies,[7] and the treatment starts before birth with the foods and
supplements the mother eats. Eating more naturally lowers the pain
experienced when the disease is minor and needs no doctor visit. More
serious diseases will become more obvious when you are eating naturally, and the problem doesn't fix itself. There won't be a pile up of
other symptoms masking the symptoms of the serious disease. Eating
with organic spices like curry, turmeric, cumin, ginger, garlic, holy basil,
and onions lowers inflammation. Eating less meat and more vegetables
also lowers inflammation.

If you are in pain, excessive sugar intake can trigger so much more in-flammation, prevent healing, or prevent properly prescribed medicines from working. When your body is hamstrung by excess sugar intake, health problems tend to multiply faster than your doctor can figure them out. It can lead to the development metabolic syndrome, diabetes, hypertension, abdominal weight gain, high cholesterol, heart disease, or many other secondary diseases, all from eating too much sugar in the first place. So abandoning the I-need-something sweet tooth, and get-ting rid of added sugar and excessive fruit consumption will go a long way to calming inflammation outright and preventing serious disease from developing later.

People who eat a lot of fish and curry in their regular diets have less swelling than the average person with the same injuries. What is it in these foods that protects against abnormal inflammation? The omega-3 fatty acids found in fish, walnuts, flax seed, and other foods have been recommended for many scientific reasons for heart patients.[8] They help the body shift inflammatory pathways to cause less severe inflammation. In the case of a heart patient, this may mean the difference between life and death when a plaque ruptures and causes inflammatory swell-ing and blockage of the coronary arteries. Less sudden blockage from swelling means less chance of complete blockage and death of the heart muscle or patient. Italians who have diabetes, obesity, hypertension, and other diseases at the same rates that we do in America don't have sudden death from heart attack at the same high rate that we do. The Mediterranean diet they eat, which is loaded with omega-3 fatty acids, protects their heart vessels from all this inflammation.

Anciently, inland cultures ate grass-fed goats, sheep, and cattle. Since omega-3 was in grass, the grazing cow incorporated omega-3 into their fat. And the humans who ate these animals got enough omega-3 this way. Since they weren't eating processed food with rancid seed oils in them, they had healthy omega-3/omega-6 balance. Omega-6, nowadays, is 98% of what Americans consume for fatty acids. Omega-6 is found in a healthy way in nuts and in a bad way in all rancid seed oils such as canola oil, safflower oil, sunflower oil, soybean oil, Crisco, margarine, low fat dairy, condiments, processed foods, and non-organic meat which has mostly omega-6 in the fat. Historically, seed oils were 2% of our fat intake. That small amount was enough to produce the right amount of inflammation for healing. Presently, we are consuming 80 grams per day of inflammatory seed oils compared to 1 to 2 grams per day in the early 1800s.[9] So basically, the food we eat can cause intense inflammation. For example, a single meal or snack with high density carbs and fat will cause a rise in the inflammatory cytokine IL6 within six hours creating intense inflammation in numerous areas of the body.

Ideally, there's a one-to-one ratio between omega-3 and omega-6. Omega-3 is anti-inflammatory, and omega-6 is inflammatory. Both are needed for the routine maintenance of the body. Whenever we get acute inflammation, we need omega-6 fatty acids to make the inflammatory molecules that help heal the infection or injury. The actual omega-3 and omega-6 ratio for most Americans has increased by 42% since the early 1900s because we eat so many seed oils and have very few sources of omega-3 fatty acids in our diet.[10] The sources of omega-3 are fatty fish such as salmon, sardines, and mackerel. You can also get special breeds of omega-3 eggs produced by a specific feed given to the chickens.

If you move further east from Italy, you'll find that nearly every Indian curry from India contains turmeric which is another anti-inflammatory. In fact, some elderly people in India will put a table-spoon of turmeric in their milk every day. The other lovely aspect of taking herbal or food-based remedies is that their "side effects" usually cause you to be healthier in multiple other ways as well.[11] If you can't incorporate turmeric into your cooking, quality supplements like those from pharmaceutical grade vitamin companies are available in health food stores.[12]

So the key to avoiding the overbearing buildup of symptoms and rapid aging is to establish a diet and lifestyle that allows energy, food, and nutrients to flow throughout the body without obstruction. By arrang-ing the diet just so, the body aligns itself for optimal healing responses.

With a better understanding of the delicate and intricate pathways of every system in the body, we see how vital to health the overall flow and alignment of the body is. We also see how we are linked and completely dependent on our environment down to the microscopic level. When we root out the poisons and toxins in our home environments and balance our diets with a mindful eye on our inflammation response, we set ourselves up for a purer and unencumbered lifestyle. By letting the right nutrients in and by balancing the diet with freshness and life, we let this life enter our internal world. It's like opening the windows in the spring after a long winter and we realize that renewal is possible yet again.

27

Katrina's Handkerchief

Understanding and honoring connection both within and without ourselves is essential for practicing flow nutrition. Being alive is a constant communication from all parts of your mind, body, and soul. I can't understate the connectedness of every aspect of the human body. This intercellular communication is the system with which the body heals itself. When a part of your body is in distress, the blood flow to that area naturally increases. The capillaries at that site will widen to aid the extra flow of blood to the injury. When this happens, you'll see or feel the inflammation symptoms of heat and redness in the affected area. The capillaries will actually become leaky in this process as the fluid is released into the tissues and causes swelling. The main symptoms arising from this are heat, redness, swelling, tenderness, and pain. And while this all seems negative, it's actually allowing leukocytes, white blood cells, to migrate through the leaky capillary into the area of injury. Once there, they release cytokines to assist with the immune response which creates tenderness in the area. This causes a larger systemic healing response with the proliferation of even more leukocytes. People often recognize this as an intense pain or fever, but without the increased swelling and blood flow, healing wouldn't be possible.

Our bodies have more pipes than we have any idea. The expanse just keeps growing once we contemplate adding the microtubules and ion channels in cell membranes to the length of the larger arteries and veins. We also have lymphatic channels just as numerous as the blood vessels, if not more. We have thirty feet of alimentary canal including the esophagus, stomach, duodenum, small intestine, large intestine, and rectum. The lungs have a large tree of bronchi, bronchioles, and alveoli. The kidneys have many pipes to collect urine. Fortunately, we have short water pipes after the kidneys. Women and men each have their own reproductive plumbing. Every lymph node has channels that tend to become plugged. Our brain cells have axons and dendrites that are chemical pipelines for neurotransmitters to travel in order to stimulate other cells.

Every one of these pipelines are subject to blockage by various insults, most of which are caused by inflammation. When we get a migraine, our brains ignite with inflammation. The blood vessels first constrict and then dilate. The dilation causes excess amounts of blood to go into the bony fixed cavity and the brain swells with nowhere to go. This puts pressure on delicate nerve endings in the blood vessels, shutting down the flow of nutrients to the information processing centers in the brain. Thus, inflammation is the cause of migraines. You might wonder what the cause of the inflammation is, and with migraines, the answer isn't always as clear as it is with other health problems. There are many self-help books describing migraines that were not cured by aggressive medical therapy.[1]

While the source of the problem may be elusive, doctors and health practitioners in the West are starting to wise up. We are continually finding the root problems of these mysterious illnesses. One such discovery lies in a better understanding of the evolution of human genetics. Many organisms have the ability to fight off viruses with the simple immune system called the innate immune system. This system causes inflammation which is hostile to the virus or bacterium. All advanced species on the planet have developed a second immune system called the adaptive immune system. The white blood cells in the adaptive immune system make magic bullets called antibodies that directly attack only the bacterium or virus while sparing healthy tissue. Both fortunately and unfortunately for humans, we have the evolved adaptive and the primitive innate immune systems. The differences between the two are night and day. One is a sniper rifle that can take out a single infectious terrorist without causing collateral damage. The other is a nuclear bomb that kills both friend, foe, and everything else in between.

If you had a choice, you'd use the adaptive immune system to fight off these viruses and bacterium. However, roughly 22% of the American population has a genetic defect in their basic recognition system that differentiates between friendly cells, harmless viruses, friendly gut bacterium (normal flora), and biotoxins from dangerous bacteria and toxic molds (mycotoxins). In effect, the part of their adaptive immune system that is supposed to catch these intruders is paralyzed. The bacterial or mold poisons are never recognized by the adaptive immune system so that they can be targeted and destroyed. These actinobacteria biotoxins and mycotoxin mold poisons are called, as a group, biotoxins. They slip through the paralyzed fingers of these people's immune systems and wreak havoc on their bodies unabated.

The biotoxins accumulate over time poisoning mitochondria by inhibiting their energy production. In this way, they damage the brain and muscles creating widespread inflammation in nearly every part of the body. So instead of clearing out the biotoxin poison as it accumulates, the body succumbs to the biotoxin disease called Chronic Inflammatory Response Syndrome (CIRS). The body's only recourse in this situation is to pull out the nuclear bomb of the innate immune system and cause widespread inflammation.[2] The widespread inflammation does not clean out the biotoxins. But it does make the body's environment hostile to viruses, bacteria, and fungi. And this might lead you to ask, what happens when the outside environment of such a person is continuously reinfecting them with these biotoxins that their immune system can't keep up with?

According to OSHA, 55% of the buildings in the United States are water damaged. Water damaged buildings grow actinobacteria, a mold-like filamentous bacterium, and toxic molds.[3] The toxic organisms create the biotoxins and mycotoxins which get into every part of the house: on every piece of furniture, on clothing, in the carpet, on the upholstery, on the walls, the duct system, and many other places. After the actinobacteria and mold is cleaned up at its source, the house is still poisonous. The effort to clean up the house completely is called remediation. There are many companies that do this. There are ways to test a house to see if the bad bacteria and toxic molds are gone and the house is safe to live in again.[4]

So when you do the math, you'll see that twenty-two percent of the population have defective mycotoxin clearance and fifty-five percent of the buildings they could possibly live in are full of actinobacteria and toxic molds with all of their nasty biotoxins. Obviously, the chances for these particular patients to develop Chronic Inflammatory Response Syndrome (CIRS) is quite high. These biotoxins and mycotoxins can persist in the body for decades long after the poor unsuspecting patients have moved away from the water damaged buildings they occupied at work and home.

Many patients look like they have fibromyalgia, or have chronic fatigue syndrome, memory problems, bladder problems, bowel problems, frequent infections in the nose and lungs, anxiety disorders, and a general malaise that is disabling.[5] Fortunately, there is a treatment that can cure these patients with several drugs that bind the biotoxins and mycotoxins to remove them from the body. There are other natural therapy medicines that repair the brain and immune system damage returning everything back to normal according to objective testing.[6]

This issue is so huge and widespread. It explains many of the treatment failures for chronic diseases in Americans. When a patient has inflammation anywhere in their body, there is no treatment that will be effective if it was caused by biotoxin illness (CIRS). The inflammation caused by the adaptive immune system fighting viruses and bacteria can be treated effectively with steroids. The misery of a COVID-19 patient is reduced with steroids and antibiotics in the average outpatient treatment setting. The blood tests for inflammation, Erythrocyte

Sedimentation Rate (ESR) and C-Reactive Protein (CRP), are elevated in people with normal immune systems exposed to infectious agents. They are also elevated in trauma and flu patients. When fighting mold illness (CIRS), the innate immune system won't trigger these two well-known inflammatory markers. So when a doctor sees this innate inflamed patient with an unknown problem, they'll order these two tests, and they'll both be negative. The treatments they would normally use for inflammation won't work because it is the innate immune system that is defective and overactive.[7]

Although very few doctors are aware of them, there are tests for the innate immune system that will show elevations in mold illness (CIRS) patients. Since steroids can't help a patient with innate immune system inflammation, a different approach is used. These treatments involve clearing out the mold poison with special drugs and then turning off the genes that make these inflammatory markers active. A significant portion of the inflamed people in the US will fail every treatment modality known to modern science until the mycotoxin is taken out of their environment and their body and the innate immune system inflammatory markers are returned to normal with specialized treatments.[8] This is a nationwide problem of misdiagnosis. These patients can go from doctor to doctor spending a hundred thousand dollars or more trying to get better. So if someone has inflammation and responds poorly to treatments, they should see a certified mold illness practitioner who knows how to fix this very specific issue.

There are about thirty-seven symptoms that indicate mold illness (CIRS). If you have eleven or more in the right areas, then you'll have 95% chance of being diagnosed. These symptoms include fatigue, weakness, aching, muscle cramps that debilitate, unusual pains, headaches, sensitivity to bright light, red eyes, blurred vision, tearing, sinus congestion, cough, shortness of breath, abdominal pain, diarrhea, joint pain, memory loss, focus and concentration problems, word finding problems in conversations, decreased simulation of new knowledge, confusion, disorientation, skin sensitivity, mood swings, appetite swings, sweats, trouble controlling body temperature regulation, excessive thirst, increased urination, susceptibility to static shocks, numbness, tingling, vertigo, metallic taste in the mouth, and tremors.[9] So as you can see, a broad range of symptoms could lead a patient and their doctor on a wild goose chase unless their doctor is clued in to where to look and what tests to administer.

Some of these findings happened as a result of the massive flooding that occurred in the 9th Ward of New Orleans during the aftermath of Hurricane Katrina. Many residents of these flooded areas used remediation to replace their drywall and flooring so they could move back into their homes. Billions of dollars went into remediating these homes, and as people started moving back in, a portion of them began coughing. OSHA did a study and found that these symptoms were related to mold illness in genetically susceptible people. We now have diagnostic criteria to find if a person has mold illness. These findings were published by OSHA in direct response to the "Katrina Cough."[10] Until 2008, the EPA would not recognize that water damaged homes made people sick. The World Health Organization (WHO) had already recognized that flooded and water damaged homes caused mold illness (CIRS) in some people.

Other discoveries into the causes and symptoms of Chronic Inflammatory Response Syndrome (CIRS) actually began with the discovery of biotoxin, rather than mycotoxin or mold, infection. It began with a family doctor, Ritchie C. Shoemaker MD, investigating illnesses that were springing up in people who had fished in the Pocomoke River in Maryland.[11] The fish were eating a biotoxin and giving it to the people who at the fish. Dr. Shoemaker also discovered a similar biotoxin in raw barracuda off the Florida Keys. People ingesting it would become violently ill and stay sick long afterwards. A similar situation occurred when there was a large algae bloom over a lake in Orlando, Florida. Everyone nearby got mysteriously sick with the biotoxin.

There is a broad field of initial causes for Chronic Inflammatory Response Syndrome. A paper was published recently showing that post-acute or long haul COVID-19 Syndrome was nearly identical to mold illness (CIRS). And the same treatments that cure biotoxin illness patients are working.[12] The victims of Lyme disease, which is also elusive and notoriously difficult to diagnose, often suffer from CIRS in addition to their Lyme infection.[13] In the broad view of CIRS, it's helpful to understand that this designation was specifically made to differentiate it from patients who nearly died from sepsis and were treated with antibiotics. Some of these patients develop Systemic Inflammatory Response Syndrome (SIRS) and run into similar runaway problems with the out-of-control fires of inflammation.

As I mentioned earlier, we can't understate the importance of regulating a healthy immune system response. When we understand better how the body heals itself, as doctors and as humans going about our daily lives, we can develop new ways to help the body fix itself. Evolution has only taken us so far physically. We can't discount what the body can do for itself, but we can use our scientific and medical evolution to boost the body's healing power to new heights. It's an exciting time to be alive in terms of the future possibilities of curing diseases. Hopefully this new research is continued by doctors and scientists who are looking for actual solutions to true healing rather than trying to find new ways to line their pocketbooks. Hopefully patients who have these chronic health issues can find doctors with this knowledge so that they can finally find the peace and happiness of unencumbered and natural health.

28

The Anti-Inflammation Diet

The art of healing comes from nature, not from the physician. Therefore, the physician must start from nature, with an open mind.

—PARACELSUS

If you have inflammation and have already seen the appropriate doctors for each disease causing or arising from it, then an anti-inflammatory diet is something you can do right now to take responsibility for your disease. So many doctors know that their efforts can be futile without the patient doing all they can to follow the doctor's advice and take some personal responsibility for their own health.

Right now, at least two paradigms of healing exist in our society. One paradigm, which centers on diagnosing and treating disease, takes a mechanistic approach to illness in which the patient's symptoms are combated with pharmaceuticals and possibly surgery. This approach assumes that if the patient's symptoms improve via painkillers, antibiotics, steroids, or other suppressive treatments, then the patient is cured.

A second paradigm, the one embraced by naturopathic medicine, looks at a person as a whole and acts to stimulate his or her healing even before disease is apparent. This paradigm, of which prevention is the cornerstone, strives to maintain homeostasis within the body allowing it to function optimally and thereby promoting improved health. Disease symptoms function as messengers to tell us what is going on in the body and can direct the practitioner to treat certain systems to bring about better health. Symptoms merely indicate the existence of a "dis" "ease" in the body—that is, an imbalance. When symptoms appear, they are only the tip of the proverbial iceberg that for some time has been developing beneath the surface. The holistic medicine paradigm approaches symptoms as indicators of something going on deeper in the body. So rather than merely suppressing the symptom, naturopathic medicine strives to find and remove the inflammation's true cause.[1]

Lately, each major medical center has developed an alternative medicine program for teaching medical students how to look beyond the symptoms, look at diet and exercise as adjuvant therapies, and for offering the patient an adjuvant therapy when the drugs are not achieving 100% of the desired effect. This approach has improved doctor patient relationships and also puts the patient in charge of doing something more to help themselves. Many medical studies by major institutions have been pouring out recently on natural therapies for common diseases to help doctors have more tools in their toolbox to fight disease on every front. For example, a 2003 JAMA study showed that soy protein, viscous fiber, and nuts can be as effective as statins and a low saturated fat diet in treating high cholesterol.[2]

More astounding was a NEJM 2002 study demonstrating that diet and exercise were more effective at preventing heart disease than drug therapy for those with impaired glucose tolerance.[3] Once you have exhausted traditional medical treatments for a disease, you can then add natural therapies as long as your primary care doctor knows the full nature of alternative therapies and herbs. Some herbs cause problems and interactions with certain drugs and should be avoided. So what are the principles of naturopathy if you are wanting to add a holistic approach to your present treatment regimen? A simplified approach is found in traditional allopathic medicine as well.

We ultimately aim to not harm the patient when treating them. With this established, we look to identify and treat the cause of the health problem while focusing on treating the whole person. We impact the healing power of nature for the most fluid results. We emphasize prevention of full-blown diseases to avoid the more drastic forms of treatment which include surgeries and medications with side effects. Through this, the doctor becomes more of a teacher guiding the patient toward a healthier way of being.

In February of 2004, Time magazine published an article on inflammation.[4] They summarized quite well the causes of chronic inflammation as listed below:

- Chronic infection
- Foreign material in the body
- Latent viruses, bacteria, parasites, fungus
- Poor blood supply
- Radiation
- Locally applied drugs (steroids)
- Age
- Vitamin C deficiency
- Zinc deficiency
- Protein deficiency
- Chronic food allergies
- Metabolic diseases
- Diabetes
- Renal failure
- Cancer
- Systemic drugs[5]

Since our bodies make both inflammatory chemicals to fight health problems and anti-inflammatory substances to quell unnecessary pain and swelling, it would be good to review the different prostaglandin families which are made from vegetable oils and fish oils:

- PGE1 helps to reduce allergies, prevents inflammation, increases mucous production in the stomach, decreases blood pressure, improves nerve function, and also helps to promote immune response. Linoleic acid from sunflower oil and seeds, safflower oil, sesame oil and seeds, and mother's breast milk is the precursor to the formation of PEG1.
- PGE2 stimulates the allergy response, promotes inflammation, increases platelet aggregation, increases smooth-muscle contraction, and suppresses immune function. Meat, dairy, and breast milk make PEG2.
- PGE3 blocs the release of pro-inflammatory prostaglandins (PGE2), promotes immune function, decreases platelet aggregation, increases HDL cholesterol, decreases triglycerides, and inhibits inflammation. Alpha Linoleic Acid (ALA) from pumpkin seeds, flaxseeds, walnuts, soybeans, and breast milk is converted into PGE3. ALA is converted to EPA and DHA which we also get from cold water fish such as salmon, sardines, mackerel, and trout.

Understanding how different foods affect your immune responses is the basis of the anti-inflammatory diet as outlined by Jessica K. Black in her book, *The Anti-Inflammation Diet and Recipe Book*. By gaining an understanding of a low inflammation diet, you can better find your nutritional flow state. This is the zone where you are at your naturally optimum state of wellness. The flow happens when you fully understand how to modify your diet and you are now almost instinctively adjusting it as you go. Some health problems and diagnoses require very specific diets. The diet outlined below is a simple one that can be modified for specific allergies or health issues. Only strictly adhere to this diet if you are suffering from inflammation as variance in your diet is beneficial in other ways.

Foods that Reduce or Prevent Inflammation

- Essential fatty acids found in oily cold-water fish such as salmon, mackerel, tuna (only small less than three-year-old tuna that is mercury free), sardines, and halibut
- Pineapple (contains bromelain which is anti-inflammatory)
- Fruits and lemon (but not other citrus fruits or dried fruits)
- Non-starchy vegetables: asparagus, bean sprouts, beet greens, broccoli, red and green cabbage, cauliflower, celery, Swiss chard, cucumber, endive, lettuce varieties, mustard and dandelion greens, radishes, spinach, and watercress
- Slightly starchy vegetables: string beans, beets, bok choy, brussels sprouts, chives, collards, eggplant, kale, kohlrabi, leeks, onion, parsley, red pepper, pumpkin, rutabagas, and zucchini
- Starchy vegetables: artichokes, parsnips, green peas, winter squash, and carrots
- Very starchy vegetables: yams and sweet potatoes (avoid potatoes and tomatoes and eat starchy vegetables only occasionally)
- Garlic, ginger, and turmeric
- Most nuts and seeds except peanuts
- Flaxseed oil
- Filtered water (drink half your body weight in fluid ounces daily)
- Eat as much organic food as possible to avoid toxic chemicals, which are very inflammatory, found in most foods today
- Organic eggs
- Small amount of rice, oat, and almond milk
- Small amounts of organic beef
- Bake with a blend of butter and coconut oil
- Nut and seed oils for salads

- Olive oil for low temperature cooking (only buy olive oil with a production date stamped on the bottle and use within a month and a half of opening)

Foods to Avoid if You Have Inflammation

- For those who are sensitive to nightshade vegetables, avoid tomatoes, tomatillos, white and red potatoes, eggplant, peppers and any red spices, paprika, tobacco, goji berries, and ashwagandha
- All wheat flours (brown and white wheat bread and wheat pasta)
- Tofu (causes inflammation in some people)
- Shellfish: shrimp, crab lobster, clams, and mussels
- Pork and commercial beef
- Citrus fruits except for lemon
- Dried fruits of all kinds
- Absolutely no sugar, NutraSweet, aspartame, sucralose, or Splenda
- Hydrogenated oils, trans fats, and partially hydrogenated oils (avoid overheating vegetable oils which can convert to trans-fat in the pan)
- Dairy products: milk, yogurt, cheese, and other animal milks
- Commercial eggs
- Peanuts and peanut butter
- Commercial drinks: coffee, caffeinated teas, sodas, and alcohol
- Processed foods: corn products and fried foods
- Canola oil[6]

Basically, the anti-inflammatory diet relies on a select group of vegetables and spices known for their anti-inflammatory properties. It focuses on avoiding inflammatory foods such as corn, soy, milk, wheat, and foods containing sugar, trans-fat, and high fructose corn syrup. Try to keep it simple when buying from a grocery store. Avoid buying anything with more than five ingredients. Hover in the vegetable department. Find real food, bring it home, cook it up, and learn to enjoy natural food.

29

Chelation with Common Foods and Natural Supplements

For many eons humans have lived on this planet. Until we started mining and digging up gold and other precious metals, we only had to deal with the naturally occurring toxic metals that were usually present in low levels. Fortunately, nature has a way of ridding our bodies of toxic metals. Selenium, for example, is a very beneficial metal that helps our thyroid function better. It also chelates, or grabs and neutralizes, toxic metals like mercury and thereby helps the body get rid of them.[1] In fact, dentists who have high selenium levels in their bodies have less symptoms of mercury toxicity later in life.

Lead is another metal that causes serious health problems in humans. For serious lead poisoning, there are many IV treatments and some oral treatments that have been used for a long time by traditional doctors. Members of ACAM, American College for Advancement in Medicine, have been using IV chelation for years for serious and less serious heavy metal poisoning. They do a challenge test. Pretreatment for a week or two with antioxidants to protect the kidney and other vital organs is mandatory. One or two strong chelators are given intravenously, orally, or both at the beginning of the test. Then the urine is collected for six to twenty-four hours after the IV chelation challenge and analyzed for toxic heavy metal levels.

In our toxic, computer-dependent, and mechanical world, many test positive to this provoked urine heavy metal test. I take care of patients from a nearby circuit board manufacturing center. Many get ill from the fumes released when they solder wires onto the board. The fumes have both heavy metals and toxic chemicals in them. They feel better on weekends off from work and when they take a leave of absence. Eventually, they have to quit for health reasons. Some of the suicides in the iPhone manufacturing plant have been blamed on intense work schedules, long hours, and little sleep. But no one in the press has mentioned heavy metal and chemical toxicity which can cause sleep problems, anxiety, and depression all by themselves. And you don't have to work at one of these plants to feel the effects of these toxic metals. Laptops and desktop computers release all kinds of toxic gases into our homes and offices while running.

Since we cannot escape the toxicity of our modern world, we need good ways to get the poisons out. Most people don't have the time and money to get IV chelation from expert ACAM chelators. Generally, thirty IV chelation sessions are recommended for heavy metal toxicity. So what can we do? Natural foods and over the counter supplements have been studied for years for their ability to rid the body of toxic metals. Some are better for one metal than another. Some are better at cleaning out the liver, some the blood, and some are better for cleaning up the brain because they can cross the blood brain barrier. Once poisoned by these metals, it usually takes a long time to get rid of them. It's like trying clean carpet that's had fingernail polish spilled on it.

One of the body's mechanisms for getting rid of toxic metals is to sequester them in bone. This is ok as long as the body is younger and still building bone. But later in life, we begin to lose our hormones and lose our bone mass as a result. When our bones are dissolving, they rerelease the toxic metals back into the blood.[2] So a whole generation of kids were poisoned by lead paint in the classroom and ended up having a lower IQ as a result of the lead dust they inhaled from the air. They got over the acute toxicity in their twenties when lead paint was banned and covered up with less toxic paint in college classrooms. As they become elderly, they get poisoned all over again by the same nasty stuff they were exposed to as children. So not only do they get osteoporosis and bone marrow disease, but they also get lead poisoning all over again. The most current form of lead toxicity in the US has happened in Flint, Michigan where whole families and community members have been poisoned by old lead water pipes. One of the many causes of Alzheimer's is a prevalence of toxic metals in the brain. Is there a way to eat enough good food and clinically proven nutraceuticals to chelate our poisonous lives as we grow older to prevent some of the diseases of aging? The research is being done on this important question now.

So how does a plant or something from a plant have the ability to remove toxins and toxic metals from our bodies? Plants live in a toxic world too. They have many of the same enzymes in their cells that we do. And they are similarly poisoned by the same metals and chemicals. So they have also evolved the machinery to rid themselves of toxic metals. When we eat these plants, we acquire their ability to remove unwanted substances from our bodies. Eating a wide variety of foods that are known to chelate and remove toxic metals is a first step. If we are ill or are tested and found to be heavy metal toxic, then consuming a diet rich in appropriate nutraceuticals is the next step. An ACAM doctor or naturopathic doctor can help consult their patients on which ones and how much of them is best for their patients, especially if the exposure was severe.

The following are lists of natural chelators with references to the research that establishes their effectiveness. You can use them as a guide for improving your daily diet and for mild metal poisoning.

VITAMINS

Ascorbic Acid Vitamin C[3]

Pyridoxine Vitamin B6[4]

D Alpha Tocopherol Natural Vitamin E[5]

B-Complex (Including Thiamine, Folate, and B12[6])

CO Q10[7]

NUTRACEUTICALS

Aged Garlic Extracts[8]

High Fiber Foods[9]

Proanthocyanidins: Pycnogenol, Grapeseed Extract, Grape/Red Wine Polyphenols[10]

Bee Pollen

Chondroitin Sulfate[11]

Flavonoids, Phenols, and Polyphenols[12]

Modified Citrus Pectin/Alginates[13]

Green Food, Drinks, and Powders

Onions[14]

L-Propionyl Carnitine[15]

Gingko Biloba[16]

Sulfur Containing Amino Acids that Chelate Mercury: Dimethylglycine, Glycine, L-Cysteine, Glutamic Acid, Taurine, Methionine, Cystine, and Glutathione made from Glycine, L-Cysteine, and Glutamic Acid[17]

Glutamine

Alpha Lipoic Acid [18]

Taurine[19]

Broken Cell Wall Chlorella[20]

Cilantro[21]

Spirulina[22]

ESSENTIAL OILS

Evening Primrose or Borage Oils: Omega 6 and Omega 3[23]

Black Currant Oil: Omega 6[24]

Flax,[25] Soy,[26] and Fish Oil:[27] Omega 3

Lecithin

MINERALS

Potassium (naturally in fruits, bananas, and vegetables)[28]

Silicon[29]

Chromium Picolinate

Zinc[30]

Selenium[31]

Calcium[32]

Magnesium[33]

Bentonite Clay

Activated Charcoal

Activated Liquid Zeolite[34]

NUTS

Almonds

Hazelnuts

Walnuts[35]

ENZYMES

Methionine Synthase Reductase[36]

Superoxide Dismutase[37]

Papain[38]

Bromelain[39]

Quercetin[40]

Glutathione Peroxidase[41]

HORMONES

Melatonin[42]

MEDITATION, FORGIVENESS, AND/OR FAITH

Letting go of bad feelings lets go of toxins.

OTHER

Aspartates[43]

Probiotics[44]

Fresh Fruit Juice[45]

Chelation mobilizes heavy metals. So using the above natural chelators without some knowledge of the process can lead to hidden away toxic metals coming out in the open to do damage a second time. So people with lots of amalgam fillings will loosen up mercury with natural chelators which will then be swallowed and absorbed. One rule of thumb that always helps is to use bentonite clay and chlorella taken orally to bind the toxic metals freed up by cilantro, for example, so that they are carried away by the digestive tract and eliminated rather than being reabsorbed. If mercury or lead are freed up, they can also hurt the kidney and liver seriously. So alpha lipoic acid preferably made in Italy will help protect the kidney. So will cilantro. Milk thistle and N-acetyl-cysteine will help protect the liver. All MDs and NDs who do chelation have a universal mantra: go slow and low. Low dose and spaced-out detox treatments over many years. I personally know patients who have ruined their kidneys having the amalgams removed from their teeth all at once which is something I don't recommend. Very few dentists can do it safely. They are hard to find, and you should only work with certified MD chelation doctors. Once the mercury is removed from the teeth, there is still a significant body burden of toxic metals. So as my patient found out after spending ten grand on amalgam mercury removal, she was no better at all. In fact, she got sicker.

The point of this chapter is not to encourage people to do their own chelation. Such an approach is hazardous at best. From all the scientific references on natural chelators that I have researched and provided; I want to show how a healthy natural diet is a protection against toxic metals. If a person has only a little accumulation of toxic metals already, they may benefit from a gradual reduction of them over decades of eating healthy. If you suspect heavy toxic metal exposure, work with professionals in both the removal of physical or external exposure and with the clearing of internalized poisoning for proper and safe healing.

Quantum Flow Healing

30 ▌

The River of Life and the Rhythm
of Sleep

Early American settlers in the Plains states earned their sleep by creating life in the soil by the sweat of their brows. They slept an average of about nine hours each night. They were mostly farmers who had a lot of hard work to do. Their journal entries showed that when the sun went down, they didn't burn the midnight oil in their lamps or candles. They went to bed early and got up early getting more sleep than just about any modern American. They were more connected with the life-giving earth and sun. They breathed fresh air and slept soundly to the noises of the earth at rest.

Nowadays, modern people waste their sleep by breaking the rhythm of life itself. Their lives often look like shattered glass too painful to step on. They have been smashing everything in a fit of rage. They shatter their sweet dreams with toxic fears. They fill their toxic and tired minds with violent images just before retiring. They listen to violence screaming at eardrum piercing sound levels all day and night and call it music. The natural music of the stars and night used to be a beautiful harmonic symphony. Our night music is now a cacophonous grating wail like someone dying a slow, agonizing, and tortuous death.

As with all things, there is a cause and effect. If sleep is a shattered dream, then perhaps the steps to actualize that dream are not being taken earlier in the day. The imbalanced lifestyle rams into the sleeping hours. It only continues the mad cycle into the next morning when sleep deprivation motivates a new day of poor life choices to compensate. This chapter will single out possible causes of the inability to get a full night's rest and how best to remedy or prevent them from occurring. It will also provide info about why sleep is so important in the bigger picture of your health and life.

Dark Room

The bedroom must be dark for sleeping well. Any yellow, green, blue, or white light, even the power light on the TV, will keep you from sleeping deeply. Red light does not affect sleep. So clocks with the wrong color or time projections of light on the ceiling can keep people half awake. Smartphones and tablets with their blue light can make insomniacs out of the heaviest of sleepers. Think of it as having the lights on while trying to fall asleep. When the moon shines through the curtains, it can keep you awake, result in insomnia, or cause sleep to be disrupted when it rises in the middle of the night.

When there is light in the room, people don't secrete the fall asleep hormone melatonin. They are left at the mercy of being so exhausted from sleep deprivation that they can finally fall asleep. Melatonin is necessary for health independent of falling asleep. It turns on the antioxidant systems in the body at night to repair the damage of the day. Shift workers and truck drivers get less sleep than average and have shorter lives than those who sleep better. A breast cancer survivor study showed high dose melatonin compared to placebo caused the women to have 43% less cancer recurrence than the placebo group after five years. This worked better than chemotherapy for preventing breast cancer recurrence. There must be something very powerful in the antioxidant stimulus of melatonin. Yet as we age, we secrete less and less melatonin and therefore sleep less and less each year. This is considered normal, but given the benefits of melatonin, the loss of regular melatonin levels seems to be related to the numerous diseases of aging as an aggravating factor. Patients ask me how much melatonin they should take. The answer is different for each person. I had one patient who couldn't even tolerate a quarter of a 1 mg tablet. So I tell patients to start low and take more and more each night till they sleep well. Some are fine with 1 mg, some 3 mg, and some require 20 mg like the breast cancer survivors in the study.[1]

Temperature

The temperature must drop while getting ready for bed and falling asleep. If it stays high, you will be less likely to sleep well. A well-placed bedroom fan will provide a cooling effect while blanketing your room in white noise. Opening windows during cooler nights is a good idea. And if nights aren't cool enough, adjusting the thermostat settings can get you to your optimal bedtime temp.

Humidity

Dry air in the winter is bad for noses. It not only causes severe nose bleeds in people on aspirin and blood thinners, but it also causes the nose to get sore, crusty, and blocked. If the humidity your area is less than 30%, you'll need humidifiers in the house and on the furnace in the winter. If the humidity is more than 40%, then mold starts to grow and causes nose problems too. A basement tends to be wetter and damper than the upstairs. A humidity gauge is only fifteen dollars and worth the investment. Get one that does twenty-four-hour humidity and temperature ranging to see the high and low numbers. Check the basement in the summer and the upstairs in the winter. Adjust the humidity with a dehumidifier or a humidifier. Hot humidifiers usually do not grow mold. Cool mist humidifiers tend to grow mold. Both need to be disinfected frequently. The furnace devices are less likely to grow mold.

Soft Beds

I remember trying to sleep on my aunt's guest bed when I was a teenager. It had a feather tick mattress. My back literally sank down two feet, and I couldn't sleep on my back or side. The springs were shot too. I obviously didn't get much sleep there. Stiffer beds tend to be better for sleep and your back. For people suffering from back injuries, getting heat treatments, physical therapy, chiropractic treatment, or massage can relieve pain and help them sleep better. Sleeping on the floor where the spine will be straight is a good idea for a temporary fix. Chiropractors have lots of good advice for fixing back problems and finding sleeping positions that are better for backs. Generally, sleeping straight on the side with a knee pillow is best. As people get older, sleeping on backs and stomachs cause obstruction and poor sleep.

Grounded to Earth

Humans used to sleep on the ground or on something touching the ground. Americans are now mostly insulated from the ground and have lost that antioxidant function of grounding that their ancestors enjoyed. They have a lot of oxidative processes that create oxidation and free radicals. Walking barefoot is grounding. Negative ions flow from the surface of the earth up through the feet neutralizing the free radicals and oxidative processes. People are healthier this way. Sheets containing silver wires plugged into the ground of the electrical socket can ground people at night and improve their sleep and health.

Dust Mites in Bedding

Dust mites like to live in beds, pillows, drapes, carpets, and couches. They live off dead skin flakes. Basically, they like to live everywhere humans park their bodies. Some beds have 100,000 mites in a finger size area. One of my patients last week said he had had the same mattress for twenty-seven years and was complaining of shoulder pain and arm numbness. Not only was his mattress loaded with mites, but it was hard, bowed, and bad for his shoulders and back.

A five-dollar dust mite proof pillow cover will prevent the inhaling of dead dust mites and the sleep disturbing congestion that follows. Mattress and box spring covers are also a good idea. You can use regular pillowcases over these covers and wash the pillowcases in hot water once a week. Getting rid of old carpet and putting wood down also helps noses. New carpet has carpet glue which is toxic to noses and livers. Boric acid powder is a more natural dust mite killer that kills mites in carpets. Allergy patients who do these things can expect a better night's sleep.

Pillows

You may really love the pillow you're using, but is it slowly causing health related problems? Having broad or small shoulders can determine what type of pillow you need. Sometimes the pillow flattens over time and the head reclines too low causing neck soreness and lower quality sleep. The pillow should make the cervical spine straight. Japanese people traditionally slept on wood pillows that never collapsed with time. And in both China and other Asian countries, sleeping on the hard floor temporarily is recommended for some back problems. Memory foam pillows last one or two years before collapsing. Feather and down pillows cause mold and allergy problems. Foam pillows in general cause chemical outgassing when new. The workers in the memory foam plants get sick from these chemicals all the time even though the factories are usually open to the outside and are often well ventilated. We can also get sick from the foam pillows. Pillows filled with beans keep their shape better, are stiffer, and are generally better for your neck. To pick the right thickness of pillow for yourself, lay on the hard floor on your side with your head on the pillow. Have someone look at your back and neck from behind. Are your spine and neck straight? If not, you need to get a different size. With the soft pillows, they crush down so much that it's hard to tell if your neck and spine are straight.

Snoring

Over 40% of sixty-five-year-old men snore badly and half of them have sleep apnea. The rate of sleep apnea is half of that for women that age and half of that for forty-year-old men. Some think that you must stop breathing to have apnea. The sleep study labs show that when snoring increases, there is often a drop in the oxygenation levels which signal a snoring apnea spell. There are too many treatments for sleep apnea to mention them all here. A trip to a sleep specialist, pulmonologist, or an ENT specialist would be a good place to start. But anyone can go to their family doctor and get a sleep study set up. Some think that only overweight people have sleep apnea, but my experience has been that thinner people also have problems with sleep apnea.

Overweight patients usually have large tongues that can fall back in the throat at night causing choking or air obstruction. I used to use a laser to cut a groove down the middle of the back side of the tongue after doing a UPPP. Now we can shrink the area with electric needles in a less morbid and painful way. When an overweight person loses even five or ten pounds, the sleep apnea lessens dramatically in some cases. I have often felt this to be because the body pulls the fat out of the airway first. I generally recommend a trial of nasal CPAP or BIPAP before surgery is considered. There are numerous operations for apnea. The least painful is turbinate cautery, followed by turbinate resection, followed by septoplasty. The other operations are painful or life changing and are not as necessary as they were before the CPAP machines were invented. So often a little weight loss, a little CPAP, and occasionally a little surgery will result in a good night's rest for the patient. For those who can't tolerate CPAP, a new surgical technique called "Inspire" has been working very well.[2] When the patient is sleeping better, exercise and a weight loss plan will be more successful because the patient has more energy from sleeping well.

Bladder Problems and Sleep

People often get the mistaken impression that they wake up because their bladder is full. So they go to the bathroom, empty themselves, feel better, and then go back to sleep. This seems to get worse with age. This disrupts sleep. Sometimes, they are waking up for other reasons, like sleep apnea. They then feel their bladder is full and go empty it. After getting up to do so, they often can't go back to sleep. The bladder can be trained to hold more. While sleeping, people release an antidiuretic hormone which slows down urine production. So most of the time, they really can wait till the morning to empty it. They need to try to go back to sleep and resist the urge to go to the bathroom. It is a habit that can be retrained. The bladder is usually noticed after waking up. It's a secondary problem blamed on the waking up. Some of my patients have food allergies that affect their bladder. Sometimes cranberry juice during the day helps the bladder at night. Caffeine is a weak diuretic causing people to urinate more. So consuming it at night can obviously cause them to urinate at night more frequently.

Leg Cramps

Leg cramps are common these days. A recent study showed that as many as 55% of Americans are deficient in magnesium.[3] We used to drink awful tasting water with lots of magnesium in it. It is now removed to make the water taste better. So many people are now deficient in it. Calcium helps muscles contract. The magnesium helps relax muscles. They both are necessary for bone formation. But taking them together causes them to compete for the same entryway into the body. So calcium wins out and the body loses magnesium. Magnesium oxide found in most pills is poorly absorbed. Milk of Magnesia (liquid magnesium oxide) is used for constipation because it causes diarrhea. Magnesium citrate pills are better absorbed but hard to find. You probably have to go to a health food store to get them. The best magnesium for absorption is magnesium glycinate. Glycine is needed for liver detox anyway, so it makes more sense to use this form of magnesium. It helps relax muscles so people can sleep better. The dose is 400 mg to 600 mg at bedtime. I see a lot of patients for dizziness. Many of them have it as a side effect of medication. The medicine for nocturnal leg cramps, Lyrica, causes dizziness. By the time these patients get to me, they usually have seen a lot of doctors for dizziness. I get out the *Physician's Desk Reference* and they are shocked to see the side effects of Lyrica matching their own symptoms to a tee. Switching them to magnesium glycinate solves both problems for the dizziness and leg cramps.

Restless Leg Syndrome

Restless leg syndrome is becoming more common as we get more and more anxious and magnesium deficient. Lyrica is often used here too. I find that Valerian root, an herb, and magnesium glycinate cure this condition better than any drug. The dose of magnesium is the same as above.

Worrying

Many of my patients wake up worried that they will forget to do something the next day. They will lay awake at night worrying about it. A good habit to get into is to have a notepad with a pen on a chain near the bed. If you wake up with something to worry about, write it down and tell yourself you will be better able to think it through clearly the next day. Then forget about it and get some rest.

Caffeine

Too much caffeine, and in some cases, too little caffeine can interfere with sleep. If people drink a lot of caffeinated drinks during the day, the caffeine withdrawal syndrome may kick in when going to bed at night and interfere with sleep. A lot of these patients have severe headaches and flu-like symptoms in the morning that are relieved by more caffeine. Caffeine detox can take one and a half to four days on average before this withdrawal syndrome goes away. Sometimes it takes longer. Some women have a liver enzyme deficiency that allows their caffeine levels to grow higher and the caffeine alertness effects can last longer interfering with sleep. Sometimes I even have them get rid of the morning coffee cup for them to get a good night's rest. Obviously drinking caffeine just before bed is bad for sleep. Sugar free caffeine drinks are the worst for sleep late at night. They have NutraSweet or aspartame. These have the amino acid phenylalanine in them which is the precursor to several alertness neurotransmitter chemicals in the brain. People can become addicted to these as well and go through withdrawal syndrome upon stopping them. Over the years, I have had two patients confess that they drank one to two gallons of coffee every day. I don't know how they even slept.

Sugar

People demolish their food groups by eating dead food and "white death" as Arnold Schwarzenegger famously called sugar and carbs back in the 70s. Eating sugar before bedtime causes nightmares in some, reactive hypoglycemia in others, drop in growth hormone production in others, drop in testosterone levels in men, and cortisol surges that keep people awake all night because cortisol must be low at night for sleep. Cortisol will increase with sugar intake and tense movies seen before bed.

Exercise

When you exercise, the body heats up one or two degrees. It then cools down slowly over several hours. The cool down promotes drowsiness and helps sleep. Although exercising too close to bedtime can keep you awake. Exercise in the early evening hours opens noses too if you have congestion problems.

Allergies

Allergies cause the nasal tissues to swell and the nose to fill up with sticky mucous that blocks it. Food allergies can also cause nasal obstruction and subsequent poor sleep. Nasal saline rinses have been promoted in the last ten years as an alternative to sinus surgery and allergy desensitization shots. My experience with thousands of allergy and sinus patients over the years have confirmed the substantial benefit of irrigating warm saline through the nose daily. Many patients swear by it preferring it above all other treatments. When all treatments, surgery, and shots have failed my patients, then we are always coming back to irrigating. For some, it seems too messy. But a gallon of salt water can be mixed up once a week, placed in the shower, and an ear bulb syringe or Neti Pot can be used to irrigate in the shower. The usual amount is one cup on each side which is five large ear bulb syringe sprays. NeilMed makes packets of preformed salt, one packet for eight ounces of water. I recommend distilled or good quality spring water. If you want to save money, one teaspoon of canning salt in a pint of water is the cheapest. Never irrigate the nose with tap water and without salt. It waterlogs the nose and makes it swell shut just like long baths in water make your feet swell up. NeilMed and Arm and Hammer make a can of pressurized saline for rinsing the nose on the go, but it's expensive. Simply Saline is a pressurized saline can that is smaller and cheaper.

Ear, Nose, and Throat Causes for Sleep Disturbance

Ear, nose, and throat problems are a common cause of disrupted sleep. Ear pain is worse because lower nighttime cortisol levels allow more inflammation. Lowering a painful part of the body while laying down causes blood to engorge in it and results in more pain. So when babies are crying in their cribs from painful ear infections, picking them up lessens the pain. It's like elevating your sprained ankle to lessen pain. Lying flat with ear pain or a sinus headache makes it worse. So sleeping with the head slightly elevated when sick is best. For adults it could take sleeping in a recliner. For babies, having them sleep in a baby chair or swing might work best.

Americans tend to over consume salt which causes them to hang on to too much fluid. It ends up accumulating in ankles, feet, and lower legs during the day. At night, this fluid flows up into nasal tissues, especially the turbinates, causing obstruction and snoring.

Mismatched jaws cause snoring and sleep problems. When the lower jaw is small and the chin recessed, retrognathia or class II malocclusion, it pushes the tongue back and causes snoring especially when sleeping on the back. Dentists make dental appliances to pull the lower jaw and tongue forward to treat this. They can be bought online in a kit form, but the homemade devices might not work as well. Also jaw advancement surgery has been quite effective in curing snoring although it is quite involved with braces and surgery and is painful.

The typical Norwegian nose is one of the many beautiful sizes and shapes of noses. I do a fair amount of cosmetic nose surgery to give patients that look. Many people want to have smaller noses, but smaller noses don't move as much air as larger noses. The epigenetics of noses is determined by how cold the climate is. If the climate is cold, then the nasal passageway is narrow in order to warm the air more quickly for the lungs which want 98° air. If the air is hot, more room is necessary for evaporation to cool the air down to 98°. Therefore, the inner passageways are roomy. A narrow nose is a disaster for allergy and sinus sufferers. Cold weather and milk are anathema to a small nose too.

Noses swell inside to warm the air better in cold weather. The narrow passageways get blocked. Milk thickens up the mucous in the nose even if you are not allergic to it and it dries out in the cold dry air blocking the passageways. The net result is a nose that is small on the outside and often dysfunctional and narrow on the inside. Poor sleep as people get older is the rule and poor sleep-in pediatric allergy sufferers is universal with small noses. In Norway and Sweden, they invented the sauna to open their noses in the winter. They sauna every day which opens their sinuses and prevents a lot of diseases like chronic wintertime sinusitis. It's aggravated by vitamin D deficiency in the northern climates where there is no direct UVB sunlight to create vitamin D in the skin. Supplementing with vitamins is now popular in northern climates. So a degree of self-care in the wintertime, including saunas and saline rinses, can have a positive ripple effect into the bedtime hours.

I've spent much of this chapter focusing on how to get to sleep. But let's explore why sleep is so important and why you need this skill set for fixing health and weight problems. Understanding the importance of sleep for your overall health gives more incentive to fix the problem. The following is a listing of research backed issues and topics that show what can go wrong when sleep takes a back seat.

Findings from Various Sleep Studies

- Reaction times in athletes and vehicle drivers slowed after periods of sleep deprivation.[4]
- Swedish train drivers hooked to EEG's while conducting trains were found to have sleep wave patterns show up in their brain waves 30% of the time. There were ten, twenty, and thirty second episodes where they were actually asleep with their eyes open.[5]
- If there is no sleep after learning something new, such as cramming all night for a test in college, there is no long-term memory storage.[6]
- Continual sleep loss can lead to obesity and diabetes.[7]

- Ghrelin, our ravenous hunger hormone, or eat-the-whole-fridge hormone, is increased substantially up to 10% after just one night of less sleep. The next day people on average consume considerably more carbohydrates.[8]
- Going to bed hungry increases delta wave sleep and growth hormone secretion. This is beneficial for weight loss.[9]
- More than 250 mg of caffeine a day can cause insomnia and worsen the quality of sleep.[10]
- Sleep deprivation leads to drop in lymphocyte levels.[11]
- Sleep deprivation changes bowel function and can lead to gastro-intestinal diseases and cancer.[12]
- Sleep deprivation causes depression, anxiety, paranoia, and aggravates bipolar disease.[13]
- Losing three hours of sleep drops the immune efficiency by 50%.[14]
- Our bodies detox while sleeping. Going to bed late disrupts the entire detox process. The lymph nodes detox from 9 p.m. to 11 p.m. The liver detoxes from 11 p.m. to 1 a.m. The gallbladder detoxes from 1 a.m. to 3 a.m. The lungs detox from 3 a.m. to 5 a.m. The colon detoxes from 5 a.m. to 7 a.m. The bowels are best able to absorb nutrients from 7 a.m. to 9 a.m. So going to bed early helps detox. It's important to relax in the hours before going to bed to allow the lymph nodes to detox.[15]
- A recent study showed that when middle-aged people get too much or too little sleep, it accelerates cognitive decline.[16]
- Teenagers stay up late, have to go to school early, and then get sleep deprived.[17]
- Power naps are best at twenty minutes. At forty-five minutes you are at your deepest sleep, and it will take a long time to wake up. And when you do wake up, you'll feel groggy. If you are going to sleep longer than twenty minutes, go for one and a half to two hours to allow for waking up refreshed instead of groggy.[18] This is the typical siesta midday nap in many parts of the world.

- Recent studies of historical peoples, indigenous tribes, and some cultures suggest biphasic sleep patterns that include awakening in middle night for a while before going back to sleep might be more normal than we think.[19]
- You can conduct your own sleep experiments at home. Try sleeping one hour longer each day for a week. Do you feel more alert? If so, you need more sleep. Try sleeping half an hour less each day. Do you feel better or worse? If you feel worse, adjust your sleep appropriately.[20]
- Nearly all the useful sleep occurs in the first three to five hours. So sleeping in does not add to restful feelings the next day. The quality of the first three to five hours is most important. Refreshing sleep occurs in the first hours of sleep. Dream sleep predominates the later pre-dawn sleep.[21]
- A bath with Epsom salts has magnesium in it, which relaxes muscles so you can relax more and sleep better. Two cups of Epsom salts and ten drops of lavender oil in the bath can set up the evening for relaxing before sleep.

As you can see from following me down this train of thought, getting a good night's rest is simple and yet complicated at the same time. Habits are tough to break. In order to find a good night flow and rhythm, it will take an honest look at your routines, products, and environment. As with every piece of advice in this book, I suggest taking on one or two goals or projects at a time. Master those and then move on to the next. Before you know it, you'll be coasting.

31

Exercise Your Dark Cloud Away

When I went to boot camp in Fort Knox, Kentucky in 1972, we had to complete a night compass course. Most of the time, it was light enough to see the compass, but not on this moonless and cloudy night. We had many check points and several miles to negotiate in wooded terrain. So we knew the starting direction from the light at the beginning and set our compasses. After pacing out the distance, we had to turn and at this point we couldn't see the compass. Here is where our training came in handy. We knew that we could turn the compass one click at a time to the new course, counting clicks and degrees, as we went. We could not see the numbers but had to guess that our click count was right and that we turned the compass dial in the right direction. If we made a mistake, even by a degree, we ended up off course and missed the final destination.

So it is in life. Initial settings on your health compass are often made in the dark by the food and exercise fads of the moment. If you have the wrong direction, even by a degree in some cases, you'll end up in health hell forty long years later. Back on that cloudless night on a Kentucky bluegrass hillside, we argued over the degrees. In life, there are many voices arguing for this or that health benefit sometimes quibbling over just how much of this or that food, vitamin, or exercise you should use. When you are healthy and life is just starting out, how do you know the course? Which of all the diets is right for you? How do you know it will end up well for you in the end? There are so many influences. Each of them making a profit on persuading you to take their course.

An example of this first step might be answering the following question: How much should you exercise and what kind of exercise should you do? The US loves the marathon look and admires that athletic ability. They get that runner's high. Some people never feel good when not running. So they get out and run till they drop. One young man in his early forties ran six marathons in a year. On the seventh marathon he dropped dead of a heart attack. The coronary arteries of heavy runners are highly calcified, and their mitochondria are depleted and dysfunctional. They tend to die younger of heart attacks and cancer compared to the rest of society. How can this happen to people who are so healthy looking and have such great muscles and trim bodies? This is also the case in all strenuous sports like football, basketball, and hockey.

So if you sign up for that sports club and begin exercising two hours a day at the crack of dawn, are you headed in the same direction? Are you slightly off course or a lot off course? The answer lies in how humans make ATP, adenosine triphosphate, in their mitochondria. A lot of research into the nuclear power plants in cells has revealed that people don't just run out of fuel, get tired, and have to quit the long exercise. When they run out of fuel, they switch to alternative energy by burning up the ADP, adenosine diphosphate, and then the AMP or adenosine monophosphate. It can take months to recover from this extreme exercise depletion of AMP. Runners call it the crash after the peak. They save their all-out peak exertion for that big race. After that, they can no longer run as fast till their body rebuilds the ATP energy production machinery in the mitochondria. What is even worse is the fact that runners burn so much oxygen that they produce more smoke (free radical oxygen) than they can get rid of.

Then the smoke damages the mitochondrial DNA and destroys it for good. The body can never repair free radical damage to mitochondrial DNA. There are only about two hundred mitochondria in a muscle cell and the body cannot make any more in most cases. There are five thousand in each heart cell. When the cardiac mitochondria are gone or dysfunctional, people get weakness, congestive heart disease, heart attacks, and even death. So extreme exertion every day is bad for your health. But you would never know that listening to all the hype about exercise being good for you. Too much can kill you. If you have fewer than normal mitochondria and have genetic defects in them from birth, you are better off being a couch potato than exercising at all.

So exercise fanaticism can not only kill your heart, but also make you addicted to adrenalin just like a speed junkie who needs his next fix to feel happy. The chemistry of reward pathways in the brain responds the same to either excessive running or taking methamphetamines. So the direction people take in life with regard to exercise is very important in order to be healthy forty years into the future. How much exercise will rejuvenate the body and produce long lasting health? The answer is simple. Just exercise till you feel invigorated and not exhausted. You should not exercise to exhaustion because it will wear out your body and cause disease and injury. If you feel invigorated after the exercise, you've found the right amount. There should be a mix of alternating days between weightlifting and aerobic exercise, usually three to five times a week.

Care should also be taken when considering the type of exercise that suits your body best. Jogging, running, and extreme road cycling can ruin people's knees. Too much stress on the joints with exercise ruins the ability to exercise later in life. This is when people need it the most to boost their immune systems, hormones, and health. Glider machines have the least impact on joints, stair steppers come next, and bicycles after that. Low repetition of heavy weights till you break a sweat are better for stamina and wear and tear on joints than high repetition low weights.

When you've established this healthy, not punishing or addictive, relationship with exercise, it opens you up more to the true psychological and hormonal benefit of exercise which primes you for a lifestyle of eating well and feeling well. A while back, I started gaining weight inexplicably. I was hurting all over and feeling cold and tired all day long. I began to wonder if I had what many of my patients have had over the expanse of my thirty years of ENT practice. I had my thyroid blood levels drawn and found that I was hypothyroid. So I researched who was the best expert on thyroid problems and read several books on the subject. I came across one of the world's experts on thyroid Dr. John Lowe. He had written a huge text on the science of thyroid therapy. He tested my basal metabolic rate with an oxygen consumption test for an hour. The basal metabolic rate is the rate at which we burn calories and oxygen into heat. He said that I had one of the lowest metabolic rates he had ever recorded. As a result of mitochondrial failure, I couldn't generate heat from burning fuel. My daily temperatures were hovering between 95° F and 97° F depending on the time of day.

I was shocked. Now I finally had an explanation for having to force myself to do any small or large task all day long. Everything seemed like a Mount Everest to climb, and it took all my willpower to accomplish any small thing. Dr. Lowe told me that I must have an immense willpower to function as a physician and surgeon with such a low metabolic rate. Thyroid hormone therapy fortunately reversed the problem. With better eating, sleeping, and meditation, I was able to get off thyroid hormone in two years and have not had to go back to it ever since.

Much later, I read Dr. Timothy Scott's monumental work on antidepressants which showed me that exercise can also raise your metabolic rate naturally. I'm sharing with you here his table showing how exercise can chase the dark clouds away and restore health:

1. Exercise raises the body's metabolic rate. (Depression lowers the body's metabolic rate.)
2. Exercise increases your energy level. (Depression lowers energy levels.)
3. Exercise brings about better sleep. (Depression hinders sleep.)
4. Exercise often involves a person with other exercisers. (Depression tends to result in more isolation and less socialization.)

5. Exercise tends to release stress and tension. (Depression increases stress and tension.)

6. Exercise gets your mind off the problem. (Depression involves an intense focus on the problem.)

7. Exercise has physical health benefits. (Depression harms physical health.)

8. Exercise often involves goals: improving strength, weight loss, etc. (Depression typically avoids goals by focusing on present problems, future fears, and the past.)

9. Group exercise requires you to get out of the house and, therefore, out of your rut. (Depression tends to keep you home and in a rut.)

10. Exercise keeps the body from getting constipated, a major stressor for older people. (Depression reduces physical activity and thus, "regularity.")[1]

One of my patients recently got a certificate for a hundred plus Jazzercise classes in less than a year. She has been so happy to lose thirty pounds in six months and go from a size fourteen to a size six. This explains how point four is true. Joining a gym, a dance workout group, or getting a personal trainer is well worth the money. It will save you from the dangerous side effects of prescription antidepressants which have no more effectiveness and maybe are even slightly less effective compared to the placebo.[2]

Our bodies are genetically wired for lots of exercise. That is how our ancestors were able to survive all these centuries doing subsistence farming and living off the land. When each mouthful of food cost a lot of work to obtain, it was hard to get fat, lazy, and sad over it. We have to invent more ways to exercise. Cleaning the house is one way to exercise. Planting a garden is another. Climbing stairs instead of taking the elevator is a healthy habit. We are all dancers inside. Our bodies love to move and twist and pump blood into dusty corners where life is dying like vascular dementia in the aging. In China, all people over sixty-five have to get out for morning exercises in the town square. There is no better way to prevent disease. So a lifelong commitment to moderation in exercise will produce the best health that lasts and lasts well into the golden years.

32

The Golden Tan Versus the Withered Tan

Humans are designed for light. Without light, people become sad and develop seasonal affective disorder (SAD). In any given country of the Northern Hemisphere, the people in the north of the country are sadder than the people in the south. This is even true in a partially arctic country like Norway where the people in Bodø, north of the Arctic Circle, are more depressed than the people in Arendal which is located in the very south. The opposite is true south of the equator. You need sunlight on your body to be happy and you need lots of it. You have this immense fiber-optic system that carries the sunlight all throughout your transparent body. Shine a flashlight through your hand in the dark. You are 50% to 70% water, and the light will stream right through your hand. You also have light channels between cells that carry information instantaneously. Inside each cell, there are laser-like tubes called microtubules that focus and transmit light. The whole system seems to be designed for light transmission. Light tickles every part of the body and mind. Alertness centers in the brain wake up with the light of the early summer day, enzymes activate, the internal factories hum with excitement, and in this state, your mood has the ability to soar.

Light is also good for bones. If people get whole body exposure, like when swimming, for an hour or two each day in the summer, they build high levels of vitamin D in their bodies. Vitamin D helps with calcium absorption. Without it, people get depressed and develop hip fractures. More women have increased health consequences, and even death, due to hip fractures than breast cancer.[1] Vitamin D deficiency is truly a national emergency. But why doesn't the vitamin D in milk and in calcium supplements protect people from hip fractures? It's because they are consuming the wrong kind of vitamin D. Many milk jugs have no vitamin D added and others have too much because of faulty machinery at the dairy plant. The proper daily dose according to recent studies varies from 2000 international units (IU) of vitamin D3 to 5000 IU, and goes even higher for extreme medical conditions, depending on which study you read.[2] Most vitamin D is sold as vitamin D2. Even the prescription vitamin D is vitamin D2. The real stuff, vitamin D3, is generally sold in health food stores not pharmacies.

When sunlight hits the skin and goes through the body, it changes cholesterol molecules into cholecalciferol. Then, the provitamin, a substance that is converted into vitamin form within the body, moves to the liver where it becomes 1-hydroxycholecalciferol and then on to the kidney where it is finished as 1,25-hydroxycholecalciferol. The final form has all the power to heal in so many ways. Not only does it help prevent one of the biggest health problems in America, hip fractures, but it also lifts depression as a powerful antidepressant. Lastly and even more importantly, it helps people fight cancer as a powerful antioxidant and anticancer molecule. So why aren't people racing for the beaches and backyards to get sun after hearing all this?

There is an epidemic of skin cancer going on at the same time that people are getting depressed from lack of sun exposure. To prevent cancer, people are using a lot of sunblock. Yet subsequently, they aren't getting enough sun. Many farmers live in the dermatologist's office getting their face removed piece by piece. Some of the farmers faces look like a basset hound's with large saggy folds of skin hanging down. A lot of people don't want to look like that either, so they avoid the sun. But this is all knee jerk medicine. Some people don't get these problems from healthy sun exposure. What is the difference between the group that does and the group that doesn't?

Plants need the sun just a bad as we do. Without it they die. In Nebraska, the farmers speak of corn in terms of growing units. It has to do with sunlight and heat. When the plants are watered and fed properly, they need a lot of sunlight to grow. On bright and hot days, you can hear them growing, making sounds as they do. I used to drive over a hundred miles into the countryside of Phillipsburg, Kansas early in the morning. I would see three-foot-tall corn stalks lining the road. On the way back late in the evening, the same corn had grown about a foot. This process is so miraculous. Photosynthesis needs lots of light to make energy for the plant to grow. Humans need lots of light to make vitamin D3. If the sun was so bad, why don't humans live in dark, damp caves eating mushrooms that never see the light of day? A study of mountain flowers could help explain why. They are so pretty, tiny, and delicate with vibrant colors. Why don't they shrivel up in seconds from the intense ultraviolet light high up in the rarified mountain air with little protection from the sun?

Delicate and brightly colored mountain plants thrive in this harsh ultraviolet storm of light because of antioxidants. Their very color comes from the pigmented antioxidants that prevent sunlight from hurting them. These colors soak up the harsh sunlight rays and turn the radiation into something useful. Could these antioxidants do the same for people? The answer is yes, they can. Not only will they protect against sunlight damage to the skin, but they will also protect from cancer and rapid aging. One of the key theories of accelerated aging is that oxidative damage rapidly builds up in body tissues. People literally rust inside from burning oxygen without enough antioxidants. They badly need the antioxidants that plants make so easily. Unfortunately, food processing ruins most of them. Several authors call this antioxidant rich and colorful food diet the rainbow diet.[3] They suggest that you eat a large variety of colorful foods in order to get the antioxidants that protect skin from rapid aging in the sun.

One of the key antioxidant ingredients found in these colorful plants is the beta carotene found in carrots, pumpkins, squash, orange tomatoes, and yellow peppers. If people eat a lot of these, they can protect their skin from sunburn and cancer. Some people eat so much beta carotene that their skin turns orange. When I was still in medical school, one of my fellow medical school students literally had orange skin. She ate carrots all day by the bag as a diet trick. She was skinny and orange because of it. Since carrots are also high in sugar, this is not a recommended diet plan for diabetics and people with hypoglycemia. There are many other colors to choose from.

Blueberries have blue pigments called anthocyanins. These antioxidants are more plentiful than those in strawberries which have flavonoids, polyphenols, and anthocyanins as well. There are six hundred carotenoid antioxidants in plants but only fourteen are found in our blood suggesting the body prefers these. Lutein is an increasingly popular carotenoid antioxidant used for protection against macular degeneration. Macular degeneration is caused by the oxidative action of years of sunlight on the retina. This is similar to the rapid aging of the skin from years of sunlight. Lutein is a carotenoid much like beta carotene. It's found in the highest concentrations in kale and spinach and is in all dark green leafy vegetables.[4] If lutein can protect the eye from sunlight damage, can it and other carotenoids protect the skin from sunlight damage? This is why these plants have antioxidants in the first place. It allows them to get the sun they need for photosynthesis and avoid being damaged by the sun. Humans don't make these antioxidants in their bodies, and like all omnivores, need to eat the plants that have them. Omnivores like bears, for example, have a berry rich diet. So, a rainbow diet helps people get the sun they need for vitamin D3 and happiness, and the antioxidants they need for cancer and aging skin protection.

33

Untying the Knot

For as he thinketh in his heart, so is he.

—PROVERBS 23:7

Why is it that people spend 80% of their time engaged in nuclear negative thinking blowing up all their well laid goals, efforts, and plans? The formulas are all the same and run on autopilot like a bad tune you can't get out of your head. The record skips over and over in the same scratched spot:

"I can't stand (blankety-blank)."
"My (blank) doesn't love me."
"I'm so stupid."
"I hate my body."
"I'll never be able to pay the bills."
"I'll never be successful at anything."

On average people think 60,000 thoughts per waking day or one per second. Amazingly, 95% of these thoughts are repetitively the same day after day. Some 80% are totally negative.[1]

Where do these thoughts come from that are so defeating? It turns out, recent research shows that the subconscious is not conscious at all but merely behaves like soundbites on a prerecorded playback loop. The repetitive messages were recorded in the first six years of life. They can't be merely erased, argued out of existence, or reasoned with. While people are conscious and aware of themselves during meditation, they can control conscious thinking. But 95% of thinking is springing up from the subconscious when they are busy, distracted, tired, or running on autopilot. Only 5% of the time are they fully aware and consciously thinking unless they are skilled in mindfulness and practice meditation.[2] So it appears that for every one step forward, nineteen steps are taken backwards. One of the best pediatric neurosurgeons in the world grew up disadvantaged in a New York brownstone being cared for by a hardworking, often absent, single mom. She kept telling him, when his subconscious mind's programs were being written, that he could be anything he wanted to be. So instead of negative programming, all he had was positive programming in his subconscious.

So how can people rerecord their subconscious programming if it's hardwired and not logical or subjective to reason? Arguing with the unthinking subconscious or hating the parents or people who helped create bad programming only strengthens the negative memory tracks. Since people can only think consciously about the problem 5% of the time, they often see the problem crop back up throughout the day from their subconscious mind. Healing the brain from early childhood or even adult-onset trauma can take years of work before real improvement takes hold in the brain. So finding the source of the problem and the right treatment method is crucial. In his book *Savor*, Thich Nhat Hanh often refers to these repeating thought patterns as mental formations or knots. He says, "If we allow knots to form and then let them grow strong, they will eventually overwhelm us, and it will be very difficult to untie them."[3] And yet, despite the difficulty, it's possible to improve, relearn, and control the brain so that a person doesn't fall into the entrapments of negative circular self-talk and subconscious self-sabotage. There are actually many ways to arrive at the same result. Some methods reach back into the depths of human history and are rooted in religious or philosophical beliefs and practices. And recently, modern medicine and psychology are homing in on what specifically works in various forms of psychotherapy to help people overcome trauma and become whole again. What's interesting to see, and this has been further proven with modern studies, is that ancient, religious, spiritual, and philosophical methods have links to modern therapies in terms of their effectiveness.

A modern psychological approach called attachment theory empha- sizes childhood relationships as a precursor to adult mental predisposi- tions. Attachment theory suggests that ". . . the repeated interactions with deficient early attachment figures can become neurally encoded and then subconsciously activated later in life, especially in stressful and intimate situations. That's how your childhood attachment patterns can solidify into a corrosive part of your personality, distorting how you see and experience the world, and how you interact with other people."[4] Children with traumatic childhood experiences suffer incredibly their whole lives and often need a lot of support from their communities and therapists in order to heal. However, people with less traumatic experi- ences can still suffer and need support while untying the knots that keep them from living a freer and more fulfilling life. It must be said also, traumatic experiences in adulthood also create mental formations that can take months or years to unravel.

You might wonder why it takes so long to heal the brain. If someone is aware there is a problem, and unfortunately many are unaware that they have a problem, why can't they just fix it and get over it? In the book *Attached*, Dr. Amir Levine writes, "Among the factors that were found to increase a child's chance of being secure were an easy tem- perament (which makes it easier for parents to be responsive), positive maternal conditions—marital satisfaction, low stress and depression, and social support—and fewer hours with a nonparental caretaker....To complicate matters further, an idea that has been gaining scientific momentum in recent years is that we are genetically predisposed toward a certain attachment style."[5] He later writes that adult relationships can have such an impact as to alter a person's attachment style which can have drastic effects on the way a person views and interacts with the world.[6]

So why is a person's style of attachment so important for their mental health? Considering that most mental health issues hinge upon being of sound mind enough to be able to navigate society and relationships with relative proficiency and ease, secure attachment, or feelings of security and belonging, are crucial. According to the theory, there are four main attachment styles. The first being a secure form of attachment. This is the ideal. A person with this style navigates relationships and the world with a generally healthy and reasonably trusting outlook. A setback isn't the end of the world, just another problem to be solved or left behind. The next style is an anxious form of attachment. This person will cling to others in an unhealthy way constantly seeking reassurance that everything is going to be ok. They tend to overact to setbacks and can self-sabotage the minute their security feels threatened. The opposite of that is the avoidant attachment style. This person has trouble committing to others and relies unhealthily on going it solo rather than integrating with partners or even society. These people will feel most secure relying on themselves, however, tend to fall apart when a real crisis strikes. And the last style is a combination of alternating anxious and avoidant. Often these people have severe trauma and have learned to survive by using whichever style seems best to navigate a situation.[7]

People with certain attachment styles are prone to developing or are dealing with ongoing mental formations that clearly affect their adult relationships and mental health. While most people would probably prefer to have that secure base to work from, it doesn't consign a person to a lifetime of misery to have a less secure outlook. There are ways to deal with those insecurities and negative mental formations so that they become manageable. It's even possible to learn how to change your brain to become more secure. Amir says, "... change can happen in both directions—secure people can become less secure and people who were originally insecure can become increasingly secure. If you are insecure, this piece of information is vital and could be your ticket to happiness in relationships. If you are secure, you should be aware of this finding because you have a lot to lose by becoming less secure."[8] It would take either a large and traumatic event or ongoing chronically traumatic events to disturb a person's secure base. However, a person seeking to become secure, or whole and balanced, would need to put some work, time, and effort into learning a new way of thinking and living.

Finding a good therapist to help discover pathways for healing is a great option for self-discovery and finding emotional stability. At times and with certain extreme mental illnesses, drug therapy will be the best option. However, drug dependence and the side effects of taking them may not be the best long-term solution. Seeking professional help is the best choice when mental health issues are leading to suicidal thoughts, self-harm, or intent to harm others. And yet, there are still ways for most people to improve and take control of their lives on a day-to-day basis. Finding your mental health flow state will help you take charge of health and wellness in all areas of your life. So finding the roots of the problem, educating yourself about how to nurture and heal it, and finding daily practices to maintain a healthier lifestyle and outlook is the approach you'll find here.

Understanding that it's common for certain emotional predispositions and traumatic events to lead people into spiraling mental vortexes is a crucial first step to healing. Embracing that you are not alone in this helps grow that sense of connection and security. The next step is becoming aware of the dangerous thought patterns so that they can be handled accordingly. In his book *Peace is Every Step*, the Vietnamese Buddhist monk Thich Nhat Hanh says that,

There are many kinds of seeds in us, both good and bad. Some were planted during our lifetime, and some were transmitted by our parents, our ancestors, and our society. In a tiny grain of corn, there is the knowledge, transmitted by previous generations, of how to sprout and how to make leaves, flowers, and ears of corn. Our body and our mind also have knowledge that has been transmitted by previous generations. Our ancestors and our parents have given us seeds of joy, peace, and happiness, as well as seeds of sorrow, anger, and so on.[9]

He likens the subconscious mind to being much like a bed of soil in which seeds have been planted. These seeds can be watered by having or not having mental awareness, by social or peer groups, or the types of media content people expose themselves to.

If negative emotional seeds are watered, they grow into the conscious mind where they become mental formations or vine-like knots that entrap and distract people from being calm, secure, and happy. In his book *Savor*, Hanh writes, "Because it is easier to avoid suffering in the short term, we have defense mechanisms that push our psychological pains, sorrows, and internal conflicts into our subconscious mind and bury them there. But occasionally they emerge and surface in our thoughts, speech, and actions, reflecting symptoms of physical and psychological disturbance."[10] So this seed that started as an emotion, a predisposition, or a catastrophic event, can grow into the conscious mind, but then become even larger and more entrenched in the mind if it's suppressed or reinforced with more negative emotion.[11] This entangled and knotted mind becomes a problem that needs addressed. Otherwise, you are stuck, just a few emotional clicks away, from falling back into the loop that paralyzes and distracts you from expressing and living fully.

The physical habits that form out of these psychological knots can be very damaging for health. Some people will turn to addictions, whether it be drugs, food, or binge-watching shows, in order to calm anxieties within. Hanh says, "Our parents and our society heavily influence how we think, feel, and behave. Our habit energies result from the way we have learned to respond to sensory perceptions. These habit energies leave indelible imprints in our mind, and they form internal knots that reside deep in our consciousness. These knots are the blocks of sadness and pain that are tied up deeply in our consciousness."[12] So in theory, if you can address the root of the problem, untying and uncluttering the mind, you can unlock the potential to clean up your life as well. This will have ripple effects on your personal relationships, family, and communities. In Western culture, people think of the mind, body, and spirit as being separate entities and that people are all distinctly carving their way out of the genius of their own individualism. However, cultures with roots that still run back centuries tend to acknowledge the interconnectedness of all things. When the feedback loops of mind, body, and spirit are not harmonious, people usually end up hurting others in the process through their own imbalance. And then it becomes the next person's responsibility to manage the mental formation that might result.

Becoming aware of mental formations allows people to become mindful of them. Mindfulness is a concept often referred to in meditation practices. Sometimes it's confused with a complete passiveness or a detached and empty way of thinking. However, it is quite engaged. Hanh writes,

> When we speak of "mindfulness," we must specify: Mindfulness of what? Mindfulness of breathing? Mindfulness of walking? Mindfulness of anger? You have to be mindful of something. If that something is not there, there is no mindfulness possible. So when we speak of observing the mind in the mind, we are speaking of the subject of cognition, the subject of our mental formations, the subject of mindfulness, of hate, of love, or of jealousy. And with every subject

there must be an object. To love means to love what? To love whom? To hate means to hate what? To hate whom? These are what is meant by the objects of the mind.[13]

Do you see how the knot begins to unravel? With each questioning and observation of the working mind, another loop is loosened. When you work your way from awareness into mindfulness, you are unlocking the power of observation to increase your control of the mind and your actions. The observer doesn't have to react to the ruminations of a runaway mind. An observer doesn't have to follow a nearly reflexive and unaware response that wreaks havoc on inner and outer peace. By observing what triggers you into a negative feedback loop and why it is so effective in dominating your mind, you can slowly, over time, start forming new habits that elicit healthier responses.

How you go about achieving that matters. As mentioned earlier, for severe problems, seeking professional help and sometimes using pharmaceuticals in addition to psychotherapy might be necessary. Anytime safety is on the line, seek professional help as soon as possible. If you or a loved one is in an abusive relationship, being severely harassed at work or online, feels threatened in any way, or has suicidal tendencies, simply meditating using the techniques described here isn't enough. In those situations, the subconscious mind will be telling these people that something is terribly wrong even if they don't want to admit it. They may end up blaming themselves entirely, which will lead to self-harm or accepting the unacceptable. While mindfulness practice could help them come to these realizations and the realization that they need to flee for safety, it may not work in time before something truly horrible happens. In these instances, getting professional help from law enforcement, lawyers, therapists, and safety shelters should be the first steps anyone takes aside from leaning on family and friends for social support.

Along with day-to-day maintenance and those hoping to improve their mental health for the sake of themselves and their loved ones, there are interesting themes that run across various methods and treatments. Only just recently have therapists and doctors come to realize why therapy is so effective. In fact, that was the focus of a recent study with the aim of finding out why different types of therapeutic approaches and methods had essentially the same success rate. What they came to realize was that it wasn't necessarily the method so much as the relationship between the therapist and patient that determined the success of the treatment.[14] Successful therapists established a secure emotional connection with their patients that laid the groundwork for healing. In her article "How You Attach to People May Explain a Lot About Your Inner Life," Elitsa Dermendzhiyska writes, "... the good therapist becomes a temporary attachment figure, assuming the functions of a nurturing mother, repairing lost trust, restoring security, and instilling two of the key skills engendered by a normal childhood: the regulation of emotions and a healthy intimacy."[15] So a good therapist is either rewriting or reconnecting those damaged or undeveloped mental pathways that are essential for mental and emotional stability. The connection with the mother or secure parental figure gives the patient a safe moment to begin the path toward balance. The early attachment with a caretaker helps an infant understand what is going on inside their head so they aren't frightened or confused by it. Dermendzhiyska writes, "The sensitive mother picks up on the infant's mental and emotional state and mirrors it; the child learns to recognize his internal experience as 'sadness' or 'anxiety' or 'joy.' Previously chaotic sensations now become coherent and integrated into the infant's sense of who he is, allowing emotions to be processed, predicted and appropriately navigated."[16] This is where security is established. The child realizes that his or her emotions and thoughts are not something to be feared or ashamed of and they now can observe their caregiver's methods for controlling themselves.

Dermendzhiyska utilizes a particular therapist/patient connection for her article. In this case, the patient Cora is suicidal and prone to self-harm. She was horribly abused by her mother and her mother's friends in her youth and most therapists were afraid to treat her because she would only accept therapy if they allowed her to continue the self-harm. When she was finally paired with the right therapist, he was able to connect with her in such a way so that she could heal and repair those broken bonds. "Cora's therapist...helped her to assimilate her most painful feelings. . . . Like a good mother, he predigested Cora's distress by making sense of it and, by giving it a meaning and explanation, he transformed it into something that could be accepted and endured. Eventually, the co-regulation of emotions between mother and infant, or therapist and client, paves the way to self-mastery and self-regulation."[17] Cora would share her grievances and fears with her therapist, and then he would mirror or absorb what she was sharing reflecting it back to her. This gave her another perspective on how to process what was still traumatizing her. As Dermendzhiyska writes, "This pattern of empathizing, then reframing and de-shaming looks uncannily like the mirroring-and-soothing exchanges between mother and infant in the first years of life. . . . After a while, clients internalize the warmth and understanding of their therapist, turning it into an internal resource to draw on for strength and support. A new, compassionate voice flickers into life, silencing that of the inner critic—itself an echo of insensitive earlier attachment figures."[18] In this way, people learn how to control their minds. In some cases, short-term or even long-term pharmaceutical use might be appropriate for treating mental health. However, it creates dependency even if the drugs aren't prone to creating addictions. The reason being that the patient never learns how to fix mental problems on their own. And it's becoming increasingly clear that the best way to learn how to do that is within a secure and trusting environment.

So therapy gives people the opportunity to repair the security issues that are a result of early neglect, abandonment, abuse, and adulthood traumatic experiences. However, it's not the only path to maintaining and re-establishing mental health and balance. For some, finding and maintaining that feeling of security and inner peace can come from a weekly or habitual religious practice where the attachment figure is a higher power. Indeed, many people have overcome addictions, childhood trauma, and adult mental health issues by finding or leaning on their religion. A belief in God gives people an ear that is always listening, a judge who will forgive, a father who will embrace and support them through their darkest trials. Religious people and communities can strengthen and support each other, giving that sense of security that humans so desperately need for peace. This is something fundamental to human nature as it has been a way humans have been coping with their existence from the dawn of their intellectual history. Various religious texts show this comforting support. I will offer some text from my own Christian religion, and also texts from other Christian religions for reference here. But the wide expanse and varying beliefs of many other religions throughout the globe are just as valid an option for those on a personal journey of self-discovery and improvement. If your personal religious faith is not represented here, feel free to fill in the blanks with your own beliefs and consult your religious texts to support your need to find inner peace.

In Christianity, there are many references to becoming like a child again so that God can help a person become whole and well. The ideal is to ". . . becometh as a child, submissive, meek, humble, patient, full of love, willing to submit to all things which the Lord seeth fit to inflict upon him, even as a child doth submit to his father."[19] Becoming as a child once again refers to that early mental state of downloading or recording. This scriptural passage refers to this change of programming as being "born again" or developing a "new heart." The child-like state mentioned in the scriptures is a prerequisite. "Jesus answered and said unto him, Verily, verily, I say unto thee, Except a man be born again, he cannot see the kingdom of God."[20] And also, "Being born again, not of corruptible seed, but of incorruptible, by the word of God, which liveth and abideth forever."[21] In the Bible, Peter mentioned "being born again . . . by the word of God." Reading the Bible in a humble, prayerful, child-like state can reprogram the subconscious mind. Returning to this child-like state and accepting the teaching that the religious texts or sermons that priests are imparting is not unlike reworking the attachment wiring in the brain during therapy sessions. This trust that through God you have the ability to heal and connect, to become secure, is the basis through which the healing power of religion works. The security comes from your own faith and opening to a higher power. It allows trust and healing back into parts of the mind that were previously disconnected by fear and pain.

One of the biggest changes I ever saw in a man came from this intense reading of the scriptures. I spent a number of hours with him and his wife teaching them about Christ. The man was so humble and child-like. He even gave up a four-pack-a-day cigarette habit because I asked him to do it for the Lord and for his sick children. He told me the secret of his spiritual power. He had been in jail for eight long years. Instead of watching a lot of television, he decided to read the Bible. He read it for hours every day for eight years. He knew the Bible in ways many of us will never know it. It became his whole life, and he became its teachings. Truly he was born again with a new heart by that experience.

The Bible completely transformed this man's life because he allowed the healing power of faith and a higher power into his life. He was able to relearn a stable foundation of security through a form of attachment to the father figure of Christ. This method was absolutely successful for him. For others who prefer to not follow a specific religion and perhaps don't have access to a good therapist, there are other ways to rerecord unhealthy internal dialogue. One of the great gifts a number of Buddhist leaders have offered the world are philosophical teachings that don't require following of the religion in order to benefit from them. They saw healthy, secure, and peaceful humans as a benefit to humanity and the world. The Dalai Lama was forced from his homeland in Tibet and as a cultural orphan used his personal tragedy to share his teachings with the world. Another Buddhist monk Thich Nhat Hanh personally saw and experienced the devastation of his homeland in Vietnam during the Vietnam War and made it a life-long pursuit to share messages of peace and authored many books on how to attain it. These books were purposefully translated into English, and he has worked tirelessly his whole life collaborating with people of similar vision, such as Martin Luther King, in order to help the world heal and overcome divisions.

The Buddhist teachings they impart don't require a faith in Buddhism or a particular religion in order to be beneficial. Their philosophies are rooted in practices dating back centuries on how to control and calm the mind. In terms of attachment theory, they are essentially helping people become secure in themselves by recognizing and observing the workings of the mind. The practice of maintaining mindfulness and spending time in mediation are employed to achieve this. In *Peace is Every Step*, Hanh writes,

> Consciousness exists on two levels: as seeds and as manifestations of these seeds. Suppose we have a seed of anger in us. When conditions are favorable, that seed may manifest as a zone of energy called anger. It is burning, and it makes us suffer a lot. It is very difficult for us to be joyful at the moment the seed of anger manifests. . . . That is why we have to be careful in selecting the kind of life we lead and the emotions we express. When I smile, the seeds of smiling and joy have come up. As long as they manifest, new seeds of smiling and joy are planted. But if I don't practice smiling for a number of years, that seed will weaken, and I may not be able to smile anymore.[22]

By observing the mind with no judgement but with compassion and a desire for understanding, you are, in a sense, becoming the attachment figure.

You reframe your own suffering, you quiet your anxious and shallow breathing enough to calm yourself, you de-shame yourself with your own self-love. In *Savor* Hanh writes, "But when we are able to maintain and increase the energy of mindfulness, we can overcome our aversion to our painful emotions. We continue to nourish mindfulness through conscious breathing and try to acknowledge our internal knots and conflicts as they emerge. We learn to receive them with the love and tenderness of a mother embracing her baby."[23] So here we find this connecting theme between various methods. Reworking the mind to find peace is about finding security again. This enables mental strength and resilience in the face of adversity. He goes on to say,

> By just observing and acknowledging our feelings and our thoughts without judgment, blame, or criticism, we have embarked on the path of emancipation from our suffering. If there is pain, sorrow, or anger, we simply acknowledge that we feel the pain, the sorrow, and the anger. When we acknowledge these feelings with mindfulness, we do not let the feelings of pain, sorrow, or anger take us over and lead us astray. Instead we try to calm them down with tenderness. Practicing like this will cause our knots to loosen up, and repeated practice will eventually help us understand their roots by identifying the sources of nutriments that have brought them into being. With this insight and understanding, we can stop the suffering at its roots.[24]

At the core of practicing flow nutrition and accessing flow states to improve life, the main aim is to always find the roots of the problem in order to find sustained and more lasting forms of health. Practicing mindfulness is not mastered overnight. It's a skill that is improved quite explicitly by accessing and maintaining a flow state. Meditating on the mind, meditating on breathing, and meditating in motion are all a part of this process. By slowing down and meditating with a breathing practice, people learn to quiet the mind and calm the heart. By meditating on the inner workings of the mind for deeper understanding and clarity, people learn to control the mind. By meditating while moving, walking, and interacting mindfully, a person learns to control their mind and breath and thereby control their actions as actions are a manifestation of the two.

Meditation can be described as an act of observation and integration. Many people will start with a completely motionless body. Some prefer to lie completely still on the floor or yoga mat while relaxing all parts of the body before finally emptying the mind and letting it float free. Sometimes soothing sounds, smells, and lighting can assist this relaxation. Some people prefer a slightly more engaged form of meditation that is performed cross-legged or kneeling. In both cases, the body is quieted so the focus can rest on breathing. Hahn offers mindful breathing practices and mantras in his many books. The mantras are often a mental chant that describes the physical aspect of breathing in and out while you're doing it. If you prefer a religious prayer or chant in place of a Buddhist mantra, repeating a single word or simple prayer can be just as effective while still adhering to your personal religious views.[25] This gives the mind something to focus on if it is running away with too many distractions. Reading more or finding a meditation guide can help fine-tune and develop these techniques. And then, ultimately, meditation moves into a flow state where you can be simultaneously mindful, meditating or observing, and interacting or moving at the same time. This would represent a flow-state mastery of manifesting internal and external security, calmness, and peace: a true presence.

So whatever your goals in life, mastery of the mind is the foundational core of the process. Finding security in relationships with others and yourself will help you get the things you most want out of life. When you find yourself in shaky mental ground seeking help through therapy, religion, or mindful practices can help you stabilize. Finding communities, friends, or family members that support this type of wellbeing will only help you move with greater ease along your path to healing.

34

Happiness Flow

The old Louisville General Hospital where I began my internal medicine rotation was formerly the Tuberculosis Sanitarium for Kentucky. The ceilings were twenty feet high and there were large windows to let in the fresh air. It was built in the early 1900s when there was no cure for tuberculosis. People would remain quarantined there for the rest of their lives. The patients of the sanitarium inevitably divided into two camps. One camp would believe and continuously talk about getting better and the other camp would fearfully believe and talk about dying. These beliefs became self-fulfilling prophecies. The people in the sanitarium would literally live or die based upon which group they associated themselves with and what they believed. Recent research shows how this happens on a molecular level.

Bruce Lipton, a pioneer in cloning and stem cells, did research establishing that what people think and believe changes their gene expression and their whole body.[1] You truly are what you believe. The previous outdated science was based on the assumption that people are prisoners of their genetic fate. However, the environment, the food people eat, and their thinking and feeling can regularly alter the way their genes are expressed for good or bad. So is the power to change your life in unbelievable ways just one belief or a few positive thoughts away? In *Anatomy of an Illness*, Norman Cousins talked about how he cured himself of a fatal and incurable illness in one month with *Laugh In* tapes and no medicine whatsoever.[2] Positive moods and thoughts really can change the entire way the body operates, and it can also reverse illnesses.

You are not simply born with defective genes that forever trap you into a state of being, feeling, and thinking. Everyone has an inborn set of genes and some of them are inherently defective. How those genes are expressed is actually much more fluid. Your beliefs can work around the defects and produce a perfect protein and functional system. There is a lot of redundancy in the body so that it can handle serious failures and still do well. The space shuttle had redundancy many times over. There were five identical guidance computers that compared results for each calculation. If one of the computers had a glitch, the other computers would shut it down. The same thing is going on inside the body. When a defective gene is read and an incorrect protein is in the process of being crudely made, epigenetic modifier systems swing into action and remove or replace the defective gene sequence product. This modifier system is under the control of your beliefs and thoughts.

One of the most important beliefs to maintain for maximum health is gratitude. A life full of gratitude and thanksgiving leads to more positive thoughts and feelings than any other perspective. This in turn alters our genetic expression by overcoming defective genes, resulting in improved physical and mental wellbeing. A newer field in psychology is called Positive Psychology. It's based in research on what really works to make people happy. Thousands of research studies have been done. The field is exploding with newfound wisdom that turns out to be scientific proof of ancient wisdom. So from the top down in psychology research and from the bottom up in genetic research on epigenetics, everything points to our thinking as the ultimate control of our mental *and* physical health.

One of the leading proponents of Positive Psychology is Joel Wade. In his book *Mastering Happiness*, Wade says,

> gratitude is also one of the crucial ingredients to a happy life. Why? We have three temporal perspectives

to our life: the past, the present, and the future. Gratitude is the embodiment of feeling good about your past. When you look back, if you look only at what you regret, at what you feel bad about, at your anger and hurt, and at those who have hurt you, you are bringing those feelings and experiences into the present. So, not only did you get to feel bad about them back then, you get the added bonus of feeling bad about them now. One could also anticipate that, without a shift of focus, you may look forward to enjoying these rotten feelings and experiences well into your future. On the other hand, when you focus on gratitude, you get to search for the good in your past. When you do this, you can bring those feelings and experiences into the present, and can enjoy extending these blessings into the future as well. It's your choice.[3]

In the end, we are masters of our destiny as anyone who has overcome a disability, cancer, major illness, or disfiguring accident can tell us. Research shows that those who live with cancer far longer than expected will often have a strong desire to live long enough to witness the birth of a grandchild, a marriage, or a reunion.

Martin Seligman, the previous head of the American Psychological Association and the founder of the Positive Psychology movement, recently published a study which showed that people who wrote letters of gratitude to others and wrote down three good things that happened every day for a week in a gratitude journal were substantially better at reversing depressive symptoms than those who performed placebo exercises in the randomized groups.[4]

These experiments were short term one-week interventions with six months of monthly follow-up testing to see the long-term consequences of gratitude exercises. If such a short-term intervention can produce dramatic reversals of depression compared to the placebo, you can only wonder what a daily gratitude journal would do for someone who was prone to depression and also had the physical illnesses associated with depression such as stomach disorders, sleeplessness, weight gain or loss, fatigue, allergies, and sinus disorders.

Gratitude practices help change a person's perspective on their life allowing for more abundance of positive thinking and its pursuant benefits. Sometimes life can become so oppressively burdensome, or the body becomes hormonally or chemically unbalanced to such a degree that other intervention is needed. If you want to attempt the more natural route, there are ways to achieve natural highs without using pills or drugs. For instance, sunlight on the skin causes endorphin release. Endorphins are natural narcotics which are produced in the brain and nerves and are used for the natural pain suppression and control of many aches and mood swings.

Vitamin D made in the skin by the action of sunlight also acts as an antidepressant. During the winter, many people from my hometown in Nebraska flee the dreary, cold, and colorless winter days by snow birding in Arizona. They come back happy and ready for a great Nebraskan summer. One patient of mine was irritable for several years until he realized that he was no longer going south for the winter golf trip he had long enjoyed. When he returned to the practice, his wintertime blues disappeared with just one week in the sun. He also did not get sick in the spring like he had been for several years.

Sleep is another way of combating the blues. Eight hours of quality sleep helps replace used up endorphins with a fresh batch. Endorphins are made when we sleep. When people get little or poor-quality sleep, too much stress, and not enough relaxation, their bodies do not make endorphins. So they are more moody, irritable, and stressed. Then they get even less sleep. To prevent this debilitating cycle, they could replace melatonin and take GABA (valerian root) to help restore healthy sleep patterns and endorphins.

As people get older, their serotonin levels decline naturally. Because of this, they become chronically depressed and grouchy old men and women. Replacing it and making their brains work well again can be a simple matter of taking St. John's Wort and 5HTP (5-hydroxytryptophan). They get their emotional pep back and can enjoy life instead of being chronically depressed.

When hormones decline with age, people end up generally feeling tired and depressed. Each hormone that declines naturally can cause an unnatural feeling to come and stay like an unwelcome guest who never leaves. Replacing each hormone that is low, according to lab tests, with the appropriate measurable dose of bioidentical hormones restores the good feelings lost with age. Finding an anti-aging functional medicine specialist or endocrinologist doctor to help with this is the best way to go. They can administer the proper tests to find exactly which hormones are low and then treat those deficiencies with the right doses. It helps to talk to your doctor about a desire to use naturally sourced hormonal therapies. They can make a world of difference in avoiding harmful side effects.

When people eat too much meat and grains while not eating enough vegetables and water, they become more acidic inside. Drinking more water, half of your body weight in ounces of water daily, helps alkalinize the blood. Eating lots of vegetables, half of total food consumption volume daily, does the same. What is lesser known is that walking barefoot on the grass can ground all the circuits in every cell and neutralize acid. Acid is basically an excess of protons and too few electrons. The grass and dirt are loaded with negative ions that can flow up through the body neutralizing the excess acid. People can feel young again after a short barefoot walk in the park.

There are many ways to experience joy again, but one of the most important of all is to forget yourself in the pursuit of working for and serving others in order to increase their happiness. Being a peacemaker while also being kind and grateful creates everlasting benefit. In the end, you'll not only feel the happiness of those you have served, but you'll also have forgotten those old negative feelings that swirled around the sinkhole of self-pity. It will give you something to write about in your gratitude journal while soaking in the sun's rays and letting the grass crinkle between your barefoot toes.

35

The Placebo Effect

How to Make Your Medical Treatment Work for You

I set out to make this book accessible to people of various beliefs and backgrounds. The hope was to encourage preventive health in all communities. I want to share with you a personal story of my faith and how I've seen it manifested in various forms of healing. I hope it has an inspirational rather than polarizing effect. In 1970, I traveled to Spain to act as a missionary for the Church of Jesus Christ of Latter Day Saints. It was during this time that I became a true believer in the healing power of faith. One of the elderly women who had recently joined our church in Barcelona went totally blind. She lived by herself, had diabetes, and had been totally blind in one eye for some time, presumably from diabetic retinopathy. Now, she had just lost eyesight in her only good eye. She asked us to give her a priesthood blessing to restore her eyesight. I was only twenty years old at the time and had never seen a healing miracle. We told her we would give her a blessing after we had fasted without food and water for twenty-four hours. The next day we visited her apartment. I rested my hands on the top of her head and gave her a priesthood blessing. I was inspired to say that her eyesight would be restored and that she would see again. We left and went back to our missionary work. That night, we prayed fervently for a miracle because one had been promised. She had a lot of faith, perhaps more than we did. The next day we went by her apartment. She was seeing again and was crying she was so happy. I could think of no rational explanation then for the miracle. When I left Spain a year later, she was still seeing well.

Some authors have equated the placebo effect to faith. This is the patient's belief that the medicine will work and their trust in the doctor who gave it to them. Most drugs are slightly better than placebo at treating a given condition. They are not wildly better than placebo as most assume. For instance, aspirin is supposed to thin the blood so people suffer fewer heart attacks. Does it prevent heart attacks in every-one who takes it? No, it does not. It is only slightly better than the placebo at doing so.[1] Most drugs are not designed to cure anything. They are designed to be slightly better than the placebo effect so that they will pass the requirements of the FDA. Then, they are marketed by pharmaceutical companies making them billions every year. A cure would make chronic pill taking a thing of the past. The drug companies would go bankrupt. The economy would perish because a large portion of the Dow Jones Industrial Average is based on drug stocks. They have been the big performers for a hundred years.

Drugs only treat symptoms because we have a medical system that is built on symptom relief. Aspirin was the first modern drug to provide symptom relief. It started the chemical approach to symptom relief that is the basis of modern medicine. It was extracted from willow bark, an herb used by native cultures for pain relief. Put another way, placebos are nearly as good as the well designed and scientifically proven drugs that have real chemical effects that are measurable in our bodies. Place-bos have been shown to cause these same measurable chemical effects. What is going on here? Why does hocus pocus have nearly as much power as real science? It costs millions of dollars to perform studies that prove a drug is slightly better than placebo.

Drug companies are researching how to minimize the strength of the placebo effect in the placebo group and maximize it in the active drug group. One trick is to do a placebo washout. Everyone in both randomized groups is given a placebo before the study starts. Those who respond well to placebos are told to leave and not participate in the study.[2] This enhances seeing a difference between the active drug group and the placebo group. Nearly all the psychotropic drugs are studied this way. However, a lot of scientists feel this is not a valid scientific method because the paradigm is so far removed from the average patient who will eventually take the drug. Even with these unscientific tricks to prejudice the results of studies in favor of drugs, a recent meta-analysis of all published SSRI (selective serotonin reuptake inhibitor) studies and unpublished studies showed the whole class of drugs to only be slightly more effective than placebo.[3]

A lot of research has been done on how to enhance the placebo effect in order to see that if by enhancing it, the effect of the drug can be enhanced. It turns out that most drugs that are only slightly better than placebos work not by scientific chemical reactions in our bodies but by the actual placebo effect itself. People believe in the drug and trust the doctor who prescribed it. This faith is what causes the chemical to have the symptom relief. This effect is enhanced if the actual drug has side effects that are noticeable like dry mouth, dizziness, and sleepiness. When people in studies feel the side effects, they believe that they are getting the actual drug. This belief, or placebo effect, causes them to report fewer of the primary symptoms being studied.[4] Doctors supposedly blind to who is on the active drug also notice these side effects and the study is no longer double blinded, but unblinded. Both the doctor and the patient know they are on the active drug. Doctors then unwittingly add their prejudiced comments to the follow up visits and enhance the faith of the patient because both the doctor and the patient have been taught to believe that only the active drug can cure someone. There is only one way to avoid this prejudice and unblinding of the trial. Doctors can use placebos that have the same side effects as the active drug. But then, the cures in the placebo group might be related to some pharmacological action of the placebo. But this advanced study design is rarely used. It would make the drug seem less effective compared to placebo. When people feel a placebo that has side effects, they believe they are taking the active drug and report more improvement than when taking empty placebos.

In the end, we see faith and belief are driving nearly all the improvement in both the placebo group and active drug group. There is another reason for active drugs working by placebo effect rather than pharmacological effect. Certain drugs only trigger pharmacological effect at certain doses. Yet many patients that are prescribed the drug in regular clinical practice are receiving much less than this activating level of the drug in order to avoid the side effects. If they are receiving less than the pharmacologically active dose, then their improvement must come from their belief that the drug will make them better. This means that the placebo effect is making them better on the under-dosed but real drug.

Placebo effects can even be seen even in sham surgery. Sham surgery is where superficial cuts are made but no surgery is done in the placebo group. Arthroscopic knee surgery and vertebroplasty injection back surgery have been studied with sham surgery being the placebo. The results show that the sham placebo surgery is just as effective in relieving the back or knee pain as the real surgery.[5]

If we are down to faith being an important part of the healing of patients, how do we account for it scientifically? The answer lies in quantum physics, the most proven and successful scientific theory of all time. It has never been proven false. Basically, quantum physics experiments show that the scientist's expectation of how an experiment will turn out alters the outcome of the experiment. This has been verified thousands of times in hundreds of studies. This sounds similar to the placebo effect. Our expectation of how the placebo will help us determines our improvement. Only in humans the result is altered approximately 30% of the time whereas with electrons and photons it is 100% of the time.[6] As Bruce H. Lipton says in his book *Biology of Belief*, "The Universe is one indivisible, dynamic whole in which energy and matter are so deeply entangled it is impossible to consider them as independent elements." So if we are so "deeply entangled," the Western attitude of rugged individualism becomes a mental knot in need of untying.

And then again, interconnected consciousness or flow between conscious entities implies that we are dependent, not only on our environment and genetics, but also dependent upon ourselves and our social groups for our own wellbeing. Lipton goes on to say, "Biological behavior can be controlled by invisible forces, including thought, as well as it can be controlled by physical molecules like penicillin, a fact that provides the scientific underpinning for pharmaceutical-free energy medicine." So how powerful is the placebo effect, personal faith, or positive social group faith and reinforcement in the healing process? Can it restore eyesight, heal a fracture faster, or get rid of metastatic cancer? Numerous studies show that it can.[7] So does this account for faith-based miracles? Are our bodies designed to respond miraculously to faith, prayer, and intention like some quantum physics experiment? Modern medical science influenced by powerful drug companies says no. To them, we are just pulleys, hinges, springs, pumps, chemical reactions, electrical circuits, computers, and sensory devices driven by genetic determination to think and feel and act a certain way.

This scientific worldview is basic Newtonian physics invented by a man who was troubled that his elegant and powerful equations took God out of science. He spent the last half of his life doing religious studies out of this deep concern over the scientific revolution he started. Quantum physics, discovered almost three hundred years later, brings back the possibility of a higher power having effects on the body that defy the Newtonian mechanistic view of how the body should work. Lipton writes, "The science of epigenetics has also made it clear that there are two mechanisms by which organisms pass on hereditary information. Those two mechanisms provide a way for scientists to study both the contribution of nature (genes) and the contribution of nurture (epigenetic mechanisms) in human behavior. If you only focus on the blueprints, as scientists have been doing for decades, the influence of the environment is impossible to fathom.[8] So if our genes are the blueprints, who or what is the architect and who or what is the builder?

Ever since mathematics was invented, mathematicians have speculated on the religious implications of its theories. Pythagoras and other ancient Greek mathematicians showed with their math that there was order and beauty, not chaos, in the world created by the Greek gods. Scientists and philosophers after Newton showed that there was no need for a higher power or unifier to be the prime mover in the universe because Newton's laws and math explained how everything in the universe moved independently. But when quantum physics brought the possibility of interconnectedness back to the actual equations, most were hesitant to leave the rationalistic mechanical worldview built on Newton's laws behind.

Modern medicine has replaced a higher power as the source of miracles in the minds of many people in the world. Yet recent research into the placebo effect shows that it is the faith and belief of the patient in the doctors, medicine, or surgery that is the real power behind the medical miracle. This faith in God used to be the source of all miracles. Now medicine has become the new deity that we trust and have faith in.

When people have no faith in anything, the placebo effect does not work very well. It's not unusual for me to see patients on three or four antihypertensive drugs or four or five antidepressants and they are still hypertensive and depressed. Weight loss surgery only works in about 20% of the patients. The rest stay the same or gain the weight back. Subliminal tapes for weight loss have the same success rate. A recent book written by Dr. Allen C. Bowling illuminates his reasoning for finding safer multiple sclerosis treatments that rely more on complementary and alternative therapies. All the traditional multiple sclerosis therapies are very toxic. He says, "Much of medicine is now focused on the body alone, instead of on the body and the mind."[9] He described the inseparable link between the brain, nervous system, and immune system and how this directly plays into the placebo effect during the healing process. If these systems are so interconnected, how could one possibly doubt the effect of the mind and belief in the healing process?[10]

So if we are really being cured by belief in the toxic drugs, might we not try faith and non-toxic therapies as well? Many alternative medicine treatments have been considered to be not only unscientific but actually fraudulent. As we have seen above, a lot of the medical research done by drug companies is unscientific and less than honest if not fraudulent. Their most grievous deception is the hiding of studies that are negative where the placebo was better than the drug. Only recently have studies been registered at the outset to prevent this scientific deception and ensure publication of all studies, both unfavorable and favorable, on a drug seeking FDA approval.

So if the local chiropractor, acupuncturist, homeopathic doctor, naturopathic doctor, or Chinese herbalist offers a treatment that works in many patients, should we call them fraudulent? Or should we understand that nontoxic therapies that invoke the placebo effect may be equal and perhaps superior in the long run to the toxic medicines that also work by placebo effect? When we look back at the history of modern medicine over the last two hundred plus years, we've seen many scientifically based treatments advanced that are now considered primitive and archaic. In those times, there was a rational scientific basis for the treatments to relieve swelling and fever that actually worked in many patients and killed others. Will people, in some future time, look back at the rise of Big Pharma and think of it in the same way we do about eighteenth-century medical treatments? Certainly. We will move on to gene therapies, enhancement of metabolic processes, hormonal anti-aging therapies, and energy therapies. But in all this scientific progress, should we downplay the power of faith and the placebo effect?

In *Biology of Belief*, Lipton writes, ". . . I truly believe that only when Spirit and Science are reunited will we be afforded the means to create a better world."[11] In this book, I'm calling for a unification of the mind-body-spirit connection for preventive healing and nutritional health. I believe that by practicing flow nutrition, you prepare your body to be ready for health defense. If you practice balanced thinking and continuously grow the mind into new areas, you keep your mental whole-health connection sound. And if you practice spiritual openness working on faith in the interconnectedness of all beings, you unify all of your defenses against internal and external threats to your overall health. We've dabbled loosely in the concepts of physics and quantum physics in this chapter and will explore them further. It is my belief, and science backs me, that our realities are so fluid and ultimately pulled upon by so many unseen forces, that with our better understanding of them, we take fear and uncertainty out of the equation enough so that we can very naturally go with the flow.

36

Physics and Medicine Then and Now

Physics was my beginning and end. Watching Sputnik cross the dark sky of the 1950s launched me towards a physics major in college. During my studies, I learned that atoms were not hard marbles but vast empty shells of energy with a small-in-size but large-in-force repelling center. This had been discovered by Niels Bohr in the 1930s by shooting atoms at each other. Werner Heisenberg working in Bohr's laboratory in Copenhagen, Denmark provided the theoretical framework of the Copenhagen interpretation of quantum mechanics which is still the dominate theory of the atom today. It replaced the Newtonian theory of the atom which resembled something closer to a billiard ball. I was told in 1968 that if you crashed a car an infinite number of times into a brick wall, quantum physics predicted that one of those times it would go right through without damage and appear on the other side.

The principles of quantum physics and its boundless potential have historically fueled the efforts to prove Newton's outdated theories were correct. One such effort was an expensive and well publicized experiment called the Michelson-Morley experiment. The scientists hoped to prove that the speed of light would become faster or slower when light was projected along different tracks. This predicted result was based on calculations using Newtonian physics.[1] When the experiment failed to show a difference in speed, it not only embarrassed the two scientists and the people who sponsored the experiment, but it doomed Newtonian physics as the solution to the universe's problems forever.

Modern medicine is failing just as spectacularly because it is also based on Newtonian physics. It was not but a few years after the failed Michelson-Morley experiment that Einstein published his shocking alternative views on the nature of the universe. He has been proven to be largely correct. In fact, the GPS system would not work without Einstein's correction of the Newtonian laws of motion. Einstein, and Maxwell before him, introduced light and energy acting from a distance to affect the way particles moved. Newton had ignored this effect in his theories by simplifying the way particles moved. Modern medicine has ignored the effects of unseen energies and the influence of non-local action at a distance in our chemistries. Modern medicine has ignored completely any reference to the spirit, the alignment of frequencies, or how the maintenance of the soul has anything to do with health. In doing so, it has made the same glaring mistake Michelson and Morley did. Energy medicine, new age physics, and many disciplines in alternative medicine have now come together to bring frequency and spirit back into the successful treatment of chronic diseases. They have brought the newer math of Einsteinian relativity with its powerful equations into the analysis and treatment of diseases.

We are now going beyond Einstein in understanding the universe. There are more powers out there that we do not understand. In certain situations, Einstein's equations are not precise enough suggesting other laws we do not know and other non-local influences we can only dream of. We now know that 95% of the energy in the universe is invisible to us, but it has a real effect on the rotation of our galaxy and the growth and development of galaxies. So much is unknowable about the outside influences on closed systems such as our heliosphere and galaxy. How can we presume to believe that there are no outside influences working on our bodies and our health?

Unfortunately, the dogma of modern medicine is so thoroughly entrenched and institutionalized to protect the profiteering of the mega-rich that it seems unshakeable in the face of overwhelming evidence to the contrary. If the body is a machine, then all you need is a mechanic with the right set of expensive tools to go in and perform an expensive surgery that may or may not be necessary. This concept is so appropriately summarized by Richard Milton,

> Using the mechanistic, reductionist approach of Victorian science, biology has not so much explained life as explained it away. The body is a machine, a matter of chemistry and electricity. Thought is merely a by-product of the computerlike brain which pulls the body's levers. Evolution is no more than a marriage of chance and chemistry. There is no ghost in the machine: human is the machine.[2]

He called it the "Frankenstein approach" because it ignores the great advances in astronomy, physics, and mathematics of the twentieth century in order to create a monster devoid of consciousness. The Newtonian medical model that ignores the outside influence of interconnected consciousness has helped to keep in place the financial extortions of mega-corporations that make huge profits from deceptive patent drugs. Recent meta-analysis of unpublished studies involving whole classes of drugs show that these drugs are no more capable of fighting disease than the placebo.[3] The apparent success of the drugs in published trials was distorted by the absence of the negative trials in publication. Is this science or is it just corporate greed hiding the truth about failed drug trials so corporations can make billions before being discovered? In fact, we have the evidence clearly on display with the recent pharmaceutical snafu of the release of non-statin cholesterol lowering drugs that were touted be the next cure-all but failed miserably after a year of studies showed them to be essentially non-effective. The publication was delayed so the company could push the failed drug for a year without negative publicity and make billions from the misery of patients who only got side effects from the drug and no benefit whatsoever.[4] How could any corporation make money and keep a significant portion of Wall Street humming with success if a healthy percentage of patients could be cured by prayer, meditation, cheap herbs, relatively cheap spinal manipulation, massage, or acupuncture?

The science of herbalism, holistic medicine, and the new field of energy medicine which combines chiropractic, Chinese, and ayurvedic medicine into one, teaches that we are nothing but energy just like the Copenhagen quantum theory says. If we are nothing but energy then every drug, herb, vitamin, and body part that is sick is also nothing but energy. Certain energies are good for us at certain levels, and certain energies are bad for us. Drugs are chemicals with energies that largely disrupt the energy processes of our bodies. They block our own natural energies that are out of balance.

There are two systems of medicine that developed from this. The most widely used in the Western world, or about a third of the human population, is allopathic medicine. Dr. Samuel Hahnemann invented the term in order to distinguish his invention, homeopathy, from ordinary medical practice which he called, "Allopathy . . . . That system of medical practice which aims to combat disease by the use of remedies which produce effects different from those produced by the special disease treated."[5] But this concept of medicine has been around much longer. Hippocrates said something similar over 2000 years ago, "They would suppose that there is some principle harmful to man; heat or cold, wetness or dryness, and that the right way to bring about cures is to correct cold with warmth, or dryness with moisture and so on. . . . These are the causes of disease, and the remedy lies in the application of the opposite principle according to the hypothesis."[6] So modern medicine is all about blocking something whether it is serotonin degradation in the synaptic cleft between neurons, angiotensin converting enzyme in the kidneys, or calcium channel blockers.

However, in blocking something, innumerable side effects are created that often make the person sicker than they were. They can actually become sicker than the disease that doctors were trying to prevent. For example, one meta-analysis study on cholesterol lowering drugs to prevent sudden death from heart attack showed eighteen fewer sudden deaths in the treatment group among the 65,000 participants compared to placebo. However, in the treatment group, there were eighteen more deaths from suicide, thousands more with depression, fatigue, leg cramps, and other symptoms that were not as frequent in the control group.[7] So which is worse? To die suddenly or to get sick from the drug? This type of reasoning can be applied to any drug with side effects that are frequent and serious.

In energy medicine, the body is seen as a collection of energies that sustain healthy life. These energies can become blocked or out of balance and negative energies (dead food, chemical poisons, toxic metals, bad thoughts, and drugs) can creep in. Herbs, homeopathy, Eastern medicine, and other systems restore the flow of chi and thus the balance of energies and health. Sweat lodges, sauna therapy, and chelation therapy are also used to rid the body of negative energies or toxins.

Energy medicine is the health equivalent of quantum physics and there is a lot of good science performed all over the world to show how extraordinarily effective it is. Allopathic medicine is still stuck playing pool in the toxic tavern. Newtonian physics is the basis of modern Western Medicine: use this drug to bounce off that chemical in the body and alter the course of the chemical process like billiard shots. This simplistic approach to medicine is not only costly but does nothing to cure the many chronic diseases unique to our modern and toxic world.

In fact, the World Health Organization has recently said that Western Medicine was too resource hungry to be extended to the rest of the world and that many native therapies in use for thousands of years were effective like using Artemisia for malaria.[8] As a result of research and consultation with world health experts, it was proposed that the traditional herbal approach to health was not only sustainable, cheap, more effective, and easier to produce and use, but better for the environment.[9]

37

Quantum Consciousness

You are the world.

—KRISHNAMURTI

Do you ever feel like you're living in multiple worlds simultaneously? We live in a physical reality and feel pains, injuries, illnesses, and cancers acutely and chronically. We also live in an emotional world where we suffer many more mental and spiritual events. They could take the form of the loss of a loved one, a failure at school or work with its associated grief, verbal or physical attacks by deceptive people, poverty and racism, or fear of death caused by war and dangerous living conditions. Many people will turn to a belief in the metaphysical to help them navigate the emotional and spiritual hardships of life. Many religious traditions will say we coexist in a spiritual world largely unseen to our eyes.

And while the physical world appears to be solid and predictable and the spiritual or emotional world more abstract and ethereal, it can be difficult to fathom how the quantum world we live in seamlessly intermeshes the two. When we study quantum physics, we discover that particles are sometimes real in particle detectors and sometimes imaginary or timeless. We find that particles can exist in two different reality states simultaneously and can literally spin both up and down at the same time. Contemplating these normally undetectable realities is certainly mind boggling. To go further and claim we can think with a quantum or subatomic consciousness is hotly debated by scientists. Many in the scientific community want to reign in quantum physics and use it more as a math tool to perform functions such as calculating GPS syncing. They want to shut down exploration into the more complex implications of these shifting reality states.

Let's consider the physical world we live in and are made from. Is it simply physical and solid with objects we can see, feel, hear, smell, taste, and manipulate? According to quantum theory, which is now proven with nearly a hundred thousand never varying experiments, the short answer is no! We are made up of microscopic atoms that are filled with mostly empty space. But if we are made up of empty space, why do we feel so solid? According to the Pauli Exclusion Principle, no two electrons can share the same space but will resist being forced together. So if you push your fingertip into a desktop, the electrons in both would resist the merging of your finger into or through the desktop.

Electrons are not solid but are essentially little bundles of energy. Protons and neutrons appear to be solid when physicists fire quantum bullets at them and the bullets bounce back. But when hit with extremely energetic quantum bullets, these same protons and neutrons break apart into the subatomic particles called quarks which are massless and have only spin, momentum, and energy. In *The Cosmic Code: Quantum Physics as the Language of Nature*, Heinz Pagel writes, "The visible world is the invisible organization of energy."[1] The atom, with all its neutrons, protons, and electrons, is made up of mostly empty space. An atom is held together by multiple agents, one of which is the strong nuclear force acting through particles called gluons. The weak nuclear force is responsible for radioactive decay. This is when an element changes into another element, like uranium converting to lead, through the release of a radioactive particle.

We like to think the universe and world we live in is stable, that everything has been going on the same way since the Big Bang. But time is subjective and not very stable. During solar flares, the rate of radioactive decay speeds up tremendously making dating of earth rocks by radioactive decay meaningless. Same goes for carbon dating. The earth's rotation is speeding up as the earth's magnetic field is weakening. Some days are quite a bit shorter than last year's average. Atomic clocks are based on things that change such as the radioactive decay of cesium atoms. Taking one clock into orbit while its synced sister clock remains on earth causes a difference in the progression of time consistent with the theory of relativity. The smallest unit of time is called Planck time. We still don't know how time moves from one Planck moment to another. In large particle accelerators, the collider particles seem to move into the future and then come back into the present to interact with observable particles. Measurable length varies too. Length used to be determined by a metal bar in France, now it's determined by so many wavelengths. The earth's gravity can't be consistently measured, and it varies in different places across the planet. This makes a fixed measurement impossible to be determined accurately.

If we don't know what we are made from and how to measure it precisely, how can we say the world is physical and the brain a computer? In *Cosmos: A Co-Creator's Guide to the Whole-World*, Ervin Laszlo and Jude Currivan write, "We are beginning to see the entire universe as a holographically interlinked network of energy and information, organically whole and self-referential at all scales of its existence. We, and all things in the universe, are non-locally connected with each other and with all other things in ways that are unfettered by the hitherto known limitations of space and time."[2] We are existentially a large collection of vibrating energetic balls of pure energy in a ground state. Since we are energy beings, we are not just solid physical objects but more like a collection of quantum objects which are all subject to quantum laws.

Quantum laws are so strange they defy normal human logic and suggest other ways of healing. The premise of the Observer Effect is so bizarre that countless experiments have been done trying to prove it wrong. It takes subjective observation and experience to an entirely new level. This phenomenon proves that whatever a person observing expects to see or is looking for in a quantum experiment, whether they're expecting to see a particle spinning in an upward direction or a downward direction, for example, then that's what they'll see. Simply watching subatomic particles with expectation changes their behavior in experiments. Millions of runs of random number generators have proven this Observer Effect to occur on a macro level. These machines randomly generate lists of numbers in different order. People are told to imagine more zeros than ones in a given list, and a 2% difference occurs following their imaginings. In some of these tests, the tapes generated by machines without observers were stored in a vault. After a year had passed, the outside of the vault would be viewed by an observer who would imagine more zeros. The result, which is mind-bogglingly ridiculous, shows that the old tapes were changed by someone's intention that happened in the future, after the tapes had already been recorded. The experiment had to be repeated many times in many different countries in the world over time to prove it was a real effect.[3]

Another mysteriously intriguing quantum law is nonlocality. This theory explores how the position of an electron belonging to an atom may be at the electron shell, or nearby it, in the room, or on the other side of the universe. Its position can only be estimated by using probability mathematic formulas such as the Schrodinger Wave Equation.[4] If we try to determine a particle's exact location, we cannot determine its momentum. This is known as the Heisenberg Uncertainty Principle. This theory ties a location to the momentum of an object or particle. So with the Heisenberg Uncertainty Principle, the more accurately we can define the location of a particle, the less accurately we can determine or predict its momentum. This effect literally makes our sun shine. Atomic fusion of hydrogen atoms into helium atoms releases pure energy in the form of photon light which warms our planet and gives us life. This is made possible by the immense gravity and mass of the sun packing atoms so tightly that their location is more precisely known as the atoms are constantly ramming into each other. Inevitably, some of these atoms are randomly and suddenly found to be in the same location at the same time and their wavelengths, and corresponding momentum, completely sync as one. This is when fusion occurs, and light is born.[5]

In quantum physics, many things are uncertain and are not as rigidly exact as the determinism of Newtonian Physics would have you believe. This uncertainty is a full shift from solely considering physics and science in terms of easily measurable pieces and parts with rigid location and comfortably predictable behaviors. Scientists who follow the style of scientific materialism, which has been the main paradigm for the last 300 years, see everything, whether it be a rock, a tree, a molecule, or a planet, as separate entities the behave exclusively differently from other entities. When scientists conduct experiments with this logic, they don't consider ways that these individual parts are interconnected and influence each other in non-measurable ways. They also don't see their part in how their own beliefs and limited measuring tools can affect the outcomes of their experiments and observations. They don't see the holist picture of the many ways that every entity in the universe is tied together by their mere existence, and thus behave as a collective whole.[6]

The quantum principle of nonlocality reveals that quantum particles can instantaneously know the states of other quantum particles even if separated by vast distances. This is often called "instantaneous action-at-a-distance."[7] Einstein, who could never quit his hold on scientific materialism, called it "spooky action at a distance." He preferred the more deterministic quanta that behaved themselves according to relativistic Einstein locality. The theory of nonlocality is closely related to the quantum concept of entanglement. If two photons are entangled by an experiment that splits them in two, each particle instantaneously knows the state of the other regardless of the limitations of the speed of light or the distance between them. They will immediately alter their behavior to match that of the other particle. Experiments have proven this with over a thousand kilometers between them.[8]

And you might ask, how do they know? What is this knowing that communicates invisibly across space and time? Across the scientific world, even edging into biology and medicine, more and more scientists are turning to embrace the concept of a quantum consciousness that spans individuals and beings, and organic and inorganic entities alike. Much like how we discussed the failings of Western Medicine earlier in this book with is mechanical piecemeal approach to the human body, the world of science is undergoing a similar spiritual awakening that looks at holistic connectedness between ourselves and the entirety of the universe.[9] In his book *The Physics of God*, Joseph Selbie writes,

> unlike most of the Western philosophers, who relied on reason and logic to arrive at an intellectual understanding of consciousness and matter, the Eastern sages relied on methodical and repeated transcendent experiences to arrive at an experiential understanding of consciousness and matter. The difference between the Western and Eastern approaches is like the difference between talking about a meal and eating one— and I soon learned that the secret to eating the meal is meditation.[10]

Being made from energy, with particles that are connected to the entire universe through nonlocality, entanglement, imprecise location, and imprecise velocity or momentum, we seem simultaneously godlike and humbly equal. In the "The Nonlocal Universe," a study published by expert biologists Andrew Lohrey and Bruce Boreham, they write, "the observer, while always a secondary feature to universal consciousness, will at the same time be the central locale for all potential and actual social exchanges. One of the important social consequences that flow from this is that all observers are equal in being at the center of the universe, with none left out."[11] With nonlocality being the point, any location is the center of the universe. As observers who have the direct power to affect with merely our imaginings and intentions, what potential lies in wait for us when we activate our universal consciousness and connectedness?

Since the tiny elementary quanta particles we are made of obey these laws on a quantum and subatomic level, we have immense possibilities when it comes to observing our body's health and the universe at large. In his book, *The Self-Aware Universe: How Consciousness Creates the Material World*, quantum physicist Amit Goswami writes, "Instead of positing that everything (including consciousness) is made of matter, this philosophy posits that everything (including matter) exists in and is manipulated from consciousness."[12] When viewed from this vantage point, what limitations are holding us back from being the true creators of our realities? Do we look for disease and experience it because of the observer effect or do we look with faith and see health experiencing the opposite? Over the ages of human experience, were our communal belief systems merely a method to tap into the void of potential and communal consciousness?

All religions and philosophical teachings have followings of people regularly behaving from their own belief systems. With my personal belief, I see this manifesting in the spiritual teaching of Jesus Christ when he says, "If ye have faith as a grain of mustard seed, ye shall say unto this mountain, remove to yonder place, and it shall remove; and nothing shall be impossible unto you."[13] When we look across the quantum collective to spiritual teachings of other faiths, they show us many other ways to achieve powerful belief. We also have individuals throughout history, like Mahatma Gandhi, who showed the whole world how thoughts become words, which becomes fasting and quiet courageous action, which changed the whole history of the Indian people and the world.[14] Certainly consciousness and divine thoughts of peace are not of this world but of the universe at large.

Quantum consciousness thus hooks our brains and positive intentions into a whole universe of possibilities. The quantum processes in our brains that produce thoughts, free will, and positive intentions can extend their influence over vast distances. Will collective movements, meditations, and prayers move civilization toward a more integrated and conscientious future? It might do us well to understand better how meditation and prayer aids us in connecting to the universe and potential at large. Joseph Selbie, a founding member of the meditation-based communities of Ananda which were inspired by the teachings of Paramhansa Yogananda, shows how the energy waves of the brain change during deep mediation,

> Meditation, too, produces an alpha-wave rhythm, which . . . is generated when people concentrate or think deeply. However, meditators often pass through the alpha-wave rhythm, like a stage in a process, to arrive at theta-wave rhythms. Theta waves have been detected when people are dreaming deeply (REM sleep), learning, visualizing, or creating. Theta-wave rhythms, also detected in deep meditation, are thus associated with what we might call motionless, but highly focused, activity, revealing that meditation is far more than a pleasant wander through one's thoughts. Deep meditation is profoundly engaging, creative, and focused.[15]

These creative and focused energies might remind you of our ongoing discussion of flow states. The practice of moving meditation, after careful and delightful skill learning, can bring the power of real creation and formation into our lives. We have the potential to engage with our healthspan by enacting subtle changes based on meditative engagement with our habits and realities. If you're still wondering if we can shape our realities by sheer belief, when you consider the power of the placebo effect, it appears we already can.

We harness the true power of our minds when we completely set them free. Steven Hawking's mentor and Physics Nobel Prize winner Roger Penrose along with Dr. Stuart Hammeroff theorize that the microtubules in the brain's neurons vibrate with a coherent quantum frequency. They suggest there is a connection between the brain's biomolecular processes and the basic structure of the universe. Many testable experiments have been conducted to validate the theory since it was first published in the 90s. Many of them have concluded with positive results.[16] We now have a testable scientific theory proposed by the top scientists in the world establishing the quantum nature of consciousness and its connection to the entire universe through quantum correlations.[17]

Since we are integral and integrated beings intrinsically connected to our planet and the universe at large, we need to revise all our outdated systems to reflect this deeper understanding of quantum reality. We are still using a paradigm of medicine built on an outdated Newtonian flawed myopic viewpoint. Allopathic medicine's flawed approach to the body as a set of pulleys, wires, and cables, with chemical reactions that need to be manipulated, and a brain much like a desktop computer has got to go. Quantum consciousness and quantum healing have the power to move us into a medical landscape light years in the future. Thoughts, meditations, prayers, and intentions are reality. The placebo effect shows us a window into quantum healing. Engaging in belief alongside effective medical treatment designed to target root causes has the potential to heal completely. What's possible with just a particle of faith, a dash of mustard seed?

38

Conclusion

Thank you for following my meandering path through the micro, the macro, the particle, and the wave. It is my greatest hope that you carry with you the essence of functional health as you discover a meaningful flow for your life that makes you feel more at peace and at ease. While we can't always escape the many pitfalls trapping us in poor health or disease, we can build a lifestyle that actively tries to avoid the worst. At my core I believe that education gives us agency to find ways of becoming less susceptible to manipulative entities, poisons, and the delusions of others. I would hope that you take with you a spirit of curiosity and a yearning to discover more hidden truths as you use flow states to fine tune the habits of your life. Health and fitness are skills in which you become more and more proficient the longer you practice them. Take your time with various aspects of this book. Take one angle and start working it. You'll find that the more you improve one area, it lights up the other areas that need work. Then, from a stronger vantage point, you are able to tackle some of the more difficult and entrenched patterns in your life.

For example, if you can't help for the moment that your job or personal life is giving you nearly unbearable amounts of stress to the point that you feel you might break, try to balance yourself out by engaging in less stressful forms of exercise that focus on breath and alignment. Perhaps you could pack or make your lunch with nutritious and unprocessed foods that make you feel satiated and comfortably full. What if you start developing odd aches and pains or develop digestive issues in the midst of all this stress? You could get your hormones or allergies tested or work with a functional health doctor to find supplementation and diet combinations that get your body back on track. By focusing on one area of the mind, body, spirit trio, you can leverage that into pulling the other aspects of your health up as you make gains in mastering the balance.

When your doctor can't find anything wrong after multiple rounds of tests and you are still feeling dis-ease, start tackling aspects of your diet one at a time while getting second or third opinions from other doctors. Replace your favorite diet soda full of aspartame with an herbal drink or low-sugared ginger ale. Switch out sugar for honey or agave in your desserts or warm drinks. Replace your mindless snack of potato chips made with hydrogenated soy, palm, or canola oils and replace it with homemade popcorn over the kitchen stove with olive oil, high quality butter, nutritional yeast, and a bit of sea salt. If you're having trouble with weight management, and you've had hormonal levels checked, start small with upgrading your exercise program. If you're at the beginning, just add one day a week and make it a habit. The more fit and healthy you become, the more you'll crave the good things that keep your life in a healthy balance. The manufactured and fake foods will eventually become more and more dissatisfying and repulsive. If your doctor ever does find a hidden health issue, you'll be more of a teammate with them as you've improved your immune system's health leading into their treatment plan.

By arming ourselves with the knowledge of where to find alignment and how to avoid discord, we create a path of abundant health for ourselves and our loved ones. The megacorporations of the world don't want an educated public that can actively fend for itself. They thrive off misinformed people blindly dependent upon them for their products and services. If people are actively consuming poor quality and highly processed, even toxic, foods, they will inevitably end up in the doctor's office with multiple inexplicable health issues and then become dependent upon multiple medications to tamp down these mysterious symptoms. With knowledge of exactly where the pitfalls lie, we can take our power back and use our precious healthspan and money to enrich our lives in more meaningful ways.

And conversely, if we have knowledge of the foodborne illnesses, the molds, and the poisons that pollute our home environments and cities, we can keep our homes and communities a source of peace and wellness. With this understanding of mindful existing, we have the obligation to call on corporations and our government to put an end to the mindless polluting of our lands and waters and to stop pawning it off onto underserved communities and poorer countries. When we get the chi or energy of our environment right, there is an underlying calmness that can grow steadier. When people aren't fighting off headaches from bleach, smoldering mold infestations, or suffocating pollution, they can focus on more important things. These changes can have ripple effects into the quality of sleep people are getting, their motivation to exercise, and can lead to personal day to day choices that enact more empowered and well-intended lives.

When we can't be manipulated or taken over by people, entities, or organisms that only want to be parasitic to our lives rather than contribute back, we can truly find our flow. We can become better creators of our realities. We can have the health and motivation to transform our communities and environment. When we take the time to nurture ourselves and our communities, we can complete the mind, body, and spiritual loop that is so necessary for a fulfilling life.

I encourage you to revisit this book from time to time to refresh or focus on a section that pertains to your current circumstance. I also encourage you to do more of your own reading and research about subjects that I touch upon briefly here. This is your flow state journey. When you decide you want to improve your health and take your personal power back, treat it like a hobby. Don't make it a hassle. Make it fun and interesting. Let it feel exciting to learn how to be the best version of yourself. Let the health and good feelings these practices produce in your life do their magic on you. Find your own center of the universe and make it the paradise you dream of visiting.

References

1. Mihaly Csikszentmihalyi, *Flow: The Psychology of Optimal Experience* (New York: First Harper Perennial, 1991), 6.
2. T. R. Reid, "Germany: 'Applied Christianity'" chap. 5 in *The Healing of America: A Global Quest for Better, Cheaper, and Fairer Health Care* (New York: Penguin Press, 2009).
3. Colette Harris and Theresa Cheung, "Your PCOS Nutrition Guide" chap. 6 in *The Ultimate PCOS Handbook: Lose Weight, Boost Fertility, Clear Skin and Restore Self-Esteem* (Berkley: Conari Press, 2008).
4. Marc David, *The Slow Down Diet: Eating for Pleasure, Energy, and Weight Loss* (Rochester: Healing Arts Press, 2005), 19-22.
5. Zel Allen, *The Nut Gourmet: Nourishing Nuts for Every Occasion* (Summertown: Book Publishing Co., 2006), 244.
6. Chris Woollams, *The Rainbow Diet: Everything You Need to Know to Help You Beat Cancer* (Buckingham: Health Issues, 2002).
7. D. W. Warnock, H. T. Delves, C. K. Campell, et al., "Toxic Gas Generation from Plastic Mattresses and Sudden Infant Death Syndrome," *The Lancet* 346, no. 8989 (December 1995): 1516-20.
8. A. Z. Elsamanoudy, M. A. M. Neamat-Allah, F. A. H. Mohammad, et al., "The Role of Nutrition Related Genes and Nutrigenetics in Understanding the Pathogenesis of Cancer," *Journal of Microscopy & Ultrastructure* 4, no. 3 (July-September 2016): 115-122, doi:10.1016/j.jmau.2016.02.002.

1. H. Selye, *The Stress of Life* (New York: The McGraw-Hill Companies, Inc., 1984), 21-25.

2. R. M. Sapolsky, *Why Zebras Don't Get Ulcers* (New York: An Owl Book, Henry Holt and Company, 2004), 45, 52-53, 84-85, 87-91, 97-99, 102-6, 109-12, 138-41, 144-238, 337, 347-38.

3. Amy Berninger, Mayris P. Webber, Justin K. Niles, et al., "Longitudinal Study of Probable Post-Traumatic Stress Disorder in Firefighters Exposed to the World Trade Center Disaster," *American Journal of Industrial Medicine* 53, no. 12 (2010): 1177-85, doi:10.1002/ajim.20894.

4. "Associations Between Repeated Deployments to Iraq (OIF/OND) and Afghanistan (OEF) and Post-Deployment Illnesses and Injuries, Active Component, U.S. Armed Forces, 2003-2010. Part II: Mental Disorders, By Gender, Age Group, Military Occupation, and "Dwell Times" Prior to Repeat (Second through Fifth) Deployments." *Medical Surveillance Monthly Report* 18, no. 9 (September 2011): 2-11, http://www.afhsc.mil/viewMSMR?file =2011/ v18_n09.pdf#Page=2.

5. B. P. Dohrenwend, J. B. Turner, N. A. Turse, et al., "The Psychological Risk of Vietnam for U.S. Veterans: A Revist with New Data and Methods," *Science* 313, no. 5789 (2006): 979-982.

6. Glenn R. Schiraldi, *The Post-Traumatic Stress Disorder Sourcebook* (New York: The McGraw-Hill Companies, Inc., 2009), 5.

7. F. B. Schoenfeld, J. C. Deviva, and R. Manber, "Treatment of Sleep Disturbances in Posttraumatic Stress Disorder: A Review," *Journal of Rehabilitation Research and Development* 49, no. 5 (July 2012): 729-52, doi:10.1682/ JRRD.2011.09.0164.

8. Ibid.

9. B. J. Morris, "How Xenohormetic Compounds Confer Health Benefits," chap. 8 in *Mild Stress: Applying Hormesis in Aging Research and Interventions*, ed. E. Le Bourg and S. Rattan (Netherlands: Springer, 2008); J. A. Baur and D.

A. Sinclair, "What is Xenohormesis?" *American Journal of Pharmacology and Toxicology* 3, no. 1 (2008): 152-159, doi:10.3844/ajptsp.2008.152.159.

10. Worthington et al. "UK Soil Association Fact Sheet," *Journal of Complimentary Medicine* 7 (2001): 2161- 2163; D. R. Davis et al. "Changes in USDA Food Composition Data for 43 Garden Crops, 1950 to 1999," *Journal of the American College of Nutrition* 23, no. 6 (2004): 669-682; R. A. McCance and E.M. Widdowson, "The Chemical Composition of Foods," *Medical Research Council Special Report Series* 235 (London: His Majesty's Stationery Office, 1940); J. D. Hyatt, P. M. Perkins Veazie, and S. Rice, "Vitamin C Content of Organically Grown Produce (abstract)," *Oklahoma Research Day*, October 26, 2007, 127; A. S. Kecka and J.W. Finley. "Database Values Do Not Reflect Selenium Contents of Grain, Cereals and Other Foods Grown or Purchased in the Upper Midwest United States," *Nutrition Research* 26 (2006): 17-22; and H. A. Schroeder, *Trace Elements and Man* (New Greenwich: Devin-Adair Publishing, 1973).

11. Pam Belluck, "Children's Life Expectancy Being Cut Short by Obesity," *New York Times*, March 17, 2005, http://www.nytimes.com/2005/03/17/health/17obese.html; and S. J. Olshansky et al., "A Potential Decline in Life Expectancy in the United States in the 21st Century," *New England Journal of Medicine* 352, no. 11 (2005): 1138-45.

12. S.M. Kwak, S.K. Myung, Y.J. Lee, and H.G. Seo, "Efficacy of Omega-3 Fatty Acid Supplements (Eicosapentaenoic Acid and Docosahexaenoic Acid) in the Secondary Prevention of Cardiovascular Disease: A Meta-Analysis of Randomized, Double-Blind, Placebo-Controlled Trials," *Archives of Internal Medicine* 172, no. 9 (May 2012): 686-94, doi:10.1001/archinternmed.2012.262.

13. James J. DiNicolantonio, James H. O'Keefe, and Carl J. Lavie, "The Big Ones That Got Away: Omega-3 Meta-analysis Flawed by Excluding the Biggest Fish Oil Trials," *Archives of Internal Medicine* 172, no.18 (2012):1427-1428, doi:10.1001/archinternmed.2012.3755.

14. Cass, Hyla. *Supplement Your Prescription: What Your Doctor Doesn't Know about Nutrition* (Laguna Beach: Basic Health Publications, 2007).

15. Eric Schlosser, *Fast Food Nation: The Dark Side of the All-American Meal* (Boston: Houghton Mifflin, 2001), 203; Marcy Lowe and Gary Gereffi, "A Value Chain Analysis of the U.S. Beef and Dairy Industries; Report Prepared for Environmental Defense Fund," (Durham: Duke University, February 2009): 15, http://www.cggc.duke .edu/environment/valuechainanalysis/CGGC_BeefDairyReport_2-16-09.pdf. The meat from culled dairy cows is primarily processed into ground beef for fast food hamburgers or supermarket retail, discussed in detail on page 44; Kenneth H. Mathews Jr., Personal communication with CGGC research staff. (USDA Economic Research Service, December 17, 2008) "An estimated 18% of total beef and veal production

originates from dairy cattle," and "Economic Opportunities for Dairy Cow Culling Management Options," Info Sheet/Veterinary Services (USDA Animal and Plant Health Inspection Service, May 1996); and Mauricio Espinoza, "Choice of Dairy-Cow Bedding Impacts E. Coli Survival, Food Safety," News Archive (Ohio State University Extension, March 18, 2005).

16.   Alessandra Tavani et al., "Red Meat Intake and Cancer Risk: A Study in Italy," *International Journal of Cancer* 86, no. 3 (2000): 425–428; Tim Birdsall, Joseph E. Pizzorno, Paul Reilly, and Michael Murray, *How to Prevent and Treat Cancer with Natural Medicine* (New York: Riverhead Books, 2003), 37.

1. Stephen Harrod Buhner, *The Lost Language of Plants: The Ecological Importance of Plant Medicines to Life on Earth* (White River Junction, VT: Chelsea Green, 2002), 153-174.
2. "Only a few of the many enzymes are destroyed by acid." Tom Bohager, *Enzymes: What the Experts Know! : Your Journey to Health and Longevity Starts Here* (Prescott: One World Press, 2006), 34.
3. Marc David, *The Slow Down Diet: Eating for Pleasure, Energy, and Weight Loss* (Rochester: Healing Arts Press, 2005), 18.
4. Tom Bohager, *Enzymes: What the Experts Know! : Your Journey to Health and Longevity Starts Here* (Prescott: One World Press, 2006), 37-38.
5. Hiromi Shinya, *The Enzyme Factor* (San Francisco: Council Oak Books, 2007), 31.
6. Tom Bohager, *Enzymes: What the Experts Know! : Your Journey to Health and Longevity Starts Here* (Prescott: One World Press, 2006), 43.
7. Ibid., 42.
8. Edward Howell, *Food Enzymes for Health and Longevity* 3rd ed. (Twin Lakes: Lotus Press, 2015); DeLeon, et al., *Philippine Journal of Science* 52 (1933): 97-127; and Humbart Santillo and Deborah Kantor, *Food Enzymes: The Missing Link to Radiant Health*, 2nd ed. (Prescott: Hohm Press, 1993), 17-20.
9. Howell, Edward, and Maynard Murray, *Enzyme Nutrition: The Food Enzyme Concept* (Wayne: Avery Publishing Group, 1985), 11-12.
10. T. F. Wang, Y. Y. Chen, Y. M. Liou, et al., "Investigating Tooth Loss and Associated Factors Among Older Taiwanese Adults," *Archives of Gerontology and Geriatrics* 58, no. 3 (May-June 2014): 446-53, doi:10.1016/j.archger.2014.01.002; Francesca De Angelis, Stefania Basili, Fratto Giovanni, et al., "Influence of the Oral Status on Cardiovascular Diseases in an Older Italian Population," *International Journal of Immunopathology and Pharmacology* 32 (January-December 2018): 394632017751786, doi:10.1177/0394632017751786; and Howard Straus and Barbara Marinacci, *Dr. Max Gerson: Healing the Hopeless* 2nd ed. (Totality Books, 2009).
11. Howell, Edward, and Maynard Murray, *Enzyme Nutrition: The Food Enzyme Concept* (Wayne: Avery Publishing Group, 1985), 138-139.

12.   Vincent A Fischetti , "Bacteriophage Lytic Enzymes: Novel Anti-Infectives," *Trends in Microbiology* 13, no. 10 (October 2005): 491-6, doi:10.1016/j.tim.2005.08.007 and B. Alberts, A. Johnson, J. Lewis, et al., *Molecular Biology of the Cell* 4th ed. (New York: Garland Science, 2002): Protein Function.

1. *The 'Kahun Medical Papyrus' or 'Gynaecological Papyrus,'* trans. Stephen Quirke (London: University College London, 2002), http://www.digitale-gypt.ucl.ac.uk/med/birthpapyrus.html.
2. Mark Blumenthal and Werner R. Busse, *The Complete German Commission E Monographs* (Austin: American Botanical Council, 1998), 230.
3. Chikako Takeshita, "Bioprospecting and Indigenous Peoples' Resistances," *Peace Review: A Journal of Social Justice* 12, no. 4 (2000): 555–562, doi:10.1080/10402650020014645.
4. R. H. Douglas and G. Jeffery, "The Spectral Transmission of Ocular Media Suggests Ultraviolet Sensitivity Is Widespread Among Mammals," *Proceedings of the Royal British Society of Biological Sciences* 281, no. 1780 (February 19, 2014), doi:10.1098/rspb.2013.2995.
5. Sylvia Dolson, *Bear-Ology: Fascinating Bear Facts, Tales & Trivia* (Masonville: PixyJack Press, 2009), 92-9; Gary Brown, *The Bear Almanac: A Comprehensive Guide to the Bears of the World*, 2nd ed. (Guilford: Lyons Press, 2009), 158-59.
6. K. Nguyen, J. Sparks, and F. Omoruyi, "Effects of Ligusticum porteri (Osha) Root Extract on Human Promyelocytic Leukemia Cells" *Pharmacognosy Research* 9, no. 2 (April-June, 2017): 156– 160, doi:10.4103/0974-8490.204641.
7. James L. Oschman, *Energy Medicine: The Scientific Basis* (Edinburgh: Churchill Livingstone, 2000), 178-79.
8. Jerry Tennant, *Healing Is Voltage: The Handbook*, (CreateSpace Independent Publishing Platform, 2010), 296-297.
9. Oschman, *Energy Medicine*, 142-43; and W. Lewandowski, M. Kalinowska, and H. Lewandowska, "The Influence of Metals on the Electronic System of Biologically Important Ligands. Spectroscopic Study of Benzoates, Salicylates, Nicotinates and Isoorotates," *Journal of Inorganic Biochemistry* 99, no. 7 (July 2005): 1407-1423.
10. Jim Oschman, "The Science Supporting the Use of Pulsing Electromagnetic Field Therapy and ONDAMED® Part 1," *The Townsend Letter* 299 (June 2008): 75-78.

11. Eldred B. Taylor, *Hormone Replacement a Scientific, Evidence Based Approach: Confessions of a Gynecologist* (Atlanta: Maximum Health Enterprises, Inc., 2006), Audio CD.

12. Barbara Starfield, "Is US Health Really the Best in the World?," *Journal of the American Medical Association* 284, no. 4 (2000): 483-485, doi:10-1001/pubs.JAMA-ISSN-0098-7484-284-4-jco00061; and Linda T. Kohn, Janet M. Corrigan, and Molla S. Donaldson, eds., *To Err Is Human: Building a Safer Health System*, by Institute of Medicine: Committee on Quality of Health Care in America (Washington D. C.: National Academy Press, 2000).

13. Steven Woloshin, Lisa M. Schwartz, Jennifer Tremmel, and H. Gilbert Welch, Direct-To-Consumer Advertisements for Prescription Drugs: What Are Americans Being Sold?," *The Lancet* 358, no. 9288 (October 6, 2001): 1141-1146, doi:10.1016/S0140-6736(01)06254-7.

14. A. P. Singh, A. Junemann, A. Muthuraman, et al., "Animal Models of Acute Renal Failure," *Pharmacology Reports* 64, no. 1 (2012): 31-44.

15. M. Hauben, S. Horn, L. Reich, and M. Younus, "Association Between Gastric Acid Suppressants and Clostridium Difficile Colitis and Community-Acquired Pneumonia: Analysis Using Pharmacovigilance Tools," *International Journal of Infectious Diseases* 11, no. 5 (September 2007): 417-22.

16. Peter Roger Breggin, *Toxic Psychiatry* (New York: St. Martin's Press, 1991), 244-49.

17. "Beta blockers deplete CoQ10. CoQ10 deficiency is a leading cause of heart failure," Ross Pelton and James B. LaValle, *The Nutritional Cost of Prescription Drugs*, 2nd ed. (Englewood: Morton Publishing Co., 2004), 58.

18. Haile T. Debas, Ramanan Laxminarayan, and Stephen E. Straus "Complementary and Alternative Medicine," in *Disease Control Priorities in Developing Countries*, 2nd ed., Dean T. Jamison, eds., et al. (New York: Oxford University Press, 2006), chap. 69.

19. Uffe Ravnskov, *The Cholesterol Myths: Exposing the Fallacy That Cholesterol and Saturated Fat Cause Heart Disease* (Washington, DC: New Trends Publishing Inc., 2000), 238-40; Barbara Starfield, "Is US Health Really the Best in the World?" *Journal of the American Medical Association* 284, no.4 (July 6, 2000): 483; and Fred Charatan, "Medical Errors Kill Almost 100000 Americans a Year," *British Medical Journal* 319, no. 7224 (December 11, 1999): 1519, doi:10.1136/bmj.319.7224.1519.

20. K. K. Ray, S. R. K. S. Seshasai, S. Erqou, et al., "Statins and All-Cause Mortality in High-Risk Primary Prevention," *Archives of Internal Medicine* 170 (2010): 1024-1031, doi:10.1001/archinternmed.2010.182.

21. Ravnskov, *The Cholesterol Myths*, 238-40; M. F. Muldoon, S. B. Manuck, and K. A. Matthews, "Lowering Cholesterol Concentrations and Mortality: A Quantitative review of Primary Prevention Trials," *British Medical Journal* 301

(1990), 309-314, doi:10.1136/bmj.301.6747.309; and G. Lindberg, L. Råstam, B. Gullberg, et al., "Low Serum Cholesterol Concentration and Short Term Mortality from Injuries in Men and Women," *British Medical Journal* 305, no. 6848 (1992), 277-279, doi:10.1136/bmj.305.6848.277.

22.   Richard Smith, "Let Food Be Thy Medicine..." British Medical Journal 328, no. 8 (January 22, 2004), doi:10.1136 /bmj.328.7433.0-g.

23.   Jacob Liberman, *Light: Medicine of the Future: How We Can Use It to Heal Ourselves Now* (Santa Fe: Bear & Company, 1991), 160-161.

24.   P. P. Mersch, H. M. Middendorp, A. L. Bouhuys, et al., "Seasonal Affective Disorder and Latitude: A Review of the Literature," *Journal of Affective Disordorders* 53, no. 1 (April 1999): 35-48.

25.   Hippocrates, Francis Adams, and Emerson Crosby Kelly, *The Genuine Works of Hippocrates*, trans. Francis Adams (Whitefish, MT: Kessinger Publishing), 104.

26.   Mark Blumenthal, *Herbal Medicine: Expanded Commission E Monographs* (Newton: Integrative Medicine Communications, 2000); and T. Efferth, S. Kahl, K. Paulus, et al., "Phytochemistry and Pharmacogenomics of Natural Products Derived from Traditional Chinese Medicine and Chinese Materia Medica with Activity Against Tumor Cell," *Molecular Cancer Theraputics* 7 (2008): 152-161, doi:10.1158/1535-7163.MCT-07-0073.

27.   Thich Nhat Hanh and Dr. Lilian Cheung, *Savor: Mindful Eating, Mindful Life* (New York: HarperCollins, 2010), 7.

1.   David Perlmutter and Carol Colman, "The Brain Workout," chap. 9 in *The Better Brain Book: The Best Tools for Improving Memory, Sharpness, and Preventing Aging of the Brain* (New York: Riverhead Books, 2004), 159-168.

2.   Daniel W.D. West and Stuart M. Phillips, "Anabolic Processes in Human Skeletal Muscle: Restoring the Identities of Growth Hormone and Testosterone," *Physician and Sportsmedicine* 38, no. 3 (October 2010): 97-104, doi:10.3810/psm.2010.10.1814.

3.   John J. Ratey and Eric Hagerman, "Hormonal Changes: The Impact on Women's Brain Health," chap. 8 in *Spark!:The Revolutionary New Science of Exercise and the Brain* (London: Quercus, 2010), 191-215.

4.   S. Fujimoto, S. Yamazaki, A. Wakabayashi, et al., "The Effects of Tai-Chi Exercise for the Prevention of Long-Term Care in Community-Dwelling Frail Elderly People: New Care-Need Certification and Mortality," *Nihon Ronen Igakkai Zasshi* 48, no. 6 (2011): 699-706, http://www.ncbi.nlm.nih.gov/pubmed /22322043.

5.   Junghee Yoo, Euiju Lee, Chungmi Kim, et al., "Sasang Constitutional Medicine and Traditional Chinese Medicine: A Comparative Overview," *Evidence-Based Complementary Alternative Medicine 2012* (2012), doi:10.1155/2012/980807.

6.   C. Scholl, B. D. Eshelman, D. M. Barnes, and P. R. Hanlon, "Raphasatin Is a More Potent Inducer of the Detoxification Enzymes Than Its Degradation Products," *Journal of Food Science* 76, no. 3 (April 2011): C504-11, doi:10.1111/j.1750-3841.2011.02078.x.

7.   L. Ferrarini, N. Pellegrini, T. Mazzeo, et al., "Anti-Proliferative Activity and Chemoprotective Effects Towards DNA Oxidative Damage of Fresh and Cooked Brassicaceae," *British Journal of Nutrition* (November 2011): 1-9, http://www.ncbi.nlm.nih.gov/pubmed/22088277.

8.   Diane C. Lagace, Michael H. Donovan, Nathan A. DeCarolis, et al., "Adult Hippocampal Neurogenesis Is Functionally Important for Stress-Induced Social Avoidance," *Proceedings of the National Academy of Sciences of the United States*

of America 107, no. 9 (February 2010): 4436-41, doi:10.1073/pnas.0910072107; and C. M. Jeckel, R. P. Lopes, M. C. Berleze, et al., "Neuroendocrine and Immunological Correlates of Chronic Stress in 'Strictly Healthy' Populations," *NeuroImmunoModulation* 17, no. 1 (2010): 9-18, doi:10.1159/000243080.

9. Firdaus S. Dhabhar, "Enhancing Versus Suppressive Effects of Stress on Immune Function: Implications for Immunoprotection and Immunopathology," *NeuroImmunomodulation* 16, no. 5 (2009): 300-17, doi:10.1159 /000216188.

10. J. M. Finlay and M. J. Zigmond, "The Effects of Stress on Central Dopaminergic Neurons: Possible Clinical Implications," *Neurochemical Research* 22, no. 11 (November 1997): 1387-94, http://www.ncbi.nlm.nih.gov /pubmed /9355111.

11. Firdaus S. Dhabhar, "A Hassle a Day May Keep the Pathogens Away: The Fight-or-Flight Stress Response and the Augmentation of Immune Function," *Integrative and Comparative Biology* 49, no. 3 (September 2009): 215-36, doi:10.1093/icb/icp045.

12. James P. Warne, "Shaping the Stress Response: Interplay of Palatable Food Choices, Glucocorticoids, Insulin and Abdominal Obesity," *Molecular and Cellular Endocrinology* 300, no. 1-2 (March 2009): 137-46, doi:10.1016/ j.mce.2008.09.036.

13. Bruce S. McEwen, "Physiology and Neurobiology of Stress and Adaptation: Central Role of the Brain," *Physiological Reviews* 87, no. 3 (July 2007): 873-904, doi:10.1152/physrev.00041.2006; Tracy L. Bale, "Stress Sensitivity and the Development of Affective Disorders," *Hormones and Behavior* 50, no. 4 (November 2006): 529-33, doi:10.1016/j.yhbeh.2006.06.033; and R. P. Hart, J. B. Wade, and M. F. Martelli, "Cognitive Impairment in Patients with Chronic Pain: The Significance of Stress," *Current Pain and Headache Reports 7*, no. 2 (April 2003): 116-26, http://www.ncbi.nlm.nih.gov/pubmed/12628053.

14. V. N. Luine, K. D. Beck, R. E. Bowman, et al., "Chronic Stress and Neural Function: Accounting for Sex and Age," *Journal of Neuroendocrinology* 19, no. 10 (October 2007): 743-51, doi: 10.1111/j.1365-2826.2007.01594.x; R. D. Marshall and A. Garakani, "Psychobiology of the Acute Stress Response and Its Relationship to the Psychobiology of Post-Traumatic Stress Disorder," *The Psychiatric Clinics of North America* 25, no. 2 (June 2002): 385-95, http://www.ncbi.nlm.nih.gov/pubmed/12136506; Bruce S. McEwen and Peter J. Gianaros, "Stress and Allostasis-Induced Brain Plasticity," *Annual Review of Medicine* 62 (February 2011): 431-45, doi:10.1146/annurev-med-052209-100430; and Dervla O'Malley, Eamonn M. M. Quigley, Timothy G. Dinan, and John F. Cryan, "Do Interactions Between Stress and Immune Responses Lead to Symptom Exacerbations in Irritable Bowel Syndrome?" *Brain, Behavior, and Immunity* 25, no. 7 (October 2011): 1333-41, doi:10.1016/j.bbi .2011.04.009.

15.	M. Frazzoni, R. Conigliaro, and G. Melotti, "Weakly Acidic Refluxes Have a Major Role in the Pathogenesis of Proton Pump Inhibitor-Resistant Reflux Oesophagitis," *Alimentary Pharmacology & Therapeutics* 33, no. 5 (March 2011): 601-606, doi:10.1111/j.1365-2036.2010.04550.x.

16.	Cathleen Colón-Emeric, Mary Beth O'Connell, and Elizabeth Haney, "Osteoporosis Piece of Multi-Morbidity Puzzle in Geriatric Care," *Mount Sinai Journal of Medicine* 78, no. 4 (July-August 2011): 515-26, doi:10.1002/msj.20269; Caroline J. Davidge Pitts and Ann E. Kearns, "Update on Medications With Adverse Skeletal Effects," *Mayo Clinic Proceedings* 86, no. 4 (April 2011): 338-43, doi:10.4065/mcp.2010.0636; B. Tepeš, "Long-Term Acid Inhibition: Benefits and Harms," *Digestive Diseases* 29, no. 5 (2011): 476-81, doi:10.1159/000331519; and Gherardo Mazziotti, Ernesto Canalis, and Andrea Giustina, "Drug-Induced Osteoporosis: Mechanisms and Clinical Implications," *The American Journal of Medicine* 123, no. 10 (October 2010): 877-84, doi:10.1016/j.amjmed.2010.02.028.

17.	Jacalyn Duffin, *History of Medicine: A Scandalously Short Introduction* (Buffalo: University of Toronto Press, 2007), 110; Robert W. Schrier, *Diseases of the Kidney & Urinary Tract*, 8th ed. (Philadelphia: Lippincott Williams & Wilkins, 2007), 1153.

18.	Marcia Angell, "The Epidemic of Mental Illness: Why?" The New York Review of Books, accessed February 2, 2012, http://www.nybooks.com/articles/archives/2011/jun/23/epidemic-mental-illness-why/?pagination =false&printpage=true; Lawrence Wilson, "Beyond Antibiotics," The Center for Development, accessed February 18, 2012, http://drlwilson.com/Articles/antibiotics.htm; S. R. Ahmad, "Adverse Drug Event Monitoring at the Food and Drug Administration: Your Report Can Make a Difference," *Journal of General Internal Medicine* 18 (2003): 56-9; Bill Sardi, "When the Cure Is Worse Than the Disease," LewRockwell.com, accessed February 18, 2012, http://www.lewrockwell .com/sardi/sardi90.html; Eric J. Thomas and Laura A. Petersen, "Measuring Errors and Adverse Events in Health Care," *Journal of General Internal Medicine* 18 (2003): 60-6, doi:10.1046/j.1525-1497.2003.20147.x; and Sidney Wolfe, "Remedies Needed in Reporting Adverse Reactions and FDA Use of Reports," *Journal of General Internal Medicine* 18, no. 1 (January 2003): 72-73, doi:10.1046/j.1525-1497.2003.t01-1-21115.x.

19.	Food and Agriculture Organization of the United Nations, *The State of Food and Agriculture*, (2009): 12, 136 Table A2 and A3, http://www.fao.org/docrep/012/i0680e/i0680e.pdf.

20.	"Why We Should Not Eat Meat," Raw Food Explained.com, accessed February 18, 2012, http://www.rawfoodexplained.com/why-we-should-not-eat-meat/flesh-foods-cause-degenerative-disease.html; and "Lack of Stomach Acid-Hypochlorhydria-Can Cause Lots of Problems," ProHealth.com, last modified December 10, 2007, http://www.prohealth.com/library/showarti-cle.cfm?libid=13388; and Ron Kennedy, "Hypochlorhydria," The Doctor's Medical Library, accessed February 18, 2012, http://www.medical-library.net/hypochlorhydria.html.

21.   W. J. Calhoun, "Nocturnal Asthma," *Chest* 123, no. 3 (March 2003): 399S-405S, http://www. ncbi.nlm.nih.gov/pubmed/12629002.

22.   J. Kwiecien, E. Machura, F. Halkiewicz, and J. Karpe, "Clinical Features of Asthma in Children Differ with Regard to the Intensity of Distal Gastro-esophageal Acid Reflux," *The Journal of Asthma* 48, no. 4 (May 2011): 366-73, http://www.ncbi.nlm.nih.gov/pubmed/21385116; R. Palmer, J. B. Anon, and P. Gallagher, "Pediatric Cough: What the Otolaryngologist Needs to Know," *Current Opinion in Otolaryngology & Head and Neck Surgery* 19, no.3 (June 2011): 204-9, http://www.ncbi.nlm.nih.gov/pubmed/21499103; Srini-vasan Ramanuja and Pramod S. Kelkar, "The Approach to Pediatric Cough," *Annals of Allergy, Asthma & Immunology* 105, no. 1 (July 2010): 3-8, 9-11, and 42, doi:10.1016/j.anai.2009.11.011; and Alaa S. Deeb, Amal Al-Hakeem, and Ghazal S. Dib, "Gastroesophageal Reflux in Children with Refractory Asthma," *Oman Medical Journal* 25, no. 3 (July 2010): 218-21, doi:10.5001 /omj.2010.60.

23.   Ibid.

24.   J. M. de Castro, "The Time of Day of Food Intake Influences Overall Intake in Humans," *The Journal of Nutrition* 134, no. 1 (January 2004): 104-11, http://jn.nutrition.org/content/134/1/104.long.

1. Myron Brin and Z. Z. Ziporin, "Evaluation of Thiamin Adequacy in Adult Humans," *Journal of Nutrition* 86 (July 1965): 319-24, http://jn.nutrition.org/content/86/3/319.long; Myron Brin, "Erythrocyte as a Biopsy Tissue for Functional Evaluation of Thiamine Adequacy," *The Journal of the American Medical Association* 187, no. 10 (March 1964): 762-6, doi:10.1001/jama.1964.03060230090022.

2. E. Isenberg-Grzeda, H. E. Kutner, and S. E. Nicolson, "Wernicke-Korsakoff-Syndrome: Under-Recognized and Under-Treated," *Psychosomatics* 53, no. 6 (November 2012):507-16, doi:10.1016/j.psym.2012.04.008.

3. E. D. Toffanello, E. M. Inelmen, N. Minicuci, et al., "Ten-Year Trends in Vitamin Intake in Free-Living Healthy Elderly People: The Risk of Subclinical Malnutrition," *The Journal of Nutrition, Health & Aging* 15, no. 2 (2011): 99-103.

4. Lyle MacWilliam, *NutriSearch Comparative Guide to Nutritional Supplements*, 4th ed. (Vernon, BC: Northern Dimensions Publishing, 2007), 28.

5. E. Isenberg-Grzeda, H. E. Kutner, and S. E. Nicolson, "Wernicke-Korsakoff-Syndrome: Under-Recognized and Under-Treated," Psychosomatics 53, no. 6 (November 2012): 507-16, doi:10.1016/j.psym.2012.04.008.

6. Linus Pauling, *Vitamin C, The Common Cold, and the Flu*, (San Francisco: W. H. Freeman, 1979), 80.

7. L. J. Dominguez and M. Barbagallo "Nutritional Prevention of Cognitive Decline and Dementia," *Acta Biomedical* 89, no. 2 (20180: 276–290, doi: 10.23750/abm.v89i2.7401.

8. Lyle MacWilliam, *NutriSearch Comparative Guide to Nutritional Supplements,* 4 ed. (Vernon, BC: Northern Dimensions Publishing, 2007).

9. Ibid.

10. Donald R. Davis, Melvin D. Epp, and Hugh D. Riordan, "Changes in USDA Food Composition Data for 43 Garden Crops, 1950 to 1999," *Journal of the American College of Nutrition* 23, no. 6 (December 2004): 669-82.

11. Lyle MacWilliam, *Comparative Guide to Nutritional Supplements*, (Vernon, BC: Northern Dimensions Publishing, 2007), 21-22 and J. Lazarou, B. H. Pomeranz, and P. N. Corey, "Incidence of Adverse Drug Reactions in

Hospitalized Patients: A Meta-Analysis of Prospective Studies," *Journal of the American Medical Association* 279, no. 15, (April 1998): 1200-5, doi:10.1001/jama.279.15.1200.

12.   Ibid., 21-22.

13.   Lyle MacWilliam, *Comparative Guide to Nutritional Supplements*, (Vernon, BC: Northern Dimensions Publishing, 2007).

14.   Ibid., 78-79, 82.

15.   NutrientRich.com, accessed February 23, 2012, http://www.nutrientrich.com/1/myth-depleted-soil-produces-less-nutritious-fruits-and-vegetables.html; David S. Ludwig, Joseph A. Majzoub, Ahmad Al-Zahrani, Gerard E. Dallal, Isaac Blanco, and Susan B. Roberts, "High Glycemic Index Foods, Overeating, and Obesity," *Pediatrics* 103, no. 3 (March 1, 1999): e26, doi:10.1542/peds.103.3.e26i; K. L. Morris and M. B. Zemel, "Effect of Dietary Carbohydrate Source on the Development of Obesity in Agouti Transgenic Mice," *Obesity Research* 13, no. 1 (January 2005): 21-35; R. Giacco, G. Della Pepa, D. Luongo, and G, Riccardi, "Whole Grain Intake in Relation to Body Weight: From Epidemiological Evidence to Clinical Trials," *Nutrition, Metabolism, and Cardiovascular Disease* 21, no. 12 (October 31, 2011): 901-8, doi:10.1016/j.numecd.2011.07.003; and Qi Sun, Donna Spiegelman, Rob M. Van Dam, Michelle D. Holmes, Vasanti S. Malik, Walter C. Willett, and Frank B. Hu, "White Rice, Brown Rice, and Risk of Type 2 Diabetes in US Men and Women," *Archives of Internal Medicine* 170, no. 11 (June 14, 2010): 961-9, doi:10.1001/archinternmed.2010.109.

16.   Walter *Crinnion, Clean, Green, and Lean: Get Rid of the Toxins that Make You Fat* (Hoboken: John Wiley, 2010), 66-68; Denham Harman, "Free Radical Theory of Aging: Nutritional Implications," *Age* 1, no. 4 (1978): 145-152, doi:10.1007/BF02432188.

17.   Gavin Menzies, *1421: The Year China Discovered America*, (New York: William Morrow, 2003); Linus Pauling, *Vitamin C, The Common Cold, and the Flu* (San Francisco: W. H. Freeman, 1979), 23.

18.   Linus Pauling, *Vitamin C, The Common Cold, and the Flu*, 33-34.

19.   I. B. Chatterjee, "Evolution and the Biosynthesis of Ascorbic Acid," *Science* 182, no. 4118 (December 1973): 1271-1272, doi:10.1126/science.182.4118.1271; and Y. Chen, C. P. Curran, D. W. Nebert, K. V. Patel, M. T. Williams, and C. V. Vorhees, "Effect of Vitamin C Deficiency During Postnatal Development on Adult Behavior: Functional Phenotype of Gulo-/-Knockout Mice," *Genes, Brain, and Behavior* 11 no. 3 (April 11, 2012): 269-77, doi:10.1111/j .1601-183X.2011.00762.x. Epub 2012 Feb 2.

20.   Linus Pauling, *Vitamin C, The Common Cold, and the Flu* (San Francisco: W. H. Freeman, 1979), 83.

21.   Joseph E. Pizzorno, Jr., and Michael T. Murray, "Vitamin Toxicities and Therapeutic Monitoring," chap. 139 in *Textbook of Natural Medicine* (Edinburgh: Elsevier Churchill Livingstone, 2005), 1391-1392.

22.   R. E. Hill, K. R. Kamath, "'Pink' Diarrhoea: Osmotic Diarrhoea from a Sorbitol-Containing Vitamin C Supplement," *The Medical Journal of Australia* 1, no. 9 (May 1, 1982): 387-9; Robert F. Cathcart, "Vitamin C, Titrating to Bowel Tolerance, Anascorbemia, and Acute Induced Scurvy," *Medical Hypotheses* 7, no. 11 (November 1981): 1359–1376, doi:10.1016/0306-9877(81)90126-2; C. J. Hoyt, "Diarrhea from Vitamin C," *Journal of the American Medical Association* 244, no. 15 (October 10, 1980): 1674; and P. M. Ferraro, G. C. Curhan, G. Gambaro, and E. N. Taylor, "Total, Dietary, and Supplemental Vitamin C Intake and Risk of Incident Kidney Stones," *American Journal of Kidney Diseases* 67, no. 3 (March 2016): 400–407, doi:10.1053/j.ajkd.2015.09.005. Some of the earlier research and the fad of the genotype diet had over-inflated the role of vitamin C in kidney stone formation. The current diet that Functional Medicine promotes is the FODMAP diet.

23.   Linus Pauling, *Vitamin C, the Common Cold, and the Flu* (San Francisco: W. H. Freeman, 1979), 45.

24.   I. B. Chatterjee, "Evolution and the Biosynthesis of Ascorbic Acid," *Science* 182, no. 4118 (1973): 1271–1272, doi:10.1126/science.182.4118.1271.

25.   Lyle MacWilliam, *NutriSearch Comparative Guide to Nutritional Supplements*, 4th ed. (Vernon, BC: Northern Dimensions Publishing, 2007), 28, 80.

26.   W. Grabowska, E. Sikora, and A. Bielak-Zmijewska, "Sirtuins: A Promising Target in Slowing Down the Ageing Process," *Biogerontology* 18, no. 4 (2017): 447-476, doi:10.1007/s10522-017-9685-9.

27.   Lyle MacWilliam, *NutriSearch Comparative Guide to Nutritional Supplements for the Americas* 6th ed. (Northern Dimensions Publishing, 2019), 115-118.

28.   Ross Pelton, *Drug-induced Nutrient Depletion Handbook* 2nd ed. (Hudson: Lexicomp, 2001) and Suzy Cohen, *Drug Muggers: Which Medications Are Robbing Your Body of Essential Nutrients—and Natural Ways to Restore Them* (New York: Rodale, 2011).

29.   Y. I. Tayem, "Therapeutic and Maintenance Regimens of Vitamin D3 Supplementation in Healthy Adults: A Systematic Review," *Cellular and Molecular Biology* 64, no. 14 (November 2018): 8-14.

30.   A. E. Czeizel, I. Dudás, L. Paput, and F. Bánhidy, "Prevention of Neural-Tube Defects with Periconceptional Folic Acid, Methylfolate, or Multivitamins?" *Annals of Nutrition and Metabolism* 58, no. 4 (October, 2011): 263–271, doi.10.1159/000330776.

31.   Fereidoon Shahidi and Adriano Costa de Camargo, "Tocopherols and Tocotrienols in Common and Emerging Dietary Sources: Occurrence,

Applications, and Health Benefits," *International Journal of Molecular Sciences* 17, no. 10 (October 2016): 1745, doi:10.3390/ijms17101745.

1.   D. Albanes, O. P. Heinonen, P. R. Taylor, et. al., "Alpha-Tocopherol and Beta-Carotene Supplements and Lung Cancer Incidence in the Alpha-Tocopherol, Beta-Carotene Cancer Prevention Study: Effects of Base-Line Characteristics and Study Compliance," *Journal of the National Cancer Institute* 88, no. 21 (November, 6, 1996): 1560-70.

2.   R. E. Patterson and D. D. Sears, "Metabolic Effects of Intermittent Fasting," *Annual Review of Nutrition* 37 (August 2017): 371-393, doi:10.1146/annurev-nutr-071816-064634.

3.   F. Wong, "Drug Insight: The Role of Albumin in the Management of Chronic Liver Disease," *Nature Clinical Practice. Gastroenterology & Hepatology* 4, no. 1 (January, 2007): 43-51; and J. Rozga, T. Piątek, and P. Małkowski, "Human Albumin: Old, New, and Emerging Applications," *Annals of Transplantation: Quarterly of the Polish Transplantation Society* 18 (May 10, 2013): 205-17, doi:10.12659/AOT.889188.

4.   R. Yu and H. E. Schellhorn, "Recent Applications of Engineered Animal Antioxidant Deficiency Models in Human Nutrition and Chronic Disease," *Journal of Nutrition* 143, no. 1 (January 2013): 1-11, doi:10.3945 /jn.112.168690.

5.   M. Shin, Y. Han, and K. Ahn, "The Influence of the Time and Temperature of Heat Treatment on the Allergenicity of Egg White Proteins," *Allergy Asthma & Immunology Research* 5, no. 2 (March 2013): 96-101, doi:10.4168 /aair.2013.5.2.96.

6.   M. A. Augustin and P. Udabage, Influence of Processing on Functionality of Milk and Dairy Proteins," *Advances in Food & Nutrition Research* 53, no. 1 (2007): 1-38.

7.   Plutarch, John Langhorne, and William Langhorne, *Plutarch's Lives of Illustrious Men: Translated from the Greek by John Dryden and Others. The Whole Carefully Revised and Corrected*, vol. 1, ed. John Dryden (Ulan Press, June 4, 2011), 659.

8.   Manuel Becana, David A. Dalton, Jose F. Moran, Iñaki Iturbe-Ormaetxe, Manuel A. Matamoros, and Maria C. Rubio, "Reactive Oxygen Species and

Antioxidants in Legume Nodules," *Physiologia Plantarum* 109, no. 4 (August 2000): 372-381, doi:10.1034/j.1399-3054.2000.100402.x.

9.   A. T. Diplock, J. L. Charuleux, G. CrozierWilli, F. J. Kok, C. RiceEvans, M. Roberfroid, W. Stahl, and J. ViñaRibes, "Functional Food Science and Defence Against Reactive Oxidative Species." *British Journal of Nutrition* 80, no. S1 (August 1998): S77S112, doi:10.1079/BJN19980106.

10.   Xin Chen, Rhian M. Touyz, Jeong Bae Park, and Ernesto L. Schiffrin, "Antioxidant Effects of Vitamins C and E Are Associated with Altered Activation of Vascular NADPH Oxidase and Superoxide Dismutase in Stroke-Prone SHR," *Hypertension* 38 (2001): 606-611, doi:10.1161/hy09t1.094005.

11.   L. E. Rikans, C. D. Snowden, and D. R. Moore, "Effect of Aging on Enzymatic Antioxidant Defenses in Rat Liver Mitochondria," *Gerontology* 38, no. 3 (1992): 133-8; and Larry W. Oberley and Garry R. Buettne, "Role of Superoxide Dismutase in Cancer: A Review," *Cancer Research* 39, (1979): 1141-1149.

12.   Frances Sienkiewicz Sizer, Leonard A. Piché, and Eleanor Noss Whitney, *Nutrition: Concepts and Controversies* (Toronto: Nelson Education, 2012), 226; and Paul E. Milbury and Alice C. Richer, *Understanding the Antioxidant Controversy: Scrutinizing the "Fountain of Youth"* (Westport: Praeger, 2008), 65-69.

13.   Jane Higdon, "Coenzyme Q10," Linus Pauling Institute, Oregon State University (February 2003), http://lpi .oregonstate.edu/infocenter/othernuts/coq10/; and A. Kalen, E. L. Appelkvist, and G. Dallner, "Age-Related Changes in the Lipid Compositions of Rat and Human Tissues," *Lipids* 24, no. 7 (1989): 579-584.

14.   Uwe Querfeld and Robert H. Mak, "Vitamin D Deficiency and Toxicity in Chronic Kidney Disease: In Search of the Therapeutic Window," *Pediatric Nephrology* 25 (2010): 2413–243, doi:10.1007500467-010-1574-2; and Lyle Dean MacWilliam, *Nutrisearch Comparative Guide to Nutritional Supplements: A Compendium of Products Available in the United States and Canada*, 4th ed. (Vernon, BC: Northern Dimensions Pub., 2007), 20-26, 48, 62-63, 78.

15.   There are many assays that do not measure the actual level of the vitamin, but measure the functional deficits, i.e., the actual effects of not enough of that vitamin to support our essential energy production in our mitochondria. Since there is a 20 fold range in how much of one vitamin is needed to make one person healthy compared to another person, it is impossible to put a general RDA for everyone. We each have our own unique RDAs for each vitamin. This can be measured several different ways. Genova Diagnostics' NutrEval measures it one way and SpectraCell's SPECTROX™ measures it another. The tests are completely different but complement one another to show functional vitamin deficits and can be found online in the following websites. "NutrEval FMV," Genova Diagnostics, accessed June 23, 2020, https://www.gdx.net/product/nutreval-fmv-nutritional-test-blood-urine and "Micronutrient Test Panel,"

SpectraCell Laboratories, accessed June 23, 2020, https://www.spectracell.com/micronutrient-test-panel.

16. "DRI Tables," United States Department of Agriculture, accessed February 5, 2013, http://fnic.nal.usda.gov /dietary-guidance/dietary-reference-intakes/dri-tables.

17. Lyle Dean MacWilliam, *Nutrisearch Comparative Guide to Nutritional Supplements: A Compendium of Products Available in the United States and Canada*, 4th ed. (Vernon, BC: Northern Dimensions Pub., 2007), 49-64, 78-79, 82.

18. H. Böhm, H. Boeing, J. Hempel, B. Raab, and A. Kroke, "Flavonols, Flavone and Anthocyanins as Natural Antioxidants of Food and their Possible Role in the Prevention of Chronic Diseases," *Deutsches Institut für Ernährungsforschung, Bergholz-Rehbrücke. Zeitschrift fur Ernahrungswissenschaft* 37, no. 2 (1998): 147-163, doi:10.1007/PL00007376.

19. F. C. Küpper, L. J. Carpenter, G. B. McFiggans, et al., "Iodide Accumulation Provides Kelp with an Inorganic Antioxidant Impacting Atmospheric Chemistry," *Proceedings of the National Academy of Sciences of the United States of America* 105, no. 19 (2008): 6954–8, doi:10.1073/pnas.0709959105.

20. P. I. Oteiza, "Zinc and the Modulation of Redox Homeostasis," *Free Radical Biology and Medicine* 53, no. 9 (November 1, 2012): 1748-59, doi:10.1016/j.freeradbiomed.2012.08.568.

21. I. N. Zelko, T. J. Mariani, and R. J. Folz, "Superoxide Dismutase Multigene Family: A Comparison of the Cuzn-Sod (Sod1), Mn-Sod (Sod2), and Ec-Sod (Sod3) Gene Structures, Evolution, and Expression," *Free Radical Biology and Medicine* 33, no. 3 (2003): 337–49, doi:10.1016/S0891-5849(02)00905-X.

22. H. Van Remmen, Y. Ikeno, M. Hamilton, M. Pahlavani, N. Wolf, S. R. Thorpe, N. L. Alderson, J. W. Baynes, C. J. Epstein, T. T. Huang, J. Nelson, R. Strong, and A. Richardson, "Life-Long Reduction in Mnsod Activity Results in Increased DNA Damage and Higher Incidence of Cancer but Does Not Accelerate Aging," *Physiological Genomics* 16, no.1 (December 2003): 29–37, doi:10.1152/physiolgenomics.00122.2003.

23. J. Nève, "Selenium as a 'Nutraceutical:' How To Conciliate Physiological and Supra-Nutritional Effects for an Essential Trace Element," *Current Opinion in Clinical Nutrition and Metabolic Care* 5, no. 6 (November 2002): 659-63; and S. Cavar, Z. Bošnjak, T. Klapec, K. Barišić, I. Cepelak, J. Jurasović, and M. Milić "Blood Selenium, Glutathione Peroxidase Activity and Antioxidant Supplementation of Subjects Exposed to Arsenic Via Drinking Water," *Environmental Toxicology and Pharmacology*, 29, no. 2 (March 2010): 138-43, doi:10.1016/j.etap.2009.12 .008.

24. R. J. Reiter, D. X. Tan, C. Osuna, and E. Gitto, "Actions of Melatonin in the Reduction of Oxidative Stress. A Review," Journal of Biomedical Science 7, no. 6 (November-December 2000): 444-58.

THE HYPE AND HAWKING OF MIRACLE
VITAMINS

1.   "Placebo Effect," Skeptic's Dictionary, last modified July 6, 2012, http://skepdic.com/placebo.html.
2.   Arthur K. Shapiro and Elaine Shapiro, *The Powerful Placebo* (Baltimore: The John Hopkins University Press, 1997), 187; Fabrizio Benedetti, *Placebo Effects*, (New York: Oxford University Press, 2009), 26-32.
3.   Ralph Moss, "A Friendly Skeptic Looks at Mangosteen," CancerDecisions.com Newsletter, accessed February 25, 2012, http://chetday.com/mangosteen.htm.
4.   C. Edward Freeman and Richard D. Worthington, "Is There a Difference in the Sugar Composition of Cultivated Sweet Fruits of Tropical/Subtropical and Temperate Origins?" *Biotropica* 21, no. 3 (September 1989), 219-22.
5.   "Hooked on Juice," Hooked on Juice.com, last modified October 2, 2006, http://www.hookedonjuice.com/.
6.   Yoshio Nagai, Shin Yonemitsu, Derek M. Erion, et al., "The Role of Peroxisome Proliferator-Activated Receptor γ Coactivator-1 β in the Pathogenesis of Fructose-Induced Insulin Resistance," *Cell Metabolism* 9, no. 3 (2009): 252-264, doi:10.1016/j.cmet.2009.01.011.
7.   Robert H. Lustig, Laura A. Schmidt, and Claire D. Brindis, "Public Health: The Toxic Truth About Sugar," *Nature* 482 (February 1, 2012): 27-9, doi:10.1038/482027a; A. A. Bremer, M. Mietus-Snyder, and R. H. Lustig, "Toward a Unifying Hypothesis of Metabolic Syndrome," *Pediatrics* 129, no. 3 (February 20, 2012): 557-70, doi:10.1542/peds.2011-2912; A. A. Bremer and R. H. Lustig, "Effects of Sugar-Sweetened Beverages on Children," *Pediatric Annals* 41, no. 1 (January 2012): 26-30, doi:10.3928/00904481-20111209-09; and Robert Lustig, "Sugar: The Bitter Truth," UCSF's Osher Center for Integrative Medicine, http://www.youtube.com/watch?v=dBnniua6-om.
8.   Scott M. Grundy, H. Bryan Brewer Jr., James I. Cleeman, et al., "Definition of Metabolic Syndrome, Report of the National Heart, Lung, and Blood Institute/American Heart Association Conference on Scientific

Issues Related to Definition," *Circulation* 109 (2004): 433-438, doi:10.1161/01.CIR.0000111245.75752.C6.

9.   S. S. Fakoor Janati, H. R. Beheshti, M. Asadi, S. Mihanparast, and J. Feizy, "Preliminary Survey of Aflatoxins and Ochratoxin A in Dried Fruits from Iran," *Bulletin of Environmental Contamination and Toxicology* 88, no. 3 (March 2012): 391-5, doi:10.1007/s00128-011-0477-7; and J. I. Pitt, J. C. Basílico, M. L. Abarca, and C. López, "Toxigenic Fungi and Mycotoxins," *Medical Mycology* 38, no. 1 (2000): 41-6.

10.   L. E. Rikans, C. D. Snowden, and D. R. Moore, "Effect of Aging on Enzymatic Antioxidant Defenses in Rat Liver Mitochondria," *Gerontology* 38, no. 3 (1992): 133-8.

11.   "NutrEval FMV," Genova Diagnostics, accessed June 23, 2020, https://www.gdx.net/product/nutreval-fmv-nutritional-test-blood-urine and "Micronutrient Test Panel," SpectraCell Laboratories, accessed June 23, 2020, https://www.spectracell.com/micronutrient-test-panel.

12.   Penny M. Kris-Etherton, William S. Harris, and Lawrence J. Appel, "AHA Scientific Statement: Fish Consumption, Fish Oil, Omega-3 Fatty Acids, and Cardiovascular Disease," *Circulation* 106 (2002): 2747-2757, doi:10.1161/01.CIR.0000038493.65177.94; and "The American Heart Association's Diet and Lifestyle Recommendations, The American Heart Association, last modified January, 13, 2014, http://www.heart.org/HEARTORG/GettingHealthy/Diet-and-Lifestyle-Recommendations_UCM_305855_Article.jsp.

13.   J. Thomas Brenna, Norman Salem Jr., Andrew J. Sinclair, and Stephen C. Cunnane, "α-Linolenic Acid Supplementation and Conversion to N-3 Long-Chain Polyunsaturated Fatty Acids in Humans," *Prostaglandins, Leukotrienes and Essential Fatty Acids* 80, no. 2–3 (February–March 2009): 85-91, doi:10.1016/j.plefa.2009.01.004.

14.   S. Mandaşescu, V. Mocanu, A. M. Dăscaliţa, R. Haliga, I. Nestian, P. A. Stitt, and V. Luca, "Flaxseed Supplementation in Hyperlipidemic Patients," *Revista Medico-Chirurgicala a Societatii de Medici si Naturalisti din Iasi* 109, no. 3 (July-September 2005): 502-6.

15.   Katherine Zeratsky, "Nutrition and Healthy Eating: Does Ground Flaxseed Have More Health Benefits Than Whole Flaxseed?," MayoClinic.com, accessed February 25, 2012, http://www.mayoclinic.com/health/flaxseed /AN01258.

16.   G. Ion, K. Fazio, J. A. Akinsete, and W. E. Hardman, "Effects of Canola and Corn Oil Mimetic on Jurkat Cells," Lipids in Health and Disease 10 (2011): 90, doi:10.1186/1476-511X-10-90.

17.   "NutrEval FMV," Genova Diagnostics, accessed June 23, 2020, https://www.gdx.net/product/nutreval-fmv-nutritional-test-blood-urine.

1.   Jennifer 8. Lee, *The Fortune Cookie Chronicles: Adventures in the World of Chinese Food*, (New York: Twelve, 2008), 14; J. R. Gates, B. Parpia, T. C. Campbell, and C. Junshi, "Association of Dietary Factors and Selected Plasma Variables with Sex Hormone-Binding Globulin in Rural Chinese Women," *The American Journal of Clinical Nutrition* 63, no. 1 (1996) 22-31; Sophie Morris, "Use Your Noodle: The Real Chinese Diet Is So Healthy It Could Solve the West's Obesity Crisis," The Independent (July 22, 2008) http://www.independent.co.uk/life-style/health-and-families/healthy-living/use-your-noodle-the-real-chinese-diet-is-so-healthy-it-could-solve-the-wests-obesity-crisis-873651.html; William B. Bateman, Noilyn F. Abesamis, and Henrietta Asjoe, *Praeger Handbook of Asian American Health Taking Notice and Taking Action*, (Santa Barbara: ABC-CLIO, 2009), 692-694; Jessie Satia-Abouta, Ruth E. Patterson, Marian L. Neuhouser, and John Elder, "Dietary Acculturation: Applications to Nutrition Research and Dietetics," *Journal of the American Dietetic Association* 102, no. 8 (August, 1 2002): 1105-1118, doi:10.1016/S0002-8223(02)90247-6); Jessie A. Satia, Ruth E. Patterson, Alan R. Kristal, T.Gregory Hislop, Yutaka Yasui, and Vicky M. Taylor, "Development of Scales to Measure Dietary Acculturation Among Chinese-Americans and Chinese-Canadians," *Journal of the American Dietetic Association* 101, no. 5 (May 1, 2001): 548-553, doi:10 .1016/S0002-8223(01)00137-7; and L. V. Nan and Katherine L. Cason, "Dietary Pattern Change and Acculturation of Chinese Americans in Pennsylvania," *Journal of the American Dietetic Association* 104, no. 5 (May 1, 2004): 771-778, doi:10.1016/j.jada.2004.02.032.
2.   "The Nutrition Source: Food Pyramids and Plates: What Should You Really Eat?" Harvard School of Public Health, accessed February 27, 2012, https://cdn1.sph.harvard.edu/wp-content/uploads/sites/30/2012/10/healthy-eating-pyramid-huds-handouts.pdf.
3.   B. Avery Ince, Ellen J. Anderson, and Robert M. Neer, "Lowering Dietary Protein to U.S. Recommended Dietary Allowance Levels Reduces Urinary Calcium Excretion and Bone Resorption in Young Women," *The Journal of Clinical Endocrinology and Metabolism* 89, no. 8 (August 1, 2004): 3801-3807, doi:10.1210/jc.2003-032016.

4. M. Almon, J. Gonzalez, A. S. Agatston, T. L. Hollar, and D. Hollar, "The Dietary Intervention of the Healthier Options for Public Schoolchildren Study - A School-Based Holistic Nutrition and Healthy Lifestyle Management Program for Elementary-Aged Children," *Journal of the American Dietetic Association* 106, no. 8 (2006): A53.

5. "Even When Eating 1,400 Mg of Calcium Daily, One Can Lose Up To 4% of His or Her Bone Mass Each Year While Consuming a High-Protein Diet," *American Journal of Clinical Nutrition* 32, no. 4 (1979).

6. Diane Feskanich, Walter C. Willett and Graham A. Colditz, "Calcium, Vitamin D, Milk Consumption, and Hip Fractures: A Prospective Study Among Postmenopausal Women," *Journal of Clinical Nutrition* 77, no. 2 (February 2003): 504-511.

7. Diane Feskanich, Walter C Willett, and Graham A. Colditz, "Calcium, Vitamin D, Milk Consumption, And Hip Fractures: A Prospective Study Among Postmenopausal Women," *American Journal of Clinical Nutrition* 77, no. 2 (February 2003), 504-511; D. Feskanich, W. C. Willett, M. J. Stampfer, and G. A. Colditz, "Milk, Dietary Calcium, and Bone Fractures in Women: A 12-Year Prospective Study," *American Journal of Public Health* 87, no. 6 (1997): 992-997; L. H. Allen, E. A. Oddoye, and S. Margen, "Protein-Induced Hypercalciuria: A Longer Term Study, *American Journal of Clinical Nutrition* 32, no. 4 (April 1979): 741-749; Jasminka Z. Ilich and Jane E. Kerstetter, "Nutrition in Bone Health Revisited: A Story Beyond Calcium," *Journal of the American College of Nutrition* 19, no. 6 (2000): 715–737, http://www.jacn.org/content/19/6/715.full; B. J. Abelow, T. R. Holford, K. L. Insogna, "Cross-Cultural Association Between Dietary Animal Protein and Hip Fracture: A Hypothesis," *Calcified Tissue International* 50, no. 1 (1992): 14–18, doi:10.1007/BF00297291; M. Hegsted, S. A. Schuette, M. B. Zemel, and H. M. Linkswiler, "Urinary Calcium and Calcium Balance in Young Men as Affected by Level of Protein and Phosphorus Intake," *The Journal of Nutrition* 111, no. 3 (1981): 553–562; and M. Hegsted, S. A. Schuette, M. B. Zemel, and H. M. Linkswiler, "Urinary Calcium and Calcium Balance in Young Men as Affected by Level of Protein and Phosphorus Intake," *The Journal of Nutrition* 111, no. 3 (1981): 553–562, http://jn.nutrition.org/content/111/3/553.long.

8. Sherry A. Rogers, *You Are What You Ate: An Rx for the Resistant Diseases of the 21st Century* (Syracuse: Prestige Pubs, 1988), 13-15.

1. David I. de Pomerai, Brette Smith, Adam Dawe, Kate North, Tim Smith, David B. Archer, Ian R. Duce, Donald Jones, E. Peter, and M. Candido, "Microwave Radiation Can Alter Protein Conformation Without Bulk Heating," *FEBS Letters* 543, no. 1 (May 2003): 93-97, doi:10.1016/S0014-5793(03)00413-7; Joanna Leszczynska, Agata Łącka, Janusz Szemraj, Jolanta Lukamowicz and Henryk Zegota, "The Effect of Microwave Treatment on the Immunoreactivity of Gliadin and Wheat Flour," *European Food Research and Technology* 217, no. 5 (2003): 387-391, doi:10.1007/s00217-003-0765-5; and Yuichi Funawatashi and Tateyuki Suzuki, "Numerical Analysis of Microwave Heating of a Dielectric," *Asian Research* 32, no. 3 (May 2003): 227 – 236, doi:10.1002/htj.10087.

2. Yves Le Loir, Florence Baron, and Michel Gautier, "Staphylococcus Aureus and Food Poisoning," *Genetics and Molecular Research* 2, no. 1 (2003): 63-76.

3. Diane Feskanich, Walter C. Willett and Graham A. Colditz, "Calcium, Vitamin D, Milk Consumption, and Hip Fractures: A Prospective Study Among Postmenopausal Women," Journal of Clinical Nutrition 77, no. 2 (February 2003): 504-511, http://ajcn.nutrition.org/content/77/2/504.full.

4. D. F. Garcia-Diaz, J. Campion, P. Quintero, and F. I. Milagro, et al., "Vitamin C Modulates the Interaction Between Adipocytes and Macrophages," Molecular Nutrition and Food Research 55, no. 2 (September 2011): S257-63, doi:10.1002/mnfr.201100296.

5. David Servan-Schreiber, *Anticancer: A New Way of Life* (New York: Penguin Books, 2008), 66-84.

6. Ibid., 66-84.

7. Ibid., 66-84.

8. World Health Organization (WHO), *Evaluation of Certain Food Additives and Contaminants: Seventy-Fourth Report of the Joint FAO/WHO Expert Committee on Food Additives* (Sterling, VA: Stylus Publishing, 2012).

9. S. P. Fowler, K. Williams, R. G. Resendez, et al., "Fueling the Obesity Epidemic? Artificially Sweetened Beverage Use and Long-Term Weight Gain," *Obesity (Silver Spring)* 16, no. 8 (August 2008): 1894-900, doi:10.1038/oby.2008.284 and M. C. Borges, M. L. Louzada, T. H. de Sa, et al., "Artificially

Sweetened Beverages and the Response to the Global Obesity Crisis," *PLOS Medicine* 14, no. 1 (2017): e1002195, doi:10.1371/journal.pmed.1002195.

10.   L. B. Link, A. J. Canchola, and L. Bernstein, et al., "Dietary Patterns and Breast Cancer Risk in the California Teachers Study Cohort," American Journal of Clinical Nutrition (October 2013); and "Too Much Sugar Turns Off Gene That Controls Effects Of Sex Steroids," *Child & Family Research Institute* (November 21, 2007).

11.   Katherine Czapp, "Magnificent Magnesium," *Wise Traditions in Food, Farming and the Healing Arts* (September 21, 2010).

12.   Humbart Santillo and Deborah Kantor, Food Enzymes: *The Missing Link to Radiant Health*, 2nd ed. (Prescott: Hohm Press, 1993), 17-25; Hiromi Shinya, *The Enzyme Factor* (San Francisco: Council Oak Books, 2007); and Tom Bohager, *Enzymes: What the Experts Know!: Your Journey to Health and Longevity Starts Here* (Prescott: One World Press, 2006).

13.   Ibid.

14.   G. E. Boeckxstaens and A. Smoot, "Systemic Review: The Role of Acid, Weakly Acidic, and Weakly Alkaline Reflux in Gastroesophageal Reflux Disease," *Alimentary Pharmacology and Therapeutics* 32 (2010): 334.

15.   "Saliva pH Test," AlkalizeforHealth.net, accessed October 13, 2013, http://www.alkalizeforhealth.net/salivaphtest.htm.

16.   "Omega 6 Omega 3 Ratio: How to Compare Omega 6 and Omega 3," WellWise.org, accessed October 17, 2013, http://omega6.wellwise.org/omega-6-omega-3-ratio.

17.   Mahinda Wettasinghe, Fereidoon Shahidi, "Iron (II) Chelation Activity of Extracts of Borage and Evening Primrose Meals," *Food Research International* 35, no. 1 (2002): 65-71; and Anna M. Bakowska-Barczak, Andreas Schieber, and Paul Kolodziejczyk, "Characterization of Canadian Black Currant (Ribes nigrum L.) Seed Oils and Residues, Journal of Agricultural Food and Chemistry 57, no. 24 (2009): 11528–11536, doi:10.1021/jf902161k.

18.   J. Eriksson and A. Kohvakka, "Magnesium and Ascorbic Acid Supplementation in Diabetes Mellitus," Annals of Nutrition & Metabolism 39, no.4 (1995): 217-23; and Ganesh N. Dakhale, Harshal V. Chaudhari, and Meena Shrivastava, "Supplementation of Vitamin C Reduces Blood Glucose and Improves Glycosylated Hemoglobin in Type 2 Diabetes Mellitus: A Randomized, Double-Blind Study," Advances in Pharmacological Sciences 2011, no. 2011 (December 28, 2011), doi:10.1155/2011/195271.

19.   Morando Soffritti, Fiorella Belpoggi, Davide Degli Esposti et al., "First Experimental Demonstration of the Multipotential Carcinogenic Effects of Aspartame Administered in the Feed to Sprague-Dawley Rats," Environmental Health Perspectives 114, no. 3 (March 2006): 379–385, doi:10.1289/ehp.871 and M. C. Borges, M. L. Louzada, T. H. de Sa, et al., "Artificially Sweetened

Beverages and the Response to the Global Obesity Crisis," *PLOS Medicine* 14, no. 1 (2017): e1002195, doi:10.1371/journal.pmed.1002195.

20.   Jane Higdon, "Micronutrient Information Center: Choline," *Linus Pauling Institute*, last modified August 8, 2009, http://lpi.oregonstate.edu/infocenter/othernuts/choline/.

21.   E. Ginter and V. Simko, "New Data on Harmful Effects of Trans-Fatty Acids," *Bratislava Medical Journal* 117, no. 5 (2016): 251-3, doi:10.4149/bll_2016_048.

22.   J. W. Anderson, L. D. Allgood, A. Lawrence, et al., "Cholesterol-Lowering Effects of Psyllium Intake Adjunctive to Diet Therapy in Men and Women with Hypercholesterolemia: Meta-Analysis of 8 Controlled Trials," *American Journal of Clinical Nutrition* 71 (2000): 472-479.

23.   Cheryle Hart and Mary Kay Grossman, *The Insulin-Resistance Diet* (New York: McGraw-Hill, 2007).

24.   Tracy Minkin and Brittani Renaud, "America's Top 5 Healthiest Fast Food Restaurants," Shine Food, last modified October 6, 2010, http://shine.yahoo.com/channel/food/americas-top-5-healthiest-fast-food-restaurants-2397396; Carol Tice, "Which Restaurant Chains Really Have Healthy Food? Consumer Picks Vs. Reality," *Forbes*, last modified October 17, 2014, https://www.forbes.com/sites/caroltice/2014/10/17/which-restaurant-chains-really-have-healthy-food/?sh=3e6cc7a3b099.

25.   "America's Restaurants: Putting Nutrition at the Center of the Plate," National Restaurant Association (2010), 2, http://web.archive.org/web/20120913180352/http://www.restaurant.org/pdfs/nutrition/center_of_the_plate.pdf.

1.   "MSG Basics," The Glutamate Association, last modified 2019, http://www.msgfacts.com/about_glutamate/msg _basics.aspx.
2.   "CFR: Code of Federal Regulations Title 21," U. S. Food and Drug Administration, last modified April 1, 2018, http://www.accessdata.fda.gov/scripts/cdrh/cfdocs/cfcfr/CFRSearch.cfm?fr=101.22.
3.   N. C. Danbolt, "Glutamate Uptake," *Progress in Neurobiology* 65, no. 1 (September 2001): 1-105, doi:10 .1016/S0301-0082(00)00067-8; and France Bellisle, "Glutamate and the UMAMI Taste: Sensory, Metabolic, Nutritional and Behavioural Considerations. A Review of the Literature Published in the Last 10 Years," *Neuroscience & Biobehavioral Reviews* 23, no. 3 (January 1999): 423-438 doi:10.1016/S0149-7634(98)00043-8.
4.   J. Nesic, T. Duka, J. M. Rusted, and A. Jackson, A Role for Glutamate in Subjective Response to Smoking and Its Action on Inhibitory Control," *Psychopharmacology (Berl)* 216, no. 1 (July 2011): 29–42, doi:10.1007/s00213-011-2189-4; and Roger F. Butterworth, Glutamate Transporter and Receptor Function in Disorders of Ammonia Metabolism," *Mental Retardation and Developmental Disabilities Research Reviews* 7, no. 4, (2001): 276–279, doi:10.1002/mrdd.1038.
5.   Zhu Guoqing, Zhong Mingkui, and Zhang Jingxing, "Effects of Microinjection of L-Glutamate and Kainic Acid into Nucleus Amygdalae on Sleep and Wakefulness," *Acta Universitatis Medicinalis Anhui* 4 (1998), http://en .cnki.com.cn/Article_en/CJFDTOTAL-YIKE804.004.htm; LI Shaodan,YANG Ming-hui, and WANG Zhen-fu, et al., "Analysis of the Level of Neurotransmitters of Sub-Healthy People with Insomnia," *Chinese General Practice* 1 (2008), http://en.cnki.com.cn/Article_en/CJFDTOTAL-QKYX200801013.htm.
6.   Sherry Rogers, *Depression Cured at Last!* (Syracuse: Prestige Publishing, 1997).
7.   Bill Misner, "Monosodium Glutamate (Msg), Glutamic Acid (Glutamate), Glutamine Review," Hammernutrition .com, accessed February 29, 2012, http://www.hammernutrition.com/downloads/msg.pdf.

8. "Patentdocs: Senomyx," Faqs.org, accessed July 1, 2013, http://www.faqs.org/patents/assignee/senomyx-inc/.

9. Peggy G. Lemaux, "Genetically Engineered Plants and Foods: A Scientist's Analysis of the Issues (Part I)," *Annual Review of Plant Biology* 59 (2008): 777, http://www.annualreviews.org/doi/pdf/10.1146/annurev.arplant.58 .032806.103840.

10. K. Cankar, M. Ravnikar, J. Zel, K. Gruden, and N. Toplak, "Real-Time Polymerase Chain Reaction Detection of Cauliflower Mosaic Virus to Complement the 35S Screening Assay for Genetically Modified Organisms," *Journal of AOAC International* 88, no. 3 (May-June 2005): 814-22.

11. K. H. Nguyen, S. A. Glantz, C. N. Palmer, and L. A. Schmidt, "Tobacco Industry Involvement in Children's Sugary Drinks Market," *British Medical Journal* 364 (March 14, 2019): l736, doi.10.1136/bmj.l736.

12. Suzanne Havala Hobbs, *Get the Trans Fat Out: 601 Simple Ways to Cut the Trans Fat Out of Any Diet* (New York: Three Rivers Press, 2006), 7.

13. J. Booyens, C. C. Louwrens, and I. E. Katzeff, "The Role of Unnatural Dietary Trans and Cis Unsaturated Fatty Acids in the Epidemiology of Coronary Artery Disease," *Medical Hypotheses* 25, no. 3 (1988): 175–182, doi:10.1016/0306-9877(88)90055-2. PMID 3367809.

14. Ibid., 7.

15. Joel M. Kauffman, *Malignant Medical Myths* (West Conshohocken, PA: Infinity Publishing, 2006); and Uffe Ravnskov, *The Cholesterol Myths: Exposing the Fallacy that Cholesterol and Saturated Fat Cause Heart Disease* (Washington, DC: New Trends Publishing, 2000).

16. Hobbs, *Get the Trans Fat Out*, 21-23.

17. "Frito-Lay Study: Olestra Causes 'Anal Oil Leakage,'" CSPI Press Releases, last modified February 13, 1997, http://www.cspinet.org/new/flaynal.html.

18. K. A. Brooks and J. G. Carter "Overtraining, Exercise, and Adrenal Insufficiency" *Journal of Novel Physiotherapy* 3, no. 125 (February 2013): 11717, doi:10.4172/2165-7025.1000.

19. Alberts B, Johnson A, Lewis J, et al., "How Cells Obtain Energy from Food," chap. 2, *Molecular Biology of the* Cell, 4th ed. (New York: Garland Science, 2002).

20. Riikka Airaksinen, Panu Rantakokko, Johan G. Eriksson, Paul Blomstedt, Eero Kajantie, and Hannu Kiviranta, "Association Between Type 2 Diabetes and Exposure to Persistent Organic Pollutants," *Diabetes Care* 34, no. 9 (September 2011): 1972–1979, doi:10.2337/dc10-2303.

21. Jérôme Ruzzin, "Public Health Concern Behind the Exposure to Persistent Organic Pollutants and the Risk of Metabolic Diseases," *BMC Public Health* 12 (2012): 290, doi:10.1186/1471-2458-12-298.

22. R. J. Jandacek, N. Anderson, M. Liu, S. Zheng, Q. Yang, and P. Tso, "Effects of Yo-Yo Diet, Caloric Restriction, and Olestra on Tissue Distribution

of Hexachlorobenzene." *American Journal of Physiology-Gastrointestinal and Liver Physiology* 288, no. 2 (February 2005): G292-9.

23.   Bernhard Hennig, Adrienne S. Ettinger, Ronald J. Jandacek, Sung Koo, Craig McClain, Harold Seifried, Allen Silverstone, Bruce Watkins, and William A. Suk, "Using Nutrition for Intervention and Prevention Against Environmental Chemical Toxicity and Associated Diseases," *Environmental Health Perspectives* 115, no. 4 (April 2007): 493–495, doi:10.1289/ehp.9549.

24.   Walter J. Crinnion, "The Role of Persistent Organic Pollutants (POPs) in Insulin Resistance, Metabolic Syndrome, and Type 2 Diabetes: Is Atlantic Salmon to Blame?" Lecture at the Medicines from the Earth Conference, June 1-4, 2012.

25.   E. Frankel, A. Bakhouche, J. Lozano-Sánchez II, et. al, "Literature Review on Production Process To Obtain Extra Virgin Olive Oil Enriched in Bioactive Compounds. Potential Use of Byproducts as Alternative Sources of Polyphenols," *Journal of Agricultural and Food Chemistry* 61, no. 22 (May 9, 2013): 5179-5188, doi:10.1021/jf400806z and J. J. Polari, M. Mori, and S. C. Wang, "Virgin Olive Oils from Super-High-Density Orchards in California: Impact of Cultivar, Harvest Time, and Crop Season on Quality and Chemical Composition" *European Journal of Lipid Science and Technology* 123, no. 2000180 (December 15, 2020): doi:10.1002/ejlt.202000180.

26.   Kaayla T. Daniel, *The Whole Soy Story: The Dark Side of America's Favorite Health Food*. (Warsaw, IN: Newtrends Publishing, 2005); Iyekhoetin Matthew Omoruyia, Grit Kabierschb, and Raimo Pohjanvirtaa, "Commercial Processed Food May Have Endocrine-Disrupting Potential: Soy-Based Ingredients Making the Difference," *Food Additives & Contaminants: Part A*, doi:10.1080/19440049.2013.817025; and M. Lefevre, R. P. Mensink, P. M. Kris-Etherton, B. Petersen, K. Smith, and B. D. Flickinger, "Predicted Changes in Fatty Acid Intakes, Plasma Lipids, and Cardiovascular Disease Risk Following Replacement of Trans Fatty Acid-Containing Soybean Oil with Application-Appropriate Alternatives," *Lipids* 47, no. 10 (October 2012): 951-62, doi:10.1007/s11745-012-3705-y.

27.   Russell L. Blaylock, *Excitotoxins: The Taste That Kills* (Albuquerque: Health Press, 1997).

28.   Bart B. Van Bockstaele, "You Are Slowly Poisoning Yourself?," *Health* (June 6, 2007), http:// digitaljournal.com/article/192321/MSG_Are_You_Slowly_Poisoning_Yourself_.

29.   C. Irvine, M. Fitzpatrick, I. Robertson, and D. Woodham, "The Potential Adverse Effects of Soybean Phytoestrogens in Infant Feeding," *New Zealand Medical Journal* 108 (May 24, 1995): 183-4; "Phytoestrogens," Purifymind.com, accessed February 29, 2012, http://www.purifymind.com/Phytoestrogens.htm.

30.   Setchell KD, Zimmer-Nechemias L, Cai J, Heubi JE. (1997) Exposure of phyto-oestrogens from soy-based formula. Lancet 350: 23-7; Tessa Martyn, "Artificial Baby Milks: How Safe Is Soya?," *The Official Journal of the Royal College of Midwives* 6, no. 5 (May 2003): 212-15, http://www.babymilkaction.org/resources/briefings /tessasoya03.html; and Ted Broer, "Does Soy Turn Little Boys Into Little Girls? The Shocking Truth!," Healthmasters.com, last modified April 5, 2010, http://www.healthmasters.com/blog/does-soy-turn-little-boys-little-girls-shocking-truth.

31.   "The Nutrition Source: Shining the Spotlight on Trans Fats," Harvard School of Public Health, http://www.hsph .harvard.edu/nutritionsource/nutrition-news/transfats/.

32.   Colin Ingram, *The Drinking Water Book*, 2nd ed. (Berkeley: Celestial Arts, 2006); and "History: Highbridge: The Bridge," http://www.highbridge-springs.com/history.

33.   Ingram, *The Drinking Water Book*.

34.   "Ferrocyanides in salt for feed use is acceptable as regards safety for target animals and human consumer...," "Opinion of the Scientific Committee for Animal Nutrition on the Safety of Potassium – and Sodium Ferrocyanide Used as Anti-Caking Agents," European Commission: Health and Consumer Protection Directorate-General, last modified December 3, 2001, https://ec.europa.eu/food/sites/food/files/safety/docs/animal-feed_additives_rules_scan-old_report_out70.pdf.

35.   David Brownstein, *Salt Your Way to Health* (West Bloomfield: Medical Alternatives Press, 2006); Jacques De Langre, *Seasalt's Hidden Powers*, 12th ed. (California: Happiness Press, 1993).

36.   David Brownstein, *Salt Your Way to Health* (West Bloomfield, MI: Medical Alternatives Press, 2006).

37.   Peter J. Reeds, "Dispensable and Indispensable Amino Acids for Humans," *The Journal of Nutrition* 130 (2000): 1835S-1840S; and Peter Furst and Peter Stehle, "What Are the Essential Elements Needed for the Determination of Amino Acid Requirements in Humans?" *The Journal of Nutrition* 134 (2004): 1558S-1565S.

38.   Georgina Gustin, "St. Louis Groups Step into Labeling Debate," *St. Louis Post-Dispatch*, June 08, 2012.

39.   J. W. Baynes and P. Gillery, "Frontiers in Research on the Maillard Reaction in Aging and Chronic Disease," *Clinical Chemistry and Laboratory Medicine* 12 (August 2013): 1-3, doi:10.1515/cclm-2013-0551.

40.   G. Sarwar Gilani, C. Wu Xiao, and K. Cockell, "Impact of Antinutritional Factors in Food Proteins on the Digestibility of Protein and the Bioavailability of Amino Acids and on Protein Quality," *British Journal of Nutrition* 108, no. S2 (2012): S315-S332, doi:10.1017/S0007114512002371.

41.   Ibid.
42.   Ibid.
43.   Ibid.
44.   Ibid.
45.   Ibid.
46.   Ibid.
47.   Ibid.
48.   H. F. Erbersdobler and V. Somoza, "Forty Years Of Furosine-Forty Years of Using Maillard Reaction Products as Indicators of the Nutritional Quality of Foods," *Molecular Nutrition and Food Research* 51, no. 4 (April 2007): 423-30.
49.   G. Spano, Biogenic Amines in Fermented Foods, *European Journal of Clinical Nutrition* 64, no. 11 (2010): S95.
50.   R. F. Hurrell and P. A. Finot, "Food Processing and Storage as a Determinant of Protein and Amino Acid Availability," *Experientia. Supplementum.* 44 (1983): 135-56.
51.   H. F. Erbersdobler and A. Hupe, "Determinatio of Lysine Damage and Calculation of Lysine Bio-Availability in Several Processed Foods," *Z Ernahrungswiss* 30, no. 1 (1991): 46-9.
52.   H. F. Erbersdobler, "Protein Reactions During Food Processing and Storage-Their Relevance to Human Nutrition," *Bibliotheca Nutritio et Dieta* 43 (1989): 140-155.
53.   Hurrell, ibid.
54.   H. E. Sauberlich, "Studies on the Toxicity and Antagonism of Amino Acids for Weanling Rats," *Journal of Nutrition* 75 (1961): 61-72.
55.   *Arizona Diet Manual*, Arizona Dietetic Association, Inc. (Arizona Dietetic Association: Phoenix, Arizona, 1992).
56.   H. P. Til, et al., "Acute and Subacute Toxicity of Tyramine, Spermidine, Spermine, Putrescine and Cadaverine in Rats," *Food and Chemical Toxicology* 35, no. 3-4 (March-April 1997): 337-348.
57.   Andrew Stern, "'Pink Slime' Producer Allows Tour of Plant to Bolster Image," *Reuters*, ed. Greg McCune, last modified March 29, 2012.
58.   Ellen Kamhi, *Alternative Medicine Magazine's Definitive Guide to Weight Loss* (Berkeley: Celestial Arts, 2007), 14.
59.   Ibid.
60.   Teodoro Bottiglieri, "S-Adenosyl-L-Methionine (SAMe): From the Bench to the Bedside-Molecular Basis of a Pleiotrophic Molecule," *American Journal of Clinical Nutrition* 76 (2002): 1151S-&S.
61.   Steven Clarke and Kelley Banfield, "S-Adenosylmethionine-Dependent Methyltransferases," chap. 7, *Homocyteine in Health and Disease*, eds. Ralph Carmel and Donald W Jacobsen (Cambridge: Cambridge University Press, 2001), 63-78.

62.   Ehab R. El-Harouna and Dominique P. Bureaub, "Comparison of the Bio-availability of Lysine in Blood Meals of Various Origins to that of L-Lysine HCL for Rainbow Trout (Oncorhynchus Mykiss)," *Aquaculture* 262, no. 2-4 (February, 28 2007): 402–409, doi.10.1016/j.aquaculture.2006.10.032.

63.   Martin Feldman and Gary Null, "Vegetarianism—Part 2: Nutritional Aspects of a Vegetarian Diet," Townsend Letter (August-September, 2011): 74.

64.   Michael W. King, "Amino Acid Metabolism," The Medical Biochemistry Page, accessed May 6, 2013, http://themedicalbiochemistrypage.org/amino-acid-metabolism.php.

65.   L. N. Chen and E. S. Parham, "College Students' Use of High-Intensity Sweeteners Is Not Consistently Associated with Sugar Consumption," *Journal of the American Dietetic Association* 91, no. 6 (June 1991): 686-690.

66.   L. N. Chen, et. al., "College Students' Use of High-Intensity Sweeteners Is Not Consistently Associated with Sugar Consumption," 686-690.

67.   Michael G. Tordoff, and Mark I. Friedman, "Drinking Saccharin Increases Food Intake and Preference—I. Comparison with Other Drinks," *Appetite* 12, no. 1 (February, 1989): 1-10.

68.   Joseph Mercola and Kendra Degen Pearsall, *Sweet Deception: Why Splenda®, Nutrasweet®, and the FDA May Be Hazardous to Your Health* (Nashville: Nelson Books, 2006): 37, 65.

69.   J. W. Olney, L. G. Sharpe, and R. D. Feigin, "Glutamate Induced Brain Damage in Infant Primates,"*Journal of Neuropathology and Experimental Neurology* 31 (1972): 464-88.

70.   J. W. Olney, et al. "Increasing Brain Tumor Rates: Is There a Link to Aspartame?"*Journal of Neuropathology and Experimental Neurology* 55 (1996): 1115-23.

71.   M. Soffritti, F. Belpoggi, D. Degli, et al., "First Experimental Demonstration of the Multipotential Carcinogenic Effects of Aspartame Administered in the Feed to Sprague-Dawley Rats," *Environmental Health Perspective* 114, no. 3 (March 2006): 379-85.

72.   D. Woods, "U.S. Scientists Challenge Approval of Sweetener," *British Medical Journal* 313, no. 7054 (1996): 386.

73.   Joseph Mercola, et. al., Sweet Deception: Why Splenda®, Nutrasweet®, and the FDA May Be Hazardous to Your Health," 74-75.

74.   S. W. Mann and M. M. Yuschak, et al., "A Combined Chronic Toxicity/Carcinogenicity Study of Sucralose in Sprague-Dawley Rats," *Food and Chemical Toxicology* 38, no. 2 (2000): S71-S89, see their other similar study in same Journal S91-7.

75.   Ibid., S71-S89.

76. "FDA Urged to Determine Safe Limits on High-Fructose Corn Syrup and Other Sugars in Soft Drinks," *Center for Science in the Public Interest*, last modified February 13, 2013, http://www.cspinet.org/new/201302131.html.

77. George A. Bray, Samara Joy Nielsen, and Barry M. Popkin, "Consumption of High-Fructose Corn Syrup in Beverages May Play a Role in the Epidemic of Obesity1, 2," *American Society for Clinical Nutrition* 79, no. 4 (April 2004): 537-543.

78. "What Happens to Food in Your Body?" BreastCancer.org, last modified on May 8, 2013, http://www .breastcancer.org/tips/nutrition/healthy_eat/ what_happens.

79. Guenther Boden, "45Obesity, Insulin Resistance and Free Fatty Acids," *Current Opinion in Endocrinology, Diabetes and Obesity* 18, no. 2 (April 2011): 139–143, doi:10.1097/MED.0b013e3283444b09.

80. C. McGartland, P. J. Robson, L. Murray, et al., "Carbonated Soft Drink Consumption and Bone Mineral Density in Adolescence: The Northern Ireland Young Hearts Project," *Journal of Bone and Mineral Research* 18 (2003): 1563-1569 and K. L. Tucker, K. Morita, N. Qiao, et al., "Colas, but not Other Carbonated Beverages, Are Associated with Low Bone Mineral Density in Older Women: The Framingham Osteoporosis Study, *American Journal of Clinical Nutrition* 84 (2006): 936 -942.

81. Veronique Douard, Yves Sabbagh, Jacklyn Lee, et al., "Excessive Fructose Intake Causes 1,25-(OH)2D3-Dependent Inhibition of Intestinal and Renal Calcium Transport in Growing Rats," *American Journal of Physiology-Endocrinology and Metabolism* 304 (April 2013): E1303-E1313, doi:10.1152/ ajpendo.00582.2012.

1.   Undo Erasmus, *Fats that Heal, Fats that Kill* (England: Alive Publishing, 1993), 35.
2.   ALA has to be converted in the body to omega 3 which makes it slightly harder than DHA or EPA for the body to use. "Why Not Flaxseed Oil?" *Harvard Health Publishing*, last modified July 29, 2019, https://www.health.harvard.edu/heart-health/why-not-flaxseed-oil.
3.   "Omega-9 – The Fatty Acids Your Body Makes Itself," Mollers.com, accessed October 16, 2022, https://www.mollers.com/omega-9-the-fatty-acids-your-body-makes-itself/#:~:text=You%20find%20Omega%2D9%20fatty,supplements%20of%20these%20fatty%20acids.
4.   K. C. Hayes and A. Pronczuk, "Replacing Trans Fat: The Argument for Palm Oil with a Cautionary Note on Interesterification," *Journal of the American College of Nutrition* 29, no. 3 (June 2010): 253S-284S.
5.   K. Agrawal, E. Melliou, X. Li, et al., "Oleocanthal-Rich Extra Virgin Olive Oil Demonstrates Acute Anti-Platelet Effects in Healthy Men in a Randomized Trial," *Journal of Functional Foods* 36 (2017): 84-93 and M. Flynn and S. Wang, "Olive Oil as Medicine: The Effect on Blood Pressure," *UC Davis Olive Center* (2015).
6.   E. Frankel, A. Bakhouche, J. Lozano-Sánchez II, et. al, "Literature Review on Production Process To Obtain Extra Virgin Olive Oil Enriched in Bioactive Compounds. Potential Use of Byproducts as Alternative Sources of Polyphenols," *Journal of Agricultural and Food Chemistry* 61, no. 22 (May 9, 2013): 5179-5188, doi:10.1021/jf400806z and J. J. Polari, M. Mori, and S. C. Wang, "Virgin Olive Oils from Super-High-Density Orchards in California: Impact of Cultivar, Harvest Time, and Crop Season on Quality and Chemical Composition" *European Journal of Lipid Science and Technology* 123, no. 2000180 (December 15, 2020): doi:10.1002/ejlt.202000180.
7.   Brown, Simon, and Steven Saunders, *Feng Shui Food* (New York: Lyons Press, 2000), 14.
8.   Jaques de Langre, *Seasalt's Hidden Powers*, 12th ed. (California: Happiness Press, 1993); and Lawrence Wilson, "Sodium and Salt-Eating," The Center for Development, last modified November 2012, http://drlwilson .com/Articles/

salt.htm; and "Health and Nutrition," Soloseasaltusa.com, accessed February 29, 2012, http://www .soloseasaltusa.com/industrial/health-nutrition.asp.

9. David Brownstein, *Salt: Your Way to Health* (Medical Alternatives Press, 2006); and Jacques De Langre, *Seasalt's Hidden Powers* (Happiness Press, 1987).

10. *Introduction to DASH Diet: With One Week Sample Menu and Recipes*, U.S. Department of Health and Human Services, (New York: Fountainhead Publications, 2011).

11. J. M. Jones, "Dietary Fiber Future Directions: Integrating New Definitions and Findings to Inform Nutrition Research and Communication," *Advance in Nutrition* 4, no. 1 (January 1, 2013): 8-15, doi:10.3945/an.112.002907.

12. L. Servillo, A. Giovane, D. Cautela, et al., "Where Does Nε-Trimethyllysine for the Carnitine Biosynthesis in Mammals Come from?" *PLoS One* 9, no. 1 (January 13, 2014): e84589, doi:10.1371/journal.pone.0084589.

13. According Michael W. King, "Lysine is also important as a precursor for the synthesis of carnitine, required for the transport of fatty acids into the mitochondria for oxidation. Free lysine does not serve as the precursor for this reaction, rather the modified lysine found in certain proteins. Some proteins modify lysine to trimethyllysine using SAMe as the methyl donor to transfer methyl groups to the ε-amino of the lysine side chain. Hydrolysis of proteins containing trimethyllysine provides the substrate for the subsequent conversion to carnitine." Michael W. King, "Lysine Catabolism," The Medical Biochemistry Page, accessed May 6, 2013, http://themedicalbiochemistrypage.org/amino-acid-metabolism.php.

14. "What is the Delgado Protocol?," DelgadoProtocol.com, accessed April 15, 2012, http://delgadoprotocol.com /about-us/.

15. Sallie Morris and Leslie Mackley, *Choosing and Using Spices: A Definitive Guide to Spices and Aromatic Ingredients and How to Use Them-with 100 Exciting Recipes* (London: Anness Publishing Limited, 1997), 16.

16. Ibid., 36.

17. Priyanga Ranasinghe and Sanja Perera et al., "Effects of Cinnamomum Zeylanicum (Ceylon Cinnamon) on Blood Glucose and Lipids in a Diabetic and Healthy Rat Mode," *Pharmacognosy Research* 4, no. 2 (April-June 2012): 73–79, doi:10.4103/0974-8490.94719.

18. Robert C. G. Martin, Harini S. Aiyer, and Yan Li, et al., "Effect on Pro-inflammatory and Antioxidant Genes and Bioavailable Distribution of Whole Turmeric vs. Curcumin: Similar Root but Different Effects," *Food Chemical Toxicology* 50, no. 2 (February 2012): 227–231, doi:10.1016/j.fct.2011.10.070.

19. C. M. Lin, J. F. Preston, and C. I. Wei, "Antibacterial Mechanism of Allyl Isothiocyanate," *Journal of Food Protection* 63, no. 6 (June 2000): 727–734.

20. Zaleha Shafiei, Nadia Najwa Shuhairi, Nordiyana Fazly Shah Yap, Carrie-Anne Harry Sibungkil, and Jalifah Latip, "Antibacterial Activity of Myristica

Fragrans Against Oral Pathogens," Evidence Based Complementary and Alternative Medicine (2012): 825362, doi:10.1155/2012/825362.

21.   Muchtaridi, Anas Subarnas, Anton Apriyantono, and Resmi Mustarichie, "Identification of Compounds in the Essential Oil of Nutmeg Seeds (Myristica fragrans Houtt.) That Inhibit Locomotor Activity in Mice," *Internation Journal of Molecular Sciences*, 11, no. 11 (2010): 4771–4781, doi:10.3390/ijms11114771.

22.   Bharat B. Aggarwal, Sahdeo Prasad, et al., "Identification of Novel Anti-inflammatory Agents from Ayurvedic Medicine for Prevention of Chronic Diseases: 'Reverse Pharmacology' and 'Bedside to Bench' Approach," *Current Drug Targets* 12, no. 11 (October 2011): 1595–1653.

23.   S. Selim, "Antimicrobial Activity of Essential Oils Against Vancomycin-Resistant Enterococchi (VRE) and Escherichia Coli O157, H7 in Feta Soft Cheese and Minced Beef Meat," *Brazilian Journal of Microbiology* 42 (2011): 187–196; and Annalisa Lucera, Cristina Costa, Amalia Conte, and Matteo A. Del Nobile, "Food Applications of Natural Antimicrobial Compounds," Frontiers in Microbiology 3 (2012): 287, doi:10.3389/fmicb.2012.00287.

24.   A. Alqareer , A. Alyahya, and L. Andersson, "The Effect of Clove and Benzocaine Versus Placebo as Topical Anesthetics," *Journal of Dentistry* 34, no. 10 (November 2006): 747-50.

25.   "Clean, Safe Spices: Guidance from the American Spice Trade Association," The American Spice Trade Association (Washington, D.C.: ASTA, 2011), 17, http://www.astaspice.org/i4a/pages/index.cfm?pageid=4200.

1.   Barry Sears and Bill Lawren, *The Anti-Aging Zone* (New York: Regan Books, 1999); Barry Sears and Bill Lawren, *The Zone: A Dietary Road Map* (New York: Regan Books, 1995).

2.   Loren Cordain, The Paleo Diet: Lose Weight and Get Healthy by Eating the Food You Were Designed to Eat (New York: J. Wiley, 2002).

3.   Loren Cordain and Joe Friel, *The Paleo Diet for Athletes: A Nutritional Formula for Peak Athletic Performance* (Emmaus, PA: Rodale, 2005); and Mike Carlson, "Get Caveman Big", *Muscle & Body* 4, no. 8 (August 2013): 60-65.

4.   D. Van Camp, N. H. Hooker, and C. T. Lin, "Changes in Fat Contents of US Snack Foods in Response to Mandatory Trans Fat Labelling," *Public Health Nutrition* 15, no. 6 (June 2012): 1130-7, doi:10.1017/S1368980012000079.

5.   Teresa Pearson, "Glucagon as a Treatment of Severe Hypoglycemia: Safe and Efficacious but Underutilized," *The Diabetes Educator* 34, no. 1 (January 2, 2008): 128, doi:10.1177/0145721707312400.

6.   P. E. Cryer, "Symptoms Of Hypoglycemia, Thresholds For Their Occurrence, And Hypoglycemia Unawareness," *Endocrinology and Metabolism Clinics of North America* 28, no. 3 (September 1999): 495-500, v-vi.

7.   "Evolutionary Conservation Of Fat Metabolism Pathways," Nutrition Review.blog, last modified May 23, 2011, http://www.nutritionreview.org/wp/2011/05/evolutionary-conservation-of-fat-metabolism-pathways/; and Biao Wang, Noel Moya, Sherry Niessen, Heather Hoover, Maria M. Mihaylova, Reuben J. Shaw, Yates, et al., "A Hormone-Dependent Module Regulating Energy Balance," *Cell* 145, no. 4 (May 13, 2011): 596-606, doi:10.1016/j.cell.2011.04.013.

8.   R. Giacco, G. Della Pepa, D. Luongo, and G. Riccardi, "Whole Grain Intake in Relation to Body Weight: From Epidemiological Evidence to Clinical Trials," *Nutrition, Metabolism, and Cardiovascular Diseases* 21, no. 12 (December 2011): 901-8, doi:10.1016/j.numecd.2011.07.003; and S. S. Jonnalagadda, L. Harnack, R. H. Liu, N. McKeown, C. Seal, S. Liu , and G. C. Fahey, "Putting the Whole Grain Puzzle Together: Health Benefits Associated with Whole Grains—Summary of American Society for Nutrition 2010 Satellite

Symposium," *The Journal of Nutrition* 141, no. 5 (May 2011): 1011S-22S, doi:10.3945/jn.110.132944.

9.   Thomas S. Wolever and Claudia Bolognesi, "Prediction of Glucose and Insulin Responses of Normal Subjects After Consuming Mixed Meals Varying in Energy, Protein, Fat, Carbohydrate and Glycemic Index," *The Journal of Nutrition* 126 (1996): 2807–2812, http://jn.nutrition.org/content/126/11/2807.full.pdf.

10.   Jette Bertelsen, Christian Christiansen, Claus Thomsen, et al., "Effect of Meal Frequency on Blood Glucose, Insulin, and Free Fatty Acids in NIDDM Subjects," *Diabetes Care* 16, no. 1 (January 1993): 4-7, doi:10.2337/diacare.16.1.4; and J. T. Powell, P. J. Franks, and N. R. Poulter, "Does Nibbling or Grazing Protect the Peripheral Arteries from Atherosclerosis?," *Journal of Cardiovascular Risk* 6 (1999), 19-22.

11.   Barry Sears, and Bill Lawren, *The Zone: A Dietary Road Map* (New York: Regan Books, 1995), 7-10.

12.   Xiaosen Ouyang et al., "Fructose Consumption as a Risk Factor for Non-Alcoholic Fatty Liver Disease," *Journal of Hepatology* 48, no. 6 (June 2008): 993-999, http://dx.doi.org/10.1016/j.jhep.2008.02.011.

13.   Ibid.

14.   Dee McCaffrey, "The Truth about Evaporated Cane Juice, Processed Free America," ProcessFreeAmerica.org, Last modified November 01, 2010, http://www.processedfreeamerica.org/resources/health-news/405-the-truth-about-evaporated-cane-juice.

15.   Regina M. McDevitt, Sally D. Poppitt, Peter R. Murgatroyd, and Andrew M .Prentice, "Macronutrient Disposal During Controlled Overfeeding with Glucose, Fructose, Sucrose, or Fat in Lean and Obese Women," *American Journal of Clinical Nutrition* 72, no. 2 (August 2000): 369-377.

16.   David Mendosa, "GI GL Carb Data," Mendosa.com, accessed August 2013, http://www.mendosa.com/GI_GL_Carb_data.xls.

17.   Jennie Brand-Miller, Kate Marsh, and Nadir R. Farid, *The New Glucose Revolution Guide to Living Well with PCOS* (New York: Marlowe and Company, 2004).

18.   P. A. Davis and W. Yokoyama, "Cinnamon Intake Lowers Fasting Blood Glucose: Meta-Analysis," *Journal of Medicinal Food* 14, no. 9 (September 2011): 884-9, doi:10.1089/jmf.2010.0180.

19.   Richard A. Anderson, Anne-Marie Roussel, Nouri Zouari, Sylvia Mahjoub, Jean-Marc Matheau , and Abdelhamid Kerkeni, "Potential Antioxidant Effects of Zinc and Chromium Supplementation in People with Type 2 Diabetes Mellitus," *Journal of the American College of Nutrition* 20, no. 3 (June 2001): 212-218, http://www.jacn.org/content/20/3/212.full.pdf.

20.   J. A. Nettleton, P. L. Lutsey, Y. Wang, J. A. Lima, E. D. Michos, Dr. Jacobs Jr., "Diet Soda Intake and Risk of Incident Metabolic Syndrome and Type 2 Diabetes in the Multi-Ethnic Study of Atherosclerosis," *Diabetes Care* 32, no. 4 (2009): 688, doi:10.2337/dc08-1799.

21.   Paul Rozin, Kimberly Kabnick, Erin Pete, Claude Fischler, and Christy Shields, "The Ecology Of Eating: Smaller Portion Sizes in France Than in the United States Help Explain the French Paradox," *Psychological Science* 14, no. 5 (September 2003): 450-54, doi:10.1111/1467-9280.02452.

22.   S. S. Fakoor Janati, H. R. Beheshti, M. Asadi, S. Mihanparast, and J. Feizy, "Preliminary Survey of Aflatoxins and Ochratoxin a in Dried Fruits From Iran," *Bulletin of Environmental Contamination and Toxicology* 88, no. 3 (March 2012): 391-5, doi:10.1007/s00128-011-0477-7.

1. Michael Pollan, *The Omnivore's Dilemma: A Natural History of Four Meals* (New York: Penguin Press, 2006), 70-90.

2. Louise E. Lee, Diane Met, Maria Giovanni, and Christine M. Bruhn, "Consumer Knowledge and Handling of Tree Nuts: Food Safety Implications," *Food Protection Trends* 31, no. 1 (2011): 18–27.

3. "Science on the Farm," The University of Waikato, accessed March 1, 2012, http://sci.waikato.ac.nz/farm/content/microbiology.html.

4. E. A. Pastorello, L. Farioli, and A. Conti et al., "Wheat Ige-Mediated Food Allergy in European Patients: Alpha-Amylase Inhibitors, Lipid Transfer Proteins and Low-Molecular-Weight Glutenins. Allergenic Molecules Recognized by Double-Blind, Placebo-Controlled Food Challenge," *International Archives of Allergy and Immunology* 144, no. 1 (2007): 10–22, doi:10.1159/000102609; Isabel Skypala and Carina Venter, *Food Hypersensitivity: Diagnosing and Managing Food Allergies and Intolerance*, (Chichester, U.K.: Wiley-Blackwell Publishing, 2009), 183-202.

5. A. Pusztai, *Plant Lectins* (New York: Cambridge University Press, 1991), 40-70; Mary G. Enig and Sally Fallon, *Nourishing Traditions: The Cookbook that Challenges Politically Correct Nutrition and the Diet Dictocrats*, 2nd ed. (Washington, DC: New Trends Publishing, 2001), 456; and Sandor Ellix Katz and Sally Fallon, *Wild Fermentation: The Flavor, Nutrition, and Craft of Live-Culture Foods* (White River Junction: Chelsea Green Publishing Company, 2003), 7.

6. Katz, *Wild Fermentation*, 5-9.

7. M. Le Gall, A. Serena, H. Jørgensen, P. K. Theil, and K. E. Bach Knudsen, "The Role of Whole-Wheat Grain and Wheat and Rye Ingredients on the Digestion and Fermentation Processes in the Gut—A Model Experiment with Pigs," *The British Journal of Nutrition* 102, no. 11 (December 2009): 1590-600, doi:10.1017/S0007114509990924; and A. M. Stephen, "Whole Grains—Impact Of Consuming Whole Grains on Physiological Effects of Dietary Fiber and Starch," *Critical Reviews in Food, Science, and Nutrition*, 34, no. 5-6 (1994): 499-511, doi:10.1080/104083994095 27677.

8. Katz, *Wild Fermentation*, 5-9.

9.   "Discover the Incredible Health-Promoting Benefits of Kefir," Mercola.com, accessed September 9, 2009, http://www.mercola.com/forms/kefir.htm.

1.   "Foods that Trigger Migraine Headaches," Health and Beyond Online, accessed January 25, 2009, http://www.chetday.com/migrainetriggers.htm.

2.   Cara B. Ebbeling et al., "Childhood Obesity: Public-Health Crisis, Common Sense Cure," *The Lancet* 360, no. 9331 (August 10, 2002): 473–482, http://dx.doi.org/10.1016/S0140-6736(02)09678-2.

3.   Ibid.

4.   Ibid. See figure 2 page 475 for a diagram of the 23 diseases caused by childhood obesity.

5.   Ebbeling, "Childhood Obesity: Public-Health Crisis, Common Sense Cure," 475, Table 2.

6.   Barry M. Popkin, "Global Nutrition Dynamics: The World Is Shifting Rapidly Toward a Diet Linked With Noncommunicable Diseases," *American Journal of Clinical Nutrition* 84, no. 2 (August 2006): 289-298.

7.   "Obesity and Overweight," World Health Organization, last modified April 2020, https://www.who.int/news-room/fact-sheets/detail/obesity-and-overweight.

8.   "Report Finds Obesity Rates Rise in States, Southeastern States Are Heaviest; National Policy Paralysis Threatens to Make Problem Worse," Trust for America's Health, last modified August 23, 2005, http://healthyamericans .org/newsroom/releases/release082305.pdf.

9.   Eleanor West, "Michelle Obama Announces New Food Program," *Food Republic* (last modified July 20, 2011), https://www.foodrepublic.com/2011/07/20/michelle-obama-announces-new-food-program/.

LIFE BEGETS LIFE WHILE ANTI-LIFE DESTROYS ALL LIFE

1.   Michael A. Schmidt, *Beyond Antibiotics: Strategies for Living in a World of Emerging Infections and Antibiotic-Resistant Bacteria* (Berkeley: North Atlantic Books, 2009), 66.

2.   Michael W. King, The Medical Biochemistry Page, last modified November 5, 2012, http:// themedicalbiochemistrypage.org/nerves.html#5ht; M. Berger, J. A. Gray, and B. L. Roth, "The Expanded Biology of Serotonin," *Annual Review of Medicine* 60, (2009): 355–66, doi:10.1146/annurev.med.60.042307.110802.

3.   "Why Is the National U.S. Cesarean Section Rate So High?," Childbirth Connection, accessed February 14, 2009, http://www.childbirthconnection.org/article.asp?ck=10456.

4.   Ibid.

5.   M. T. E. Suller and A. D. Russell, "Triclosan and Antibiotic Resistance in Staphylococcus Aureus," *Journal of Antimicrobial Chemotherapy*, 46, no. 1 (2000): 11-18, doi:10.1093/jac/46.1.11.

6.   M. F. De La Cochetière, T. Durand, P. Lepage, A. Bourreille, J. P. Galmiche, and J. Doré, "Resilience of the Dominant Human Fecal Microbiota upon Short-Course Antibiotic Challenge," *Journal of Clinical Microbiology* 43, no. 1 (November 2005): 5588-5592, doi:10.1128/JCM.43.11.5588-5592.2005.

7.   Dionysios A. Antonopoulos, Susan M. Huse, Hilary G. Morrison, Thomas M. Schmidt, Mitchell L. Sogin, and Vincent B. Young, "Reproducible Community Dynamics of the Gastrointestinal Microbiota Following Antibiotic Perturbation," *Infection and Immunity* 77, no. 2 (June 2009): 10-11, doi:10.1128/IAI.01520-08.

8.   "Comprehensive Digestive Stool Analysis 2.0 (CDSA 2.0), Genova Diagnostics, accessed March 2, 2012, http://www.gdx.net/product/10006.

9.   T. M. Chapman, G. L. Plosker, D. P. Figgitt, "Spotlight on VSL#3 Probiotic Mixture in Chronic Inflammatory Bowel Diseases," *BioDrugs* 21, no. 1, (2007): 61-3; Paolo Gionchetti, Fernando Rizzello, Karen M. Lammers, et al., "Antibiotics and Probiotics in Treatment of Inflammatory Bowel Disease," *World Journal of Gastroenterology* 12, no. 21 (June 2006): 3306-3313; and V. Gupta

and R. Garg, "Probiotics," *Indian Journal of Medical Microbiology* 27, no. 3 (July-September 2009): 202-9, doi:10.4103/0255-0857.53201.

10.   Sherry Rogers, Total Wellness Newsletter (February 2009): 2; F. Castex, G. Corthier, S. Jouvert, G. W. Elmer, F. Lucas, and M. Bastide, Prevention of Clostridium Difficile-Induced Experimental Pseudomembranous Colitis by Saccharomyces Boulardii: A Scanning Electron Microscopic and Microbiological Study," *Journal of General Microbiology* 136, no. 6 (June 1990): 1085-9, doi:10.1099/00221287-136-6-1085.

11.   Martin J. Blaser, "Who Are We? Indigenous Microbes and the Ecology of Human Diseases," *EMBO Reports* 7, no. 10 (2006): 956-960, doi:10.1038/sj.embor.7400812.

12.   M. E. Sanders, D. J. Merenstein, G. Reid, et al., "Probiotics and Prebiotics in Intestinal Health and Disease: From Biology to the Clinic," *Nature Reviews. Gastroenterology & Hepatology* 16, no. 10 (October 2019): 605-616, doi:10.1038/s41575-019-0173-3.

13.   M. Alsan, N. Morden, J. Gottlieb, et al., "Antibiotic Use in Cold and Flu Season and Prescribing Quality: A Retrospective Cohort Study," *Medical Care* 53, no. 12 (December 2015): 1066-71, doi:10.1097/MLR.0000000000000440.

14.   A. Langdon, N. Crook, G. Dantas, "The Effects of Antibiotics on the Microbiome Throughout Development and Alternative Approaches for Therapeutic Modulation," *Genome Medicine* 8, no. 1 (April 2016):39, doi:10.1186/s13073-016-0294-z.

15.   John M. Hickner, John G. Bartlett, Richard E. Besser, et al., "Principles of Appropriate Antibiotic Use for Acute Rhinosinusitis in Adults: Background," *Annals of Internal Medicine* 134, no. 6 (2001): 498-505, doi:10.7326/0003-4819-134-6-200103200-00017.

16.   M. Lawson and A. L. Lawson, "Investigating the Antibiotic Resistance Problem," *The American Biology Teacher* 60, no. 6 (June 1998): 412-417, doi:10.2307/4450512.

17.   Hickner, et al., "Principles of Appropriate Antibiotic Use for Acute Rhinosinusitis in Adults: Background," 498-505.

18.   "Vitamin C and the Common Cold," Linus Pauling Institute, last modified December 2006, http://lpi.oregonstate.edu/ss06/cold.html; Jane Higdon and Victoria J. Drake, "Micronutrient Information Center: Vitamin C," Linus Pauling Institute, last modified November 2009, http://lpi.oregonstate.edu/infocenter/vitamins/vitaminC/; S. Hickey and H. Roberts, "Misleading Information on the Properties of Vitamin C," *Plos Medicine* 2, no. 9 (September 2005): e307, doi:10.1371/journal.pmed.0020307; and R. M. Douglas, H. Hemila, R. D'Souza, E. B. Chalker, and B. Treacy, "Vitamin C for Preventing and Treating the Common Cold," *Cochrane Database of Systematic Reviews* 4 (October 2004), doi:10.1002/14651858.CD000980.pub2.

19.   S. Sasazuki, S. Sasaki, Y. Tsubono, S. Okubo, M. Hayashi, and S. Tsugane, "Effect of Vitamin C on Common Cold: Randomized Controlled Trial," *European Journal of Clinical Nutrition* 60, no. 1 (January 2006): 9-17, doi:10.1038/ sj.ejcn.1602261.

1.   T. S. Eliot, *The Complete Poems and Plays: 1909-1950* (Orlando: Houghton Mifflin Harcourt, 1971), 58.

2.   Sherry Rogers, *Detoxify or Die*, (Sarasota, FL: Sand Key Co., 2002).

3.   "There is ample evidence worldwide to support the notion that food self-sufficiency among peasant communities is an essential prerequisite for their physical well-being." David Barkin, "Mexican Peasant Strategies: Alternatives in the Face of Globalization," accessed May 21, 2011, http://lasa.international.pitt.edu/LASA98/barkin.pdf; David Barkin, Rosemary Batt, and Billie DeWalt, *Food Crops Vs. Feed Crops: The Global Substitution of Grains in Production* (Boulder: Lynne Rienne, 1990).

4.   "Between 1986 and 1995 (figures are available for these years), developed land increased by 222,390 acres. This loss was at the expense of farmland, that decreased by 123,390 acres; forest land, by 44,620 acres; and freshwater wetlands, by 51,860 acres.... New Jersey will likely be the first state to run out of land sometime in the twenty-first century." "Rethinking Farmland Preservation in New Jersey," New Jersey Future, May 2001, http://www.njfuture.org/research-publications/research-reports/rethinking-farmland-preservation-in-new-jersey/.

5.   Edgar Hertwich, ed., "Interim Report IR-02-073 Life-cycle Approaches to Sustainable Consumption Workshop Proceedings," International Institute for Applied Systems Analysis, Laxenburg, Austria, November, 22, 2002, 11-19, accessed August 2013, http://citeseerx.ist.psu.edu/viewdoc/download?doi=10.1.1.203.2531&rep=rep1&type=pdf#page=15.

6.   John Prine "Paradise," JPShrine.org, accessed March 26, 2011, http://www.jpshrine.org/lyrics/songs/jpparadise.html.

7.   Jonathan Swift, "Chapter X" in *Gulliver's Travels* (Mineola, NY: Dover Publications, 2011), 154.

8.   Claudia Luther, Jack Lalanne Dies at 96; Spiritual Father of U.S. Fitness Movement, Los Angeles Times, last updated January 23, 2011, http://articles.latimes.com/2011/jan/23/local/la-me-jack-lalanne-20110124.

9.   John Robbins, "Jack Lalane Dies: Who the Fitness Guru Really Was," The Huffington Post. posted January 24, 2011, http://www.huffingtonpost.com/john-robbins/jack-lalanne-dies-who-the_b_812902.html.

10.   Michael d'Estries, "Jack Lalanne: The First Fitness Superhero," posted January 24, 2011, http://www.mnn.com/health/fitness-well-being/blog9s/jack-lalanne-the-first-fitness-superhero.

11.   S. Wachtel-Galor and I. F. F. Benzie, eds., "Herbal Medicine: An Introduction to Its History, Usage, Regulation, Current Trends, and Research Needs," chap. 1 in *Herbal Medicine: Biomolecular and Clinical Aspects* (Boca Raton: CRC Press, 2011), http://www.ncbi.nlm.nih.gov/books/NBK92773/.

12.   Gregory A. Petsko, "When Failure Should Be the Option," *BMC Biology* 8 (2010): 61, doi:10.1186/1741-7007-8-61; K. Lock, J. Pomerleau, L. Causer, D. R. Altmann, and M. McKee, "The Global Burden of Disease Attributable to Low Consumption of Fruit and Vegetables: Implications for the Global Strategy on Diet," *Bull World Health Organization* 83, no. 2 (February 2005):100-8, doi:10.1590/S0042-96862005000200010; D. J. Newman and G. M. Cragg, "Natural Products as Sources of New Drugs Over the Last 25 Years," Journal of Natural Products 70 (2007): 461–77, doi:10.1021/np068054v; P. Ertl and A. Schuffenhauer, Cheminformatics Analysis of Natural Products: Lessons from Nature Inspiring the Design of New Drugs, *Progress in Drug Research* 66 (2008): 217, 219-35; G.Tan, C. Gyllenhaal, and D. D. Soejarto, "Biodiversity as a Source of Anticancer Drugs," *Current Drug Targets* 7, no. 3 (March 2006): 265-77, doi:10.2174/138945006776054942; and C. Cordier, D. Morton, S. Murrison, A. Nelson, and C. O'Leary-Steele, "Natural Products as an Inspiration in the Diversity-Oriented Synthesis of Bioactive Compound Libraries," *Natural Product Reports* 25, no. 4 (August 2008): 719-37, doi:10.1039/b706296f.

1. James Gleick, *Chaos: Making a New Science* (New York: Penguin Books, 2008).

2. Borut Poljsak, Dušan Šuput, and Irina Milisav, "Achieving the Balance between ROS and Antioxidants: When to Use the Synthetic Antioxidants," *Oxidative Medicine and Cellular Longevity* (2013), http://dx.doi.org /10.1155/ 2013 /956792.

3. Stefan D. Anker, Tuan Peng Chua, Piotr Ponikowski, et al., "Hormonal Changes and Catabolic/Anabolic Imbalance in Chronic Heart Failure and Their Importance for Cardiac Cachexia," *Circulation* 96 (1997): 526-534, doi:10.1161/01.CIR.96.2.526.

4. Jeremy M. Berg, John L. Tymoczko, and Lubert Stryer, "Hemoglobin Transports Oxygen Efficiently by Binding Oxygen Cooperatively," chap. 10, *Biochemistry*, 6th ed., (New York: W. H. Freeman, 2006).

5. Harvinder S. Sandhu, "Osteoporosis: Calcium and Magnesium," *Spine-Universe* (last modified May 11, 2019), https://www.spineuniverse.com/conditions/osteoporosis/osteoporosis-calcium-magnesium.

6. "Dilprit Bagga, Ling Wang, Robin Farias-Eisner, et al., "Differential Effects of Prostaglandin Derived from Ω-6 and Ω-3 Polyunsaturated Fatty Acids on COX-2 Expression and IL-6 Secretion," *Proceedings of the National Academy of Sciences* 100, no. 4 (February 18, 2003) 1751-1756, doi:10.1073/ pnas.0334211100.

7. J. J. DiNicolantonio and J. H. O'Keefe, "Omega-6 Vegetable Oils as a Driver of Coronary Heart Disease: The Oxidized Linoleic Acid Hypothesis," *Open Heart* 5, no. 2 (2018): e000898, doi: 10.1136/openhrt-2018-000898.

WHO WANTS TO EAT LIKE A CAVEMAN?

1. Michael J. Crumb, "World Food Conference Focuses on Subsistence Farming," Associated Press, Lubbock Avalanche-Journal, last modified October 16, 2010, http://lubbockonline.com/agriculture/2010-10-17/world-food-conference-focuses-subsistence-farming.

2. Michael Rabinoff, Nicholas Caskey, Anthony Rissling, et al., "Pharmacological and Chemical Effects of Cigarette Additives," *American Journal of Public Health* 97, no. 11 (November 2007): 1981–1991, doi:10.2105/AJPH.2005.078014.

3. Kelly D. Brownell and Kenneth E. Warner, "The Perils of Ignoring History: Big Tobacco Played Dirty and Millions Died. How Similar Is Big Food?" *The Milbank Quarterly* 87, no. 1 (2009): 259–294.

4. R. D. Mattes and B. M. Popkin, "Nonnutritive Sweetener Consumption in Humans: Effects on Appetite and Food Intake and Their Putative Mechanisms," *American Journal of Clinical Nutrition* 89, no. 1 (January 2009): 1-14; P. Dominguez-Salas, S. E. Cox, A. M. Prentice, et al., Maternal Nutritional Status, C(1) Metabolism and Offspring DNA Methylation: A Review of Current Evidence in Human Subjects," *The Proceedings of the Nutrition Society* 71, no. 1 (February 2012): 154-65, doi:10.1017/S0029665111003338.

5. David J. P. Barker, "The Malnourished Baby and Infant Relationship with Type 2 Diabetes, *British Medical Bulletin* 60, no. 1 (2001): 69-88, doi:10.1093/bmb/60.1.69.

6. V. Roos, M. Rönn, S. Salihovic, et al., "Circulating Levels of Persistent Organic Pollutants in Relation to Visceral and Subcutaneous Adipose Tissue by Abdominal MRI," *Obesity (Silver Spring)* 21, no. 2 (February 2013): 413-8, doi:10.1002/oby.20267.

7. Natasha Turner, *The Hormone Diet: Lose Fat. Gain Strength. Live Younger Longer* (New York: Rodale, 2009), 171, 361, 403.

8. Ünüvar Tolga, "Fetal and Neonatal Endocrine Disruptors," *Journal of Clinical Research in Pediatric Endocrinology* 4, no. 2 (June 2012): doi:10.4274/Jcrpe.569.

9. D. K. Li, Z. Zhou, M. Miao, et al., "Urine Bisphenol-A (BPA) Level in Relation to Semen Quality," *Fertility and Sterility* 95, no. 2 (February 2011):

625-30, doi:10.1016/j.fertnstert.2010.09.026; Lang IA, et al. "Association of Urinary Bisphenol A Concentration with Medical Disorders and Loratory Abnormalities in Adults," *Journal of the American Medical Association* 300, no. 11 (September, 17, 2008): 1303-10.

10. Turner, *The Hormone Diet*, 403.

11. "Organic Musts," InspirationGreen.com, http://www.inspirationgreen.com/ food-organic-choices.

12. Theo Stein and Miles Moffeit, "Mutant Fish Prompt Concern—Study Focuses on Sewage Plants," *Jersey Coast Anglers Association Newsletter*, (November 2004), http://www.jcaa.org/jcnl0411/MutantFish.htm.

13. Stein and Moffeit, "Mutant Fish Prompt Concern."

14. C. Desbrow, E. J. Routledge , G. C. Brighty, et al., "Identification of Estrogenic Chemicals in STW Effluent. 1. Chemical Fractionation and in Vitro Biological Screening," *Environmental Science and Technology* 32, no. 11 (1998): 1549–1558, doi:10.1021/es9707973.

15. D. K. Li, et al., "Urine Bisphenol-A (BPA) Level in Relation to Semen Quality," 625-30; Turner, *The Hormone Diet: Lose Fat. Gain Strength. Live Younger Longer*, 77-109.

16. "The Nutrition Source: Fats and Cholesterol: Out with the Bad, In with the Good," Harvard School of Public Health, http://www.hsph.harvard.edu/ nutritionsource/fats-full-story/; and Melinda Wenner Moyer, "Carbs against Cardio: More Evidence that Refined Carbohydrates, not Fats, Threaten the Heart," *Scientific American* (May 2010), http://www.scientificamerican.com/ sciammag/?contents=2010-05.

17. Dr. Mercola, "Avoid This if You Want to Keep Your Thyroid Healthy," Mercola.com, Last modified September 05, 2009, http://articles.mercola.com/sites/articles/archive/2009/09/05/another-poison-hiding-in-your-environment.aspx.

18. J. Eisenstein, S. B. Roberts, G. Dallal, et al., "High-Protein Weight-Loss Diets: Are They Safe and Do They Work? A Review of the Experimental and Epidemiologic Data," *Nutrition Reviews* 60, no. 7 (July 2002): 189-200, http://dx.doi.org/10.1301/00296640260184264.

19. D. J. Pattison, D. P. Symmons, M. Lunt, et al., "Dietary Risk Factors for the Development of Inflammatory Polyarthritis: Evidence for a Role of High Level of Red Meat Consumption," *Arthritis & Rheumatism* 50, no. 12 (December 2004): 3804–3812, http://dx.doi.org/10.1002/art.20731.

20. Alan E. Norrish, Lynnette R. Ferguson, Mark G. Knize, et al., "Heterocyclic Amine Content of Cooked Meat and Risk of Prostate Cancer," Journal of the National Cancer Institute 91, no. 23 (1999): 2038-2044, doi:10.1093/jnci/ 91.23.2038.

21.   Kristin E. Anderson, Rashmi Sinha, Martin Kulldorff, et al., "Meat Intake And Cooking Techniques: Associations with Pancreatic Cancer," *Mutation Research/Fundamental and Molecular Mechanisms of Mutagenesis* 506–507 (September, 30 2002): 225-231, http://dx.doi.org/10.1016/S0027-5107(02)00169-0.

22.   Ai Kubo, T. R. Levin, Gladys Block, et al., "Dietary Patterns and the Risk of Barrett's Esophagus," *American Journal of Epidemiology* 167, no. 7 (2008): 839-846, doi:10.1093/aje/kwm381.

23.   "Side Effects of Antacids and Acid Blockers," RefluxDefense.com, accessed January 18, 2014, http://refluxdefense.com/heartburn_GERD_articles/side-effects-antacids-and-acid-blockers.html.

24.   B. S. Reddy, S. Mangat, J. H. Weisburger, et al., "Effect of High-Risk Diets for Colon Carcinogenesis on Intestinal Mucosal and Bacterial Beta-Glucuronidase Activity in F344 Rats," *Cancer Research* 37, no. 10 (October 1977): 3533-6.

25.   Mark Bittman, "Rethinking the Meat-Guzzler," *The New York Times* (January 27, 2008), http://www.nytimes .com/2008/01/27/weekinreview/27bittman.html?pagewanted=all&_r=0.

26.   J. R. Crawford and D. Say, "Vitamin B12 Deficiency Presenting as Acute Ataxia," *BMJ Case Reports* 2013 (March 26, 2013): pii, doi:10.1136/bcr-2013-008840.

27.   Mayo Clinic Staff, "Mediterranean Diet: A Heart-Healthy Eating Plan," *Mayo Clinic* (June 14, 2013) http://www.mayoclinic.org/mediterranean-diet/art-20047801; and V. Demarin, M. Lisak, and S. Morović, "Mediterranean Diet in Healthy Lifestyle and Prevention of Stroke," *Acta Clinica Croatica* 50, no. 1 (March 2011): 67-77.

28.   B. C. Pereira, J. R. Pauli, C. T. Souza, et al., "Eccentric Exercise Leads to Performance Decrease and Insulin Signaling Impairment," *Medicine and Science in Sports and Exercise* (August 30, 2013); and A. C. Hackney, K. J. Koltun, "The Immune System and Overtraining in Athletes: Clinical Implications," *Acta Clinica Croatica* 51, no. 4 (December 2012): 633-41.

29.   K. A. Brooks and J. G. Carter, Overtraining, Exercise, and Adrenal Insufficiency," *Journal of Novel Physiotherapies* 3, no. 125 (February 16, 2013): 11717, doi:10.4172/2165-7025.1000125; and A. Urhausen, H. Gabriel, and W. Kindermann, "Blood Hormones as Markers of Training Stress and Overtraining, *Sports Medicine* 20, no. 4 (October 1995): 251-76.

30.   E. Fosslien, "Cancer Morphogenesis: Role of Mitochondrial Failure," Annals of Clinical and Laboratory Science 38, no. 4 (2008): 307-29.

31.   K. A. Brooks and J. G. Carter, Overtraining, Exercise, and Adrenal Insufficiency," Journal of Novel Physiotherapies 3, no. 125 (February 16, 2013): 11717, doi:10.4172/2165-7025.1000125; and A. Urhausen, H. Gabriel, and W. Kindermann, "Blood Hormones as Markers of Training Stress and Overtraining, Sports Medicine 20, no. 4 (October 1995): 251-76.

32.   Harriet V. Kuhnlein and Nancy J. Turner, "Descriptions and Uses of Plant Foods by Indigenous Peoples," chap. 4 in *Traditional Plant Foods of Canadian Indigenous Peoples: Nutrition, Botany and Use* (Amsterdam: Overseas Publishers Association, 1991).

33.   A. P. Hills, N. M. Byrne, and R. Lindstrom, "'Small Changes' to Diet and Physical Activity Behaviors for Weight Management," *Obesity Facts* 6, no. 3 (2013): 228-38, doi:10.1159/000345030.

34.   "The American Heart Association's Diet and Lifestyle Recommendations, The American Heart Association, last modified January, 13, 2014, http://www.heart.org/HEARTORG/GettingHealthy/Diet-and-Lifestyle-Recommendations_UCM_305855_Article.jsp.

35.   "Create Your Plate," American Diabetes Association, last modified January 2, 2014, http://www.diabetes.org/food-and-fitness/food/planning-meals/create-your-plate/.

36.   "Shopping List: Basic Ingredients for a Healthy Kitchen," American Cancer Society, last modified July, 9, 2013, http://www.cancer.org/healthy/eathealthyge-tactive/eathealthy/shopping-list-basic-ingredients-for-a-healthy-kitchen.

THE MONTE CARLO DIET: BUT THE HOUSE
ALWAYS WINS

1. M. Lenoir, F. Serre, L. Cantin, and S. H. Ahmed, "Intense Sweetness Surpasses Cocaine Reward," *Plos One* 2, no. 8 (2007): e698, doi:10.1371/journal.pone.0000698.

2. S. L. Parylak, G. F. Koob, and E. P. Zorrilla, "The Dark Side of Food Addiction," *Physiology & Behavior* 104, no. 1, (July, 25, 2011): 149-56, doi:10.1016/j.physbeh.2011.04.063.

3. A. Iemolo, M. Valenza, L. Tozier, et al., "Withdrawal from Chronic, Intermittent Access to a Highly Palatable Food Induces Depressive-Like Behavior in Compulsive Eating Rats," Behavioral Pharmacology 23, no. 5-6 (September 2012): 593-602, doi:10.1097/FBP.0b013e328357697f.

4. Elizabeth A. Smith and Ruth E. Malone, "Altria Means Tobacco: Philip Morris's Identity Crisis," *American Journal of Public Health* 93, no. 4 (April 2003): 553–556; "Boycott Tobacco-Company Owned Products," Medicolegal, last modified June 2001, http://medicolegal.tripod.com/boycott.htm.

5. This reference contains several hundred food additives with the toxic ones highlighted and the side effects noted. "Food Additives 'E' Numbers," Cure-Zone.org, accessed August 2013, http://curezone.com/foods/enumbers.asp.

6. M. Stefanidou, G. Alevisopoulos, A. Chatziioannou, et al., "Assessing Food Additive Toxicity Using a Cell Model," Veterinary & Human Toxicology 45, no. 2 (March 2003): 103-5.

7. 86% celebrate with family and 51% celebrate at home. Julie Ray "The Gallup Brain: Americans and Thanksgiving," Gallup.com, last modified November 26, 2002, http://www.gallup.com/poll/7291/Gallup-Brain-Americans-Thanksgiving.aspx.

8. Philippa Ellwood, M. Innes Asher, Luis García-Marcos, et al., "Do Fast Foods Cause Asthma, Rhinoconjunctivitis and Eczema? Global findings from the International Study of Asthma and Allergies in Childhood (ISAAC) Phase Three," *Thorax* 68, no. 4 (2013): 351-360, doi:10.1136/thoraxjnl-2012-202285.

9. "Lymphoma: Nutritional Considerations," NutritionMD.org, accessed August 2013, http://www.nutritionmd.org/consumers/oncology/lymphoma_nutrition.html.

10. John E. Huxsahl, "ADHD Diet: Do Food Additives Cause Hyperactivity? What Does the Research Say about the Relationship Between Food Additives and ADHD?" MayoClinic.org, accessed Aug 2013, http://www.mayoclinic.com/health/adhd/AN01721.

11. Lisa Baertlein, "California County Wants to Ban Toys in Kids' Meals, Reuters.com, last modified Apr 27, 2010, http://www.reuters.com/article/2010/04/27/us-obesity-toys-idUSTRE63Q5RJ20100427.

12. *Super-Size Me*, directed by Morgan Spurlock (United States, Kathbur Pictures, 2004), DVD.

13. Mahshid Dehghan, Noori Akhtar-Danesh, and Anwar T. Merchant, "Childhood Obesity, Prevalence and Prevention," *Nutrition Journal* 4, no. 24 (2005), doi:10.1186/1475-2891-4-24.

14. Rita Mae, *Sudden Death* (New York: Bantam, 1984), 68.

15. "Insanity is repeating the same mistakes and expecting different results." *Basic Text of Narcotics Anonymous* 6th ed., Narcotics Anonymous (November 1981): 23.

16. This is derived from the written works of Hippocrates and is not worded exactly the same, yet follows in the same vein. Hippocrates and Emerson Crosby Kelly, Francis Adams, and Emerson Crosby Kelly, *The Genuine Works of Hippocrates*, trans. Francis Adams (Whitefish, MT: Kessinger Publishing), 3.

1.   R. D. McCracken, "Lactase Deficiency: An Example of Dietary Evolution," *Current Anthropology* 12, no. 4/5, (October-December, 1971): 479-517.

2.   Tim Kenny, "Gastroenteritis in Children," Patient.co.uk, last modified November, 17, 2012, http://www.patient.co.uk/health/gastroenteritis-in-children; and "Review: Could the Flu Cause Lactase Deficiency?" eHealthme.com, accessed August 2013, http://www.ehealthme.com/cs/the+flu/lactase+deficiency.

3.   Joseph M. Miller, Irving Freeman, and William H. Heath, "Calcinosis Due to Treatment of Duodenal Ulcer," *JAMA* 148, no. 3 (1952): 198-199, doi:10.1001/jama.1952.62930030003009a.

4.   L. E. Targownik, L. M. Lix, C. J. Metge, et al., "Use of Proton Pump Inhibitors and Risk of Osteoporosis-Related Fractures," *Canadian Medical Association Journal*, 179, no. 4 (August, 12, 2008): 319-26. doi:10.1503/cmaj.071330.

5.   Will Brink, "New Longevity Benefits of Whey Protein," *Life Extension Magazine* (September 2013), http://www.lef.org/magazine/mag2013/sep2013_New-Longevity-Benefits-of-Whey-Protein_01.htm; and L. S. Mortensen, M. L. Hartvigsen, L. J. Broader, et al., "Differential Effects of Protein Quality on Postprandial Lipemia in Response to a Fat-Rich Meal in Type 2 Diabetes: Comparison of Whey, Casein, Gluten, and Cod Protein," *American Journal of Clinical Nutrition* 90, no. 1 (July 2009): 41-8, doi:10.3945/ajcn.2008.27281.

6.   Jay R. Hoffman and Michael J. Falvo, "Protein—Which Is Best?" *Journal of Sports Science and Medicine* 3 (2004): 118-130.

7.   S.G. Srikantia, "The Use Of Biological Value Of A Protein In Evaluating Its Quality For Human Requirements," *Joint FAO/WHO/UNU Expert Consultation on Energy and Protein Requirements* (Rome: October 5-17, 1981) accessed August 2013, http://www.fao.org/docrep/meeting/004/m2835e/m2835e00.htm.

8.   Many research studies say that whey reduces overall metabolic syndrome parameters while one recent one with a small cohort size suggests it may spike insulin levels which, in an athlete, would be a good thing to store nutrients in muscles depleted of them by exercise. G.I. Smith, J. Yoshino, K.L. Stromsdorfer, et al., "Protein Ingestion Induces Muscle Insulin Resistance Independent of Leucine-Mediated Mtor Activation," *Diabetes* 64, no. 5 (May

2015): 1555-63, doi:10.2337/db14-1279. Epub 2014 Dec 4; G.T.D. Sousa, F.S. Lira, J.C. Rosa, et al., "Dietary Whey Protein Lessens Several Risk Factors for Metabolic Diseases: A Review," *Lipids in Health and Disease* 11, no. 67 (July 10, 2012): doi:10.1186/1476-511X-11-67; and F. K. Haraguchi, M. L. Pedrosa, and H. D. Paula, et al., "Evaluation of Biological and Biochemical Quality of Whey Protein," *Journal of Medicinal Food* 13, no. 6 (December 2010): 1505-9, doi:10.1089/jmf.2009.0222.

9. J.L. Frestedt, J.L. Zenk, M.A. Kuskowski, et al., "A Whey-Protein Supplement Increases Fat Loss and Spares Lean Muscle in Obese Subjects: A Randomized Human Clinical Study," *Nutrition & Metabolism* 5, no. 8 (2008), doi:10.1186/1743-7075-5-8.

10. T. S. Sathyanarayana Rao, M. R. Asha, K. S. Jagannatha Rao, et al., "Understanding Nutrition, Depression And Mental Illnesses," *Indian Journal of Psychiatry* 50, no. 2 (April-June 2008): 77-82; and Séverin Sindayikengera and Wen-shui Xia, "Nutritional Evaluation of Caseins and Whey Proteins and their Hydrolysates from Protamex," *Journal of Zhejiang University Science B* 7, no. 2 (February 2006): 90-98.

11. Michael McEvoy, "Raw Dairy Is a Nutritional Powerhouse: Pasteurized Dairy Is Dead," MetabolicHealing.com, last modified December 11, 2011, http://metabolichealing.com/raw-dairy-is-a-nutritional-powerhouse-pasteurized-dairy-is-dead/.

12. "General Properties of Casein," Sigmaaldrech.com, accessed November 24, 2012, http://www.sigmaaldrich.com/life-science/metabolomics/enzyme-explorer/enzyme-reagents/casein.html.

13. R. Nagpala, P. V. Behareb, M. Kumarb, et al., "Milk, Milk Products, and Disease Free Health: An Updated Overview," *Critical Reviews in Food Science and Nutrition* 52, no. 4 (2012): 321-33, doi:10.1080/10408398.2010.500231]pages 321-333.

14. McEvoy, "Raw Dairy Is a Nutritional Powerhouse."

15. Mike Hughlett, "General Mills Sued over Whether Yoplait Greek Yogurt Is Yogurt," *Star Tribune*, last modified July 12, 2012, http://www.startribune.com/business/162301436.html.

16. Stacey J. Bell, Gregory T. Grochoskib, and Andrew J. Clarkec, "Health Implications of Milk Containing β-Casein with the A2 Genetic Variant," *Critical Reviews in Food Science and Nutrition* 46, no. 1 (2006): 93-100, doi:10.1080/10408390591001144.

17. S. Kamiński, A. Cieslińska, and E. Kostyra, "Polymorphism of Bovine Beta-Casein and Its Potential Effect on Human Health," *Journal of Applied Genetics* 48, no. 3 (2007): 189-98.

18. "General Properties of Casein," Sigmaaldrech.com, access November 24, 2012, http://www.sigmaaldrich.com/life-science/metabolomics/enzyme-explorer/enzyme-reagents/casein.html.

19. S. Benedé, I. López-Expósito, G. Giménez, et al., "In Vitro Digestibility of Bovine B-Casein with Simulated and Human Oral and Gastrointestinal Fluids. Identification and Ige-Reactivity of the Resultant Peptides," *Food Chemistry* 143 (January 15, 2014): 514-21, doi:10.1016/j.foodchem.2013.07.110.

20. Robert Walter Henningson, *Factors Affecting the Germicidal Property of Raw Milk* (New York: Cornell University Press, 1956), 34.

21. Bennett Anthony, and James Edge, *Benefits and Potential Risks of the Lacto-peroxidase System of Raw Milk Preservation: Report of an FAO/WHO Technical Meeting, FAO Headquarters, Rome,* (Rome: Food and Agriculture Organization of the United Nations, 2006), 28, http://www.fao.org/3/a-a0729e.pdf.

1.   Appleton, *Lick the Sugar Habit*, 69.

2.   Kathleen DesMaisons, *The Sugar Addict's Total Recovery Program* (New York: Ballantine Books, 2000), 25.

3.   Michael Murray and Michael Lyons, *How To Prevent And Treat Diabetes With Natural Medicine* (New York: Riverhead Trade, 2004), 16-17.

4.   Carol Simontacchi, *The Crazy Makers: How the Food Industry Is Destroying Our Brains and Harming Our Children* (Los Angeles: Tarcher, 2007), 195-96.

5.   Nancy Appleton, *Lick the Sugar Habit* (New York: Avery Trade, 1988), 141.

6.   Connie Bennett and Stephen T. Sinatra, *Sugar Shock!: How Sweets and Simple Carbs Can Derail Your Life* (New York: Berkley Trade, 2006), 177.

7.   Ibid., 42, 151, 160, 166.

8.   Metin Basaranoglu, Gokcen Basaranoglu, Tevfik Sabuncu, and Hakan Sentürk, "Fructose as a Key Player in the Development of Fatty Liver Disease," *World Journal of Gastroenterology* 19, no. 8 (February 28, 2013): 1166–72, doi:10.3748/wjg.v19.i8.1166.

9.   Laura P. Musselman, Jill L. Fink, Kirk Narzinski, Prasanna V. Ramachandran, Sumitha S. Hathiramani, Ross L. Cagan, and Thomas J. Baranski, "A High-Sugar Diet Produces Obesity and Insulin Resistance in Wild-Type Drosophila," *Disease Models and Mechanisms* 4, no. 6 (November 2011): 842–849, doi:10.1242/dmm.007948.

10.   Fabrice Bonnet, Pierre-Henri Ducluzeau, Amalia Gastaldelli, Martine Laville, Christian H. Anderwald, Thomas Konrad, Andrea Mari, Beverley Balkau, and for the RISC Study Group, "Liver Enzymes Are Associated With Hepatic Insulin Resistance, Insulin Secretion, and Glucagon Concentration in Healthy Men and Women," *Diabetes* 60, no. 6 (June 2011): 1660-67, doi:10.2337/db10-1806.

11.   Michael Murray and Michael Lyons, *How To Prevent And Treat Diabetes With Natural Medicine* (New York: Riverhead Trade, 2004), 16, 138, and 233.

12.   Ibid., 16, 31, 127, 197-203; Deepashree Gupta, Charles B. Krueger, and Guido Lastra, "Over-nutrition, Obesity and Insulin Resistance in the Development of β-Cell Dysfunction," *Current Diabetes Reviews* 8, no. 2 (March 2012): 76-83, doi:10.2174/157339912799424564.

13.   Ibid.

14.   A. Tajaddini, D. L. Kilpatrick, P. Schoenhagen, E. M. Tuzcu, M. Lieber, and D. G. Vince, "Impact of Age and Hyperglycemia on the Mechanical Behavior of Intact Human Coronary Arteries: An Ex Vivo Intravascular Ultrasound Study," *American Journal of Physiology Heart and Circulatory Physiology* 288, no. 1 (January 2005): H250-5, doi:10.1152/ajpheart.00646.2004.

15.   "The Dropping Well, Knaresborough, North Yorkshire," The Journal of Antiquities, last modified March 20, 2013, http://thejournalofantiquities.com/2013/03/20/the-dropping-well-knaresborough-north-yorkshire/.

16.   J. Uribarri, S. Woodruff, S. Goodman, W. Cai, X. Chen, R. Pyzik, A.Yong, G. E. Striker, and H. Vlassara, "Advanced Glycation End Products in Foods and a Practical Guide to Their Reduction in the Diet," *Journal of the American Diet Association* 110, no. 6 (June 2010): 911-16, doi:10.1016/j.jada.2010.03.018; Melpomeni Peppa, Jaime Uribarri, and Helen Vlassara, "Glucose, Advanced Glycation End Products, and Diabetes Complications: What Is New and What Works," *Clinical Diabetes* 21, no. 4 (October 2003): 186-7, doi:10.2337/diaclin.21.4.186; and Kazuhiro Sugimoto, Minoru Yasujima, and Soroku Yagihashi, "Role of Advanced Glycation End Products in Diabetic Neuropathy," *Current Pharmaceutical Design* 14, no. 10 (2008): 953-961, doi:10.2174/138161208784139774.

17.   Steven V. Joyal, *What Your Doctor May Not Tell You About Diabetes: An Innovative Program to Prevent, Treat, and Beat This Controllable Disease* (New York: Grand Central Life & Style, 2008).

18.   C. H. Wilder-Smith, A. Materna, C. Wermelinger, and J. Schuler, "Fructose and Lactose Intolerance and Malabsorption Testing: The Relationship with Symptoms in Functional Gastrointestinal Disorders," *Alimentary Pharmacology & Therapeutics* 39, epublication ahead of print (April 9, 2013), doi:10.1111/apt.12306.

19.   Lawrence Wilson, "Sugar Addiction," last modified January 2010, www.drl-wilson.com/articles/SUGAR%20ADDICTION.htm.

20.   "Digestive Disorders," Total Health Institute, accessed April 27, 2013, http://www.totalhealthinstitute.com/digestive-disorders/.

21.   Joseph Mercola, "The First Thing to Do When a Cold or Flu Strikes," Mercola.com, last updated November 13, 2011, https://articles.mercola.com/sites/articles/archive/2011/11/13/could-a-cup-or-more-of-this-a-day-keep-the-flu-away.aspx.

22.   L. Chen, R. H. Jia, C. J. Qiu, and G. Ding, "Hyperglycemia Inhibits the Uptake Of Dehydroascorbate in Tubular Epithelial Cell," *American Journal of Nephrology* 25, no. 5 (September-October 2005): 459-65, doi:10.1159/000087853; and Cherie Calbom and John Calbom, *The Coconut Diet: The Secret Ingredient*

That Helps You Lose Weight While You Eat Your Favorite Foods (New York: Grand Central Life & Style, 2006), 22.

23.   J. Eriksson and A. Kohvakka, "Magnesium and Ascorbic Acid Supplementation in Diabetes Mellitus," *Annals of Nutrition & Metabolism* 39, no.4 (1995): 217-23; and Ganesh N. Dakhale, Harshal V. Chaudhari, and Meena Shrivastava, "Supplementation of Vitamin C Reduces Blood Glucose and Improves Glycosylated Hemoglobin in Type 2 Diabetes Mellitus: A Randomized, Double-Blind Study," *Advances in Pharmacological Sciences* 2011, no. 2011 (December 28, 2011), doi:10.1155/2011/195271.

24.   Loren Cordain, *The Paleo Diet Revised: Lose Weight and Get Healthy by Eating the Foods You Were Designed to Eat* (New Jersey: John Wiley & Sons, 2011).

25.   Loren Cordain, "Getting Started with the Paleo Diet," accessed May 4, 2013, http://thepaleodiet.com/getting-started-with-the-paleo-diet/.

26.   Loren Cordain, "The Paleo Diet Premise," accessed May 4, 2013, http://thepaleodiet.com/the-paleo-diet-premise/.

FOODBORNE ILLNESSES: REVENGE OF THE SUPERBUGS

1.   Stephen Harrod Buhner, *Herbal Antibiotics: Natural Alternatives for Treating Drug-resistant Bacteria* (North Adams: Storey Publishing, 2012), 67.
2.   "Multistate Outbreak of Salmonella Panama Infections Linked to Cantaloupe," *Centers for Disease Control and Prevention*, last modified March 29, 2011, http://www.cdc.gov/salmonella/panama0311/032911/.
3.   "Multistate Outbreak of Salmonella Agona Infections Linked to Rice & Wheat Puff Cereal (Final Update)," *Centers for Disease Control and Prevention*, last modified May 13, 2008, http://www.cdc.gov/salmonella/agona/.
4.   "Multistate Outbreak of Salmonella Infections Associated with Frozen Pot Pies," Morbidity and Mortality Weekly Report, 57, no. 47 (November 28, 2008): 1277-1280, http://www.cdc.gov/mmwr/preview/mmwrhtml/mm5747a3.htm.
5.   Paul S. Mead, Laurence Slutsker, Vance Dietz, et al., "Food-Related Illness and Death in the United States," *Emerging Infectious Dise8ase Journal* 5, no. 5 (October 1999).
6.   Ibid.
7.   Marler Clark, "Kroger, Recall Your E. Coli Contaminated Meat and Tell The Public Who Supplied It, Says William D. Marler, Food Safety Attorney," *Reuters*, last modified June 25, 2008, https://www.businesswire.com/news/home/20080625005900/en/Kroger-Recall-E.-coli-Contaminated-Meat-Public.
8.   "E. coli Infection," FamilyDoctor.org, last modified February 2011, https://familydoctor.org/condition/e-coli-infection/.
9.   "Staphylococcal (Staph) Food Poisoning," *Centers for Disease Control and Prevention*, last modified August 9, 2018, https://www.cdc.gov/foodsafety/diseases/staphylococcal.html.
10.   Y. Le Loir, F. Baron, M. Gautier, "Staphylococcus Aureus and Food Poisoning," *Genetics and Molecular Research* 2, no. 1 (March 31, 2003): 63-76.
11.   "Staphylococcal (Staph) Food Poisoning," *Centers for Disease Control and Prevention*.
12.   Y. Le Loir, F. Baron, M. Gautier, "Staphylococcus Aureus and Food Poisoning," *Genetics and Molecular Research* 2, no. 1 (March 31, 2003): 63-76.

13.   "Bad Bug Book: "Foodborne Pathogenic Microorganisms and Natural Toxins Handbook Staphylococcus aureus," U.S. Food & Drug Administration, last modified August 5, 2013, https://pdf.usaid.gov/pdf_docs/pnado152.pdf.

14.   Y. Le Loir, F. Baron, M. Gautier, "Staphylococcus Aureus and Food Poisoning," *Genetics and Molecular Research* 2, no. 1 (March 31, 2003): 63-76.

15.   *Bad Bug Book: Foodborne Pathogenic Microorganisms and Natural Toxins Handbook Staphylococcus Aureus*, 2nd ed., *U.S. Food & Drug Administration* (2012), https://www.fda.gov/food/foodborne-pathogens/bad-bug-book-second-edition.

16.   "Staphylococcal Food Poisoning," *Centers for Disease Control and Prevention*, last modified August 9, 2018, https://www.cdc.gov/foodsafety/diseases/staphylococcal.html.

1. Marshall H. Segall, Donald T. Campbell, and Melville J. Herskovit, "The Influence of Culture on Visual Perception," chap. 14, *Social Perception*, eds. Hans Toch and Henry C. Smith (New York: Van Nostrand Reinhold, 1968).

2. W. P. Koorts, "The Nature of the Dawn's Heart Star," The Astronomical Society of South Africa, accessed May 19, 2013, http://adsabs.harvard.edu/full/2007AfrSk..11...54K.

3. "The Kalahari People," Sunway Safaris, last modified April 28, 2010, https://sunwaysafaris.wordpress.com/2010/04/28/the-kalahari-people/.

4. Robert C. Brandys and Gail M. Brandys, *Worldwide Exposure Standards for Mold and Bacteria*, 7th ed. (Hinsdale: Occupational & Environmental Health Consulting Services, 2005), chap. 1.

5. Gerald W. Williams, "References on the American Indian Use of Fire in Ecosystems," USDA Forest Service (June 12, 2003), http://www.itcnet.org/file_download/5d76d377-8025-4780-8511-4dc8d0596e45.

6. Wurzbacher Christian, Kerr Janice, and Grossart Hans-Peter, "Aquatic Fungi," chap. 10 in *The Dynamical Processes of Biodiversity: Case Studies of Evolution and Spatial Distribution*, eds. Oscar Grillo and Gianfranco Venora, (InTech, 2011), 231, doi:10.5772/23029.

7. Robert C. Brandys and Gail M. Brandys, *Worldwide Exposure Standards for Mold and Bacteria*, 7th ed. (Hinsdale: Occupational & Environmental Health Consulting Services, 2005), chap. 1; and J. J. Pestka, I. Yike, D. G. Dearborn, M. D. Ward, and J. R. Harkema, "Stachybotrys Chartarum, Trichothecene Mycotoxins, and Damp Building-Related Illness: New Insights into a Public Health Enigma," *Toxicology Sciences* 104, no. 1 (2008): 4–26, doi:10.1093/toxsci/kfm284.

8. "Medical Uses of H2O2," The Truth About Food Grade Hydrogen Peroxide, accessed September 11, 2022, www.foodgrade-hydrogenperoxide.com/id43.html.

9. G. Zhu, Q. Wang, S. Lu, and Y. Niu, "Hydrogen Peroxide: A Potential Wound Therapeutic Target?" *Medical Principles and Practice* 26, no. 4 (2017): 301-308, doi:10.1159/000475501.

10.   Steven Shepherd, *Brushing Up on Gum Disease*, Department of Health and Human Services, Public Health Service, Food and Drug Administration, and Office of Public Affairs, Rockville, MD, (1990).

11.   William Shakespeare, *Hamlet* (New York: Simon & Schuster, 2003).

12.   P. M. Scott, "Ergot alkaloids: extent of human and animal exposure," *World Mycotoxin Journal* 2, no. 2 (April 28, 2009): 141-149, doi.10.3920/WMJ2008.1109.

13.   "Pharmacology: Ancient Times," Antimicrobial Resistance Learning Site, (Michigan State University: 2011), http://amrls.cvm.msu.edu/pharmacology/historical-perspectives.

14.   R. Subramani, R. Kumar, P. Prasad, W. Aalbersberg, and S. T. Retheesh, "Cytotoxic and Antibacterial Substances Against Multi-Drug Resistant Pathogens from Marine Sponge Symbiont: Citrinin, A Secondary Metabolite of Penicillium Sp.," *Asian Pacific Journal of Tropical Biomedicine* 3, no. 4 (April 2013): 291-6, doi:10.1016/S2221-1691(13)60065-9.

15.   J. W. Bennett and M. Klich "Mycotoxins," *Clinical Microbiology Reviews* 16, no. 3 (July 2003): 497–516, doi:10.1128/CMR.16.3.497–516.2003.

16.   Robert C. Brandys and Gail M. Brandys, *Worldwide Exposure Standards for Mold and Bacteria*, 7th ed. (Hinsdale: Occupational & Environmental Health Consulting Services, 2005), chap. 1.

17.   Ibid.

18.   Ibid.

19.   "Ergot of Rye - I: Introduction and History," University of Hawaii Botany, http://www.botany.hawaii.edu/faculty/wong/BOT135/LECT12.HTM.

20.   A. W. Schaafsma and D. C. Hooker, "Climatic Models to Predict Occurrence of Fusarium Toxins in Wheat and Maize," International Journal of Food Microbiology 119, no. 1–2 (2007): 116–25 doi:10.1016/j.ijfoodmicro.2007.08.006.PMID 17900733.

21.   W. P. Norred, WP. "Fumonisins—Mycotoxins Produced by Fusarium Moniliforme, *Journal of Toxicology and Environtal Health* 38, no. 3 (March 1993): 309-28.

22.   Robert C. Brandys and Gail M. Brandys, *Worldwide Exposure Standards for Mold and Bacteria*; and Aedeen Cremin, ed., *Archaeologica: The World's Most Significant Sites and Cultural Treasures* (London: Frances Lincoln, 2007), 139.

23.   Y.N. Yin, L.Y. Yan, J.H. Jiang, and Z. H. Ma, "Biological Control of Aflatoxin Contamination of Crops," *Journal of Zhejiang University of Science. B.* 9, no. 10 (2008): 787–92, doi:10.1631/jzus.B0860003. PMC 2565741.

24.   R. Mateo, A. Medina, E. M. Mateo, F. Mateo, and M. Jiménez, "An Overview of Ochratoxin A in Beer and Wine," *International Journal of Food Microbiology* 119, no. 1–2 (2007): 79–83, doi:10.1016/j.ijfoodmicro.2007.07.029; and P.

Bayman, J. L. Baker "Ochratoxins: A Global Perspective," *Mycopathologia* 162, no. 3 (2006): 215–23, doi:10.1007/s11046-006-0055-4.

25.　M. O. Moss, "Fungi, Quality and Safety Issues in Fresh Fruits and Vegetables," *Journal of Applied Microbiology* 104, no. 5 (2008): 1239–43, doi:10.1111/j.1365-2672.2007.03705.x; and M. W. Trucksess and P. M. Scott, "Mycotoxins in Botanicals and Dried Fruits: A Review," *Food Additives & Contaminants. Part A, Chemical Analysis, Control Exposure, & Risk Assessment* 25, no. 2 (2008): 181–92, doi:10.1080/02652030701567459.

26.　"Refrigeration and Food Safety," USDA.gov, last modified June 15, 2013, http://www.fsis.usda.gov/wps/portal /fsis/topics/food-safety-education/get-answers/food-safety-fact-sheets/safe-food-handling/refrigeration-and-food-safety/ct_index.

MICROWAVE MADNESS OR NUKE 'EM PUKE 'EM

1.   Paul S. Mead, Laurence Slutsker, Vance Dietz, et al., "Food-Related Illness and Death in the United States," *Emerging Infectious Disease Journal* 5, no. 5 (October 1999).
2.   F. Berrino, "Life Style Prevention of Cancer Recurrence: The Yin and the Yang," *Cancer Treatment and Research* 159 (2014): 341-51, doi:10.1007/978-3-642-38007-5_20; and M. Crovetto and R. Uauy, "Recommendations for Cancer Prevention of World Cancer Research Fund (WCRF): Situational Analysis for Chile," *Revista Médica de Chile* 141, no. 5 (May 2013): 626-36, doi:10.4067/S0034-98872013000500011.
3.   Ben Mustapha, M. Bousselmi, T. Jerbi, et al., "Gamma Radiation Effects on Microbiological, Physico-Chemical and Antioxidant Properties of Tunisian Millet (Pennisetum Glaucum L.R.Br.)," *Food Chemistry* 154 (July 2014): 154:230-7, doi:10.1016/j.foodchem.2014.01.015; B. S. Berlett and R. L. Levine, "Designing Antioxidant Peptides," *Redox Report* 19, no. 2 (March 2014): 80-6, doi:10.1179/1351000213Y.0000000078; Dr. Mercola, Nuclear Lunch: The Dangers and Unknowns of Food Irradiation, Mercola.com, accessed February 14, 2014, http://www.mercola.com/article/irradiated/nuclear_lunch.htm; F. Raul, F. Gosse, H. Delincee, et al., "Food-Borne Radiolytic Compounds (2-Alkylcyclobutanones) May Promote Experimental Colon Carcinogenesis," *Nutrition & Cancer* 44, no. 2 (2002): 189-91; and "High-Dose Irradiation: Wholesomeness of Food Irradiated with Doses above 10 Kgy," WHO Technical Report Series 890 (Geneva, Switzerland: 1997), https://www.ncbi.nlm.nih.gov/pubmed/10524010.
4.   "The Department of the Army's Food Irradiation Program—Is It Worth Continuing?" *US Government Accounting Office*, PSAD-78-146 (September 29, 1978): 6, 14.
5.   "Facts about Food Irradiation," *International Consultative Group on Food Irradiation* (Vienna: WorldLinks, 1999), 28-9.
6.   Ibid., 28-9.
7.   Ibid., 28-9.

8. Donald R. Davis, "Declining Fruit and Vegetable Nutrient Composition: What Is the Evidence?" *Horticultural Science* 44, no. 1 (February 2009): 15-19.

9. "Irradiation and Food Safety Answers to Frequently Asked Questions," USDA, last modified August 9, 2013, http://www.fsis.usda.gov/wps/portal/fsis/topics/food-safety-education/get-answers/food-safety-fact-sheets/production-and-inspection/irradiation-and-food-safety/irradiation-food-safety-faq.

10. "Public Law 107 - 171 - Farm Security and Rural Investment Act of 2002," U. S. Government Printing Office (2002), http://www.gpo.gov/fdsys/pkg/PLAW-107publ171/content-detail.html; Curt Anderson Washington, "FDA Approves Beef Irradiation," *Associated Press* (December, 02, 1997); Tony Webb, Tim Lang, and Kathleen Tucker, *Coming Soon to Your Local Meat Market; Food Irradiation: Who Wants It?* (New York: HarperCollins, 1987), 49-54; and Michael Boland and Sean Fox, "Food Irradiation and Public Health," *University of Michigan Food Policy Research Center* (November 2012), https://www.cahfs.umn.edu/sites/cahfs.umn.edu/files/brief_food-irradiation_2018.pdf.

11. "Food Irradiation," Clemson Cooperative Extension, last modified March, 2007, http://www.clemson.edu/extension/hgic/food/food_safety/other/hgic3866.html.

12. "How Does Food Irradiation Work?" The Center for Consumer Research, accessed February 27, 2014, https://ccr.ucdavis.edu/food-irradiation/how-does-food-irradiation-work.

13. "NORAD at 40: Historical Overview," Federation of American Scientists, Fas.org, accessed March 14, 2014, https://www.fas.org/nuke/guide/usa/airdef/norad-overview.htm.

14. F. Vallejo, F. A. Tomás-Barberán, and C. García-Viguera, "Phenolic Compound Contents in Edible Parts of Broccoli Inflorescences after Domestic Cooking," *Journal of the Science of Food and Agriculture* 83, no. 14 (November 2003): 1511–1516, doi:10.1002/jsfa.1585; and Kun Song and John A. Milner, "The Influence of Heating on the Anticancer Properties of Garlic," *The Journal of Nutrition* 131, no. 3 (March 1, 2001): 1054S-1057S, http://jn.nutrition.org/content/131/3/1054S.long.

15. Doaa F. George, Marcela M. Bilek, and David R. McKenzie, "Non-Thermal Effects in the Microwave Induced Unfolding of Proteins Observed by Chaperone Binding," *Bioelectromagnetics* 29, no. 4 (May 2008): 324-330, doi:10.1002/bem.20382.

16. "Food Safety Information for Consumers: Cook Foods Adequately," Washington State University, WSU.edu, accessed March 14, 2014, https://extension.wsu.edu/foodsafety/food-safety/.

17.   Hyla Cass, "A Practical Guide to Avoiding Drug-Induced Nutrient Depletion," NutritionReview.org, last modified April 22, 2013, http://nutritionre-
view.org/2013/04/practical-guide-avoiding-drug-induced-nutrient-depletion/.

18.   A. B. Miller, M. E. Sears, L. L. Morgan, et al., "Risks to Health and
Well-Being From Radio-Frequency Radiation Emitted by Cell Phones and
Other Wireless Devices," *Frontiers in Public Health* 7 (2019): 223, doi:10.3389/
fpubh.2019.00223.

1.	R. G. Shashy, E. J. Moore, and A. Weaver, "Prevalence of the Chronic Sinusitis Diagnosis in Olmsted County, Minnesota" *Archives of Otolaryngology–Head & Neck Surgery* 130, no. 3 (March 2004): 320-3, doi:10.1001/archotol.130.3.320. PMID: 15023840.

2.	N. Singh, D. Baby, J. P. Rajguru, et al., "Inflammation and Cancer," *Annals of African Medicine* 18, no. 3 (July-September 2019): 121–126, doi:10.4103/aam.aam_56_18.

3.	J. R. Daniell and O. L. Osti, "Failed Back Surgery Syndrome: A Review Article," *Asian Spine Journal* 12, no. 2 (April 2018): 372–379, doi:10.4184/asj.2018.12.2.372.

4.	"WHO Global Report on Traditional and Complementary Medicine 2019," *Geneva: World Health Organization* (2019), License: CC BY-NC-SA 3.0 IGO, https://apps.who.int/iris/bitstream/handle/10665/312342/9789241515436-eng.pdf?sequence=1&isAllowed=y.

5.	T. Reffelmann, T. Ittermann, and M. Dörr, "Low Serum Magnesium Concentrations Predict Cardiovascular and All-Cause Mortality," *Atherosclerosis* 219, no. 1 (November 2011): 280-4, doi:10.1016/j.atherosclerosis.2011.05.038 and A. Azoulay, P. Garzon, and M. J. Eisenberg, "Comparison of the Mineral Content of Tap Water and Bottled Waters," *Journal of General Internal Medicine* 16, no. 3 (March 2001): 168–175, doi:10.1111/j.1525-1497.2001.04189.x.

6.	Jonathan V. Wright, *Your Stomach: What is Really Making You Miserable and What to Do About It* (Edinburg: Axios Press, 2009).

7.	Y. Belkaid and T. Hand, "Role of the Microbiota in Immunity and Inflammation" *Cell* 157, no. 1 (2014): 121-41, doi:10.1016/j.cell.2014.03.011.

8.	"Omega-3 Fatty Acids: An Essential Contribution," *Harvard: T. H. CHAN*, 2022, https://www.hsph.harvard.edu/nutritionsource/what-should-you-eat/fats-and-cholesterol/types-of-fat/omega-3-fats/.

9.	Chris A. Knobbe, *Ancestral Dietary Strategy to Prevent and Treat Macular Degeneration* (Boulder: Cure AMD Foundation, 2016), 107-108.

10.	T. L. Blasbalg, J. R. Hibbeln, C. E. Ramsden, et al., "Changes in Consumption of Omega-3 and Omega-6 Fatty Acids in the United States During the 20th

Century," *American Journal of Clinical Nutrition* 93, no. 5 (May 2011): 950–962, doi:10.3945/ajcn.110.006643.

11. Bipasha Mukherjee, "Health Benefits of Turmeric Powder—A Complete Guide on Holy Powder," *TheFitIndian.com*, last modified October 22, 2013, http://www.thefitindian.com/health-benefits-of-turmeric-powder/.

12. Charlie Skeen, "Why I Recommend Pharmaceutical Grade Supplements Over Food Grade," *Live Well Naturally*, https://livewellnaturally.com/dispensary/Why_I_Recommend_Pharmaceutical_Grade_Supplements.html.

1.   Institute of Medicine (US) Committee on Advancing Pain Research, Care, and Education, *Relieving Pain in America: A Blueprint for Transforming Prevention, Care, Education, and Research* (Washington DC: National Academies Press, 2011), chap. 3.

2.   R. C. Shoemaker, K. Johnson, L. Jim, et al., "Diagnostic Process for Chronic Inflammatory Response Syndrome (CIRS): A Consensus Statement Report of the Consensus Committee of Surviving Mold," *Internal Medicine Review* 4, no. 5 (May 2018).

3.   R. C. Shoemaker and D. E. House, "A Time-Series Study of Sick Building Syndrome: Chronic, Biotoxin-Associated Illness from Exposure to Water-Damaged Buildings," *Neurotoxicology and Teratology* 27, no. 1 (January-February 2005): 29-46, doi:10.1016/j.ntt.2004.07.005.

4.   R. C. Shoemaker and M. Maizel, "Innate Immunity, MR Spectroscopy, HLA DR, TGF beta-1, VIP and Capillary Hypoperfusion Define Acute and Chronic Human Illness Acquired Following Exposure to Water-Damaged Buildings," *Center for Research on Biotoxin Associated Illnesses*, https://www.survivingmold.com/docs/Resources/Shoemaker%20Papers/213v1.pdf.

5.   R. C. Shoemaker and M. Maizel, "Exposure to Interior Environments of Water-Damaged Buildings Causes a CFS-like Illness in Pediatric Patients: A Case/Control Study," *Bulletin of the IACFS/ME*, https://www.survivingmold.com/docs/Exposure_to_Interior_Environments_of_Water.pdf.

6.   J. Ryan and R. C. Shoemaker, "RNA-Seq on Patients with Chronic Inflammatory Response Syndrome (CIRS) Treated with Vasoactive Intestinal Polypeptide (VIP) Shows a Shift in Metabolic State and Innate Immune Functions that Coincide with Healing," *Medical Research Archives* 4, no. 7 (2016): 1-11; R. Shoemaker, D. House, and J. Ryan, "Vasoactive Intestinal Polypeptide (VIP) Corrects Chronic Inflammatory Response Syndrome (CIRS) Acquired Following Exposure to Water-Damaged Buildings," Health 5, no. 3 (2013): 396-401, doi:10.4236/health.2013.53053; and "Mold Illness Treatment – Step By Step," SurvivingMold.com, last modified 2022, https://www.survivingmold.com/resources-for-patients/treatment/step-by-step.

7.   R. C. Shoemaker, K. Johnson, L. Jim, et al., "Diagnostic Process for Chronic Inflammatory Response Syndrome (CIRS): A Consensus Statement Report of the Consensus Committee of Surviving Mold," *Internal Medicine Review* 4, no. 5 (May 2018).

8.   R. C. Shoemaker, D. House, and J. C. Ryan, "Vasoactive Intestinal Polypeptide (VIP) Corrects Chronic Inflammatory Response Syndrome (CIRS) Acquired Following Exposure to Water-Damaged Buildings," *Health* 5 no. 3 (March 2013): doi:10.4236/health.2013.53053.

9.   Ritchie C. Shoemaker, Scott McMahan, and Andrew Hayman, *The Art and Science of CIRS Medicine* (Kindle, 2020), 40-48; S. W. McMahon, "An Evaluation of Alternate Means to Diagnose Chronic Inflammatory Response Syndrome and Determine Prevalence," *Medical Research Archives*, 5, no. 3 (March 2017); and Ashley Biscoe, "Could Your Unexplained Symptoms Actually Be Mold Toxicity?" *Attune Functional Medicine*, https://www.attunemed.com/blog/could-your-unexplained-symptoms-actually-be-mold-toxicity/.

10.   C. Romalewski, S. Nelson, M. Tang, et al., "Katrina Cough," *State of Louisiana Department of Health and Hospitals Infectious Disease Epidemiology Section* (2006), https://ldh.la.gov/assets/oph/Center-PHCH/Center-CH/stepi/specialstudies/KatrinaCoughReport.pdf. and B. Rath, et al., "Adverse Respiratory Symptoms and Environmental Exposures among Children and Adolescents Following Hurricane Katrina," *Public Health Reports* 126, no. 6 (2011): 853-60, doi:10.1177/003335491112600611.

11.   R. C. Shoemaker and W. Lawson, "Pfiesteria in Estuarine Waters: The Question of Health Risks," *Environmental Health Perspectives* 115, no. 3 (March 2007): A126-7, doi:10.1289/ehp.115-1849899.

12.   D. Brownstein, P. Galiatsatos, L. Galland, et al., "COVID-19: A Primer Update from Treatment to Long Haulers," *The George Washington University School of Medicine and Health Sciences* (July 17, 2021): https://cme.smhs.gwu.edu/content/covid-19-primer-update-treatment-long-haulers.

13.   R. C. Shoemaker, H. K. Hudnell, D. E. House, et al., "Atovaquone Plus Cholestyramine in Patients Coinfected with Babesia Microti and Borrelia Burgdorferi Refractory to Other Treatment," *Advances in Therapy* 32, no. 1 (January-February 2006): 1-11, doi:10.1007/BF02850341 and R. C. Shoemaker, P. C. Giclas, C. Crowder et al., "Complement Split Products C3a and C4a Are Early Markers of Acute Lyme Disease in Tick Bite Patients in the United States," *International Archives of Allergy and Immunology* 146, no. 3 (February 2008): doi:10.1159/000116362.

1. Jessica K. Black, *The Anti-Inflammation Diet and Recipe Book* (Alameda: N.D. Hunter House Publishing, 2006), 2-3.
2. D.J. Jenkins, C.W. Kendall, A. Marchie, D. A. Faulkner, J.M. Wong, R. de Souza, A. Emam, T.L. Parker, E. Vidgen, K.G. Lapsley, E.A. Trautwein, R.G. Josse, L.A. Leiter, and P.W. Connelly, "Effects of a Dietary Portfolio of Cholesterol-Lowering Foods vs Lovastatin on Serum Lipids and C-Reactive Protein," *Journal of the American Medical Association* 290, no. 4 (July 23, 2003): 502-10.
3. William C. Knowler, Elizabeth Barrett-Connor, Sarah E. Fowler, Richard F. Hamman, John M. Lachin, Elizabeth A. Walker, and David M. Nathan, "Reduction in the Incidence of Type 2 Diabetes with Lifestyle Intervention or Metformin," *New England Journal of Medicine* 346 (February 7, 2002): 393-40, doi:10.1056/NEJMoa012512.
4. Christine Gorman, Alice Park, and Kristina Dell, "Health: The Fires Within," *Time Magazine* (Feb. 23, 2004): http://content.time.com/time/magazine/article/0,9171,993419,00.html.
5. Christine Gorman, Alice Park, and Kristina Dell, "Health: The Fires Within" *Time Magazine* (Feb. 23, 2004): http://content.time.com/time/magazine/article/0,9171,993419,00.html.
6. Jessica K. Black, *The Anti-Inflammation Diet and Recipe Book* (Alameda: N.D. Hunter House Publishing, 2006), 41-44.

CHELATION WITH COMMON FOODS AND NATURAL SUPPLEMENTS

1. S. Yoneda and K.T. Suzuki, "Detoxification of Mercury by Selenium by Binding of Equimolar Hg-Se Complex to a Specific Plasma Protein," *Toxicology and Applied Pharmacology* 143, no. 2 (1997): 274-280.

2. H. Hu, M. Rabinowitz, and D. Smith, "Bone Lead as a Biological Marker in Epidemiologic Studies of Chronic Toxicity: Conceptual Paradigms," *Environmental Health Perspectives* 106, no. 1 (January 1998): 1-8.

3. B. Yamini and S.D. Sleight, "Effects of Ascorbic Acid Deficiency on Methyl Mercury Dicyandiamide Toxicosis in Guinea Pigs," *Journal of Environmental Pathology, Toxicology and Oncology* 5, no. 4-5 (1984): 139-50.

4. Parathyroid hormone contains tryptophan which is ruined or oxidized by iron and copper. Pyridoxine protected PTH/tryptophan from heavy metal toxicity. J.A. Ji, B. Zhang, W. Cheng, and Y. J. Wang, "Methionine, Tryptophan, and Histidine Oxidation in a Model Protein, PTH: Mechanisms and Stabilization," *Journal of Pharmaceutical Sciences* 98, no. 12 (December 2009): 4485-500. The copper induced dopamine oxidation of metallo-Beta Amyloid complexes in Alzheimer's disease model was completely inhibited by all forms of vitamin B6. A. Hashim, L. Wang, K. Juneja, Y. Ye, Y. Zhao, and L. J. Ming, "Vitamin B6s Inhibit Oxidative Stress Caused by Alzheimer's Disease-Related Cu(II)-B-Amyloid Complexes-Cooperative Action of Phospho-Moiety," *Bioorganic & Medicinal Chemistry Letters* 21, no. 21 (November 1, 2011): 6430-2.

5. L. W. Chang, M. Gilbert, and J. Sprecher, "Modification of Methylmercury Neurotoxicity by Vitamin E," *Environmental Research* 17 (1978): 356-366.

6. Children with the highest mercury levels in NHANES study had the lowest measles antibody titers and also the lowest B12 levels. C. M. Gallagher, D. M. Smith, and J. R. Meliker, "Total Blood Mercury and Serum Measles Antibodies in US Children," *The Science of the Total Environment* 410-411 (December 2011): 65-71; M. Yakub and M. P. Iqbal, "Association of Blood Lead (Pb) and Plasma Homocysteine: A Cross Sectional Survey in Karachi, Pakistan," *Public Library of Science One* 5, no. 7 (July 21, 2010): e11706. Mercury, arsenic, copper, and iron accumulate in autistic patients and alter and deplete thiols

which normally bind them. Thiols depend on Thiamine, B12, and folate to function properly in heavy metal binding. M.E. Obrenovich, R. J. Shamberger, D. Lonsdale, "Altered Heavy Metals and Transketolase Found in Autistic Spectrum Disorder," *Biological Trace Element Research* 144, no. 1-3 (December 2011): 475-86.

7. "Coenzyme Q10," Mayo Clinic, last modified Oct. 13, 2017, https://www.mayoclinic.org/drugs-supplements-coenzyme-q10/art-20362602.

8. Aged garlic extract showed significant ability to chelate copper. S. A. Dillon, R. S. Burmi, G. M. Lowe, D. Billington, and K. Rahman, "Antioxidant Properties of Aged Garlic Extract: An In Vitro Study Incorporating Human Low Density Lipoprotein," *Life Sciences* 72, no. 14 (February 21, 2003): 1583-94.

9. Fiber pretreatment reversed predisposition to the iron inducible cancers. R. L. Nelson, S. J. Yoo, J. C. Tanure, G. Andrianopoulos, and A. Misumi, "The Effect of Iron on Experimental Colorectal Carcinogenesis," *Anticancer Research* 9, no. 6 (November-December 1989): 1477-82. The following authors have found that phytic acid is a potent inhibitor of iron-mediated generation of the hazardous oxidant, hydroxyl radical. E. Graf and J. W. Eaton, "Dietary Suppression of Colonic Cancer. Fiber or Phytate?" *Cancer* 56, no. 4 (August 15, 1985): 717-8.

10. Proanthrocyanins have an important contribution in chelation of transition metals. P. Cos, T. De Bruyne, N. Hermans, S. Apers, D. V. Berghe, and A. J. Vlietinck, "Proanthocyanidins in Health Care: Current and New Trends," *Current Medicinal Chemistry* 11, no. 10 (May 2004): 1345-59 and H. Yang, Z. Xu, W. Liu, Y. Deng, and B. Xu, "The Protective Role of Procyanidins and Lycopene Against Mercuric Chloride Renal Damage in Rats," *Biomedical And Environmental Sciences* 24, no. 5 (October 2011): 550-9.

11. Chondroitin sulfate is in the glomerular basement membrane of the renal glomeruli and its sulfate group is a very strong binder of mercury. It plays a very important role in renal heavy metal detoxification. O. T. Ryaskin, *Trends in Autism Research* (New York: Nova Biomedical Books, 2004), 207.

12. L. Mira, M. T. Fernandez, M. Santos, R. Rocha, M. H. Florencio, and K. R. Jennings, "Interactions of Flavonoids with Iron and Copper Ions: A Mechanism for their Antioxidant Activity," *Free Radical Research* 36, no. 11 (2002): 1199-1208; I. F. Cheng and K. Breen, "On the Ability of Four Flavonoids, Baicilein, Luteolin, Naringenin, and Quercetin, to Suppress the Fenton Reaction of the Iron-ATP Complex," *Biometals* 13, no.1 (2000): 77-83; and Inhibition of heavy metal induced reactive oxygen species. B. Frei and J. V. Higdon, "Antioxidant Activity of Tea Polyphenols In Vivo: Evidence from Animal Studies," *The Journal of Nutrition* 133, no. 10 (2003): 3275S-3284S.

13. I. Eliaz, E. Weil, and B. Wilk, "Integrative Medicine and the Role of Modified Citrus Pectin/Alginates in Heavy Metal Chelation and Detoxification—

Five Case Reports," *Forsch Komplementmed* 14 (2007): 358-364, doi:10.1159/00010982.

14.   "Onions contain a variety of organic sulphur compounds that provide health benefits. Sulphur-containing amino acids are found as the proteins in onions as well as garlic and eggs. These specific amino acids are called methionine and cystine and, amongst other things, they are very good at detoxifying your body from heavy metals." In fact, they are able to latch on to mercury, cadmium, and lead and escort them out of the body. "Health Benefits of Onions," Foods-Healing-Power.com, accessed 23 June 2012, http://www.foods-healing-power.com/health-benefits-of-onions.html.

15.   L-propionyl carnitine binds iron and chelates it through the Fenton reaction lowering the generation of free radicals. A. Z. Reznick, V. E. Kagan, R. Ramsey, et al., "Antiradical Effects in L-Propionyl Carnitine Protection of the Heart Against Ischemia-Reperfusion Injury: The Possible Role of Iron Chelation," *Archives of Biochemistry and Biophysics* 296, no. 2 (August 1, 1992): 394–401.

16.   G. Sener, O. Sehirli, A. Tozan, A. Velioğlu-Ovunç, et al., "Ginkgo Biloba Extract Protects Against Mercury(II)-Induced Oxidative Tissue Damage in Rats," *Food and Chemical Toxicology* 45, no. 4 (April 2007): 543-50 and T. Tunali-Akbay, G. Sener, H. Salvarli, et al., "Protective Effects of Ginkgo Biloba Extract Against Mercury(II)-Induced Cardiovascular Oxidative Damage in Rats," *Phytotherapy Research* 21, no. 1 (January 2007): 26-31.

17.   Lyn Patrick, "Mercury Toxicity and Antioxidants: Part I: Role of Glutathione and Alpha-Lipoic Acid in the Treatment of Mercury Toxicity," *Alternative Medicine Review* 7, no. 6 (2002): 456-471.

18.   D. Ziegler, M. Reljanovic, H. Mehnert, and F. A. Gries, "Alpha-Lipoic Acid in the Treatment of Diabetic Neuropathy in Germany: Current Evidence from Clinical Trials," *Experimental & Clinical Endocrinology & Diabetes* 107, no. 7 (1999): 421-30; Z. Gregus, A. F. Stein, F. Varga, and C. D. Klaassen, "Effect of Lipoic Acid on Biliary Excretion of Glutathione and Metals," *Toxicology & Applied Pharmacology* 114, no. 1 (May 1992): 88-96; and J. H. Suh, R. Moreau, S. H. Heath, and T. M. Hagen, "Dietary Supplementation with (R)-Alpha-Lipoic Acid Reverses the Age-Related Accumulation of Iron and Depletion of Antioxidants in the Rat Cerebral Cortex," *Redox Report* 10, no. 1 (2005): 52-60.

19.   R. W. Chesney, et al., "Role of Taurine in Infant Nutrition," *Advances in Experimental Medicine and Biology* 442 (1998): 463-76; P. P. Stapleton, et al., "Host Defense—A Role for the Amino Acid Taurine?" *Journal of Parenteral and Enteral Nutrition* 22, no. 1 (January-February 1998): 42-8; and H. P. Redmond, et al., "Immunonutrition—The Role of Taurine," *Nutrition* 14, no. 7-8 (July-August 1998): 599-604.

20.   H. P. Carr, et al., "Characterization of the Cadmium-Binding Capacity of Chlorella Vulgaris," *Bulletin of Environmental Contamination and Toxicology* 60, no. 3 (1998): 433-440.

21.   Y. Omura, Y. Shimotsuura, A. Fukuoka, H. Fukuoka, and T. Nomoto, "Significant Mercury Deposits in Internal Organs Following the Removal of Dental Amalgam, & Development of Pre-Cancer on the Gingiva and the Sides of the Tongue and Their Represented Organs as a Result of Inadvertent Exposure to Strong Curing Light (Used to Solidify Synthetic Dental Filling Material) & Effective Treatment: A Clinical Case Report, along with Organ Representation Areas for Each Tooth," *Acupuncture & Electro-Therapeutics Research* 21, no. 2 (April-June 1996): 133-60.

22.   M. Misbahuddin, A. Z. Maidul Islam, S. Khandker, et al., "Efficacy of Spirulina Extract Plus Zinc in Patients of Chronic Arsenic Poisoning: A Randomized Placebo-Controlled Study," *Journal of Toxicology* 44, no. 2 (March 2006): 135-41 and Bill Bodri, *How to Help Support the Body's Healing After Intense Radioactive Or Radiation Exposure* (Reno, NV: Top Shape Publishing, 2004), 48.

23.   Mahinda Wettasinghe and Fereidoon Shahidi, "Iron (II) Chelation Activity of Extracts of Borage and Evening Primrose Meals," *Food Research International* 35, no. 1 (2002): 65-71, doi:10.1016/S0963-9969(01)00120-X.

24.   Anna M. Bakowska-Barczak, Andreas Schieber, and Paul Kolodziejczyk, "Characterization of Canadian Black Currant (Ribes nigrum L.) Seed Oils and Residues," *Journal of Agricultural and Food Chemistry* 57, no. 24 (2009): 11528-11536 and Marja P. Kähkönen, Anu I. Hopia, Heikki J. Vuorela, et al., "Antioxidant Activity of Plant Extracts Containing Phenolic Compounds," *Journal of Agricultural and Food Chemistry* 47, no. 10 (1999): 3954-3962.

25.   Ahmed E. Abdel-Moneim, Mohamed A. Dkhil, and Saleh Al-Quraishy, "The Potential Role of Flaxseed Oil on Lead Acetate-Induced Kidney Injury in Adult Male Albino Rats," *African Journal of Biotechnology* 10, no. 8 (February 21, 2011): 1436-1441, doi:10.5897/AJB10.1310.

26.   C. Mashilipa, Q. Wang, M. Slevin, and N. Ahmed, "Antiglycation and Antioxidant Properties of Soy Sauces," *Journal of Medicinal Food* 14, no. 12 (December 2011): 1647-53, doi:10.1089/jmf.2011.0054.

27.   H. M. Luan, L. C. Wang, H. Wu, Y. Jin, and J. Ji, "Antioxidant Activities and Antioxidative Components in the Surf Clam, Mactra Veneriformis," *Natural Product Research* 25, no. 19 (November 2011): 1838-48, doi:10.1080/14786419.2010.530268.

28.   Good for thallium poisoning, but has to be used with caution under a doctor's supervision and potassium level monitoring. A. Saddique and C. D. Peterson, "Thallium Poisoning: A Review," *Veterinary and Human Toxicology* 25, no. 1

(February 1983): 16-22 and R. S. Hoffman, "Thallium Toxicity and the Role of Prussian Blue in Therapy," *Toxicological Reviews* 22, no. 1 (2003): 29-40.

29.   N. McGillicuddy, E. P. Nesterenko, P. N. Nesterenko, P. Jones, and B. Paull, "Chelation Ion Chromatography of Alkaline Earth and Transition Metals a Using Monolithic Silica Column with Bonded N-Hydroxyethyliminodiacetic Acid Functional Groups," *Journal of Chromatography A.* 1276 (February 8, 2013): 102-11, doi:10.1016/j.chroma.2012.12.033.

30.   S. J. Flora and S. K. Tandon, "Beneficial Effects of Zinc Supplementation During Chelation Treatment of Lead Intoxication in Rats," *Toxicology* 64, no. 2 (November 1990): 129-39; R. A. Papaioannou, A. Sohler, and C. C. Pfeiffer, "Reduction of Blood Lead Levels in Battery Workers by Zinc and Vitamin C," *Orthomolecular Psychiatry* 7 (1978): 94-106; and R. Dufault, R. Schnoll, W. J. Lukiw, et al., "Mercury Exposure, Nutritional Deficiencies and Metabolic Disruptions May Affect Learning in Children," *Behavioral and Brain Functions* 27, no. 5 (October 2009): 44.

31.   S. Yoneda and K.T. Suzuki, "Detoxification of Mercury by Selenium by Binding of Equimolar Hg-Se Complex to a Specific Plasma Protein," *Toxicology and Applied Pharmacology* 143, no. 2 (1997): 274-280; K. Seppänen, M. Kantola, R. Laatikainen, et al., "Effect of Supplementation with Organic Selenium on Mercury Status as Measured by Mercury in Pubic Hair," *Journal of Trace Elements in Medicine and Biology* 14, no. 2 (June 2000): 84-7; and N. V. Ralston and L. Raymond, "Dietary Selenium's Protective Effects against Methylmercury Toxicity" *Journal of Toxicology* 278, no. 1 (November 28, 2010): 112-23.

32.   *Centers for Disease Control and Prevention. Managing Elevated Blood Lead Levels Among Young Children: Recommendations from the Advisory Committee on Childhood Lead Poisoning Prevention*, ed. Birt Harvey, chap. 4 (Atlanta: CDC, 2002).

33.   S. N. Chugh, T. Kolley, R. Kakkar, et al., "A Critical Evaluation of Anti-Peroxidant Effect of Intravenous Magnesium in Acute Aluminum Phosphide Poisoning," *Magnesium Research* 10, no. 3 (September 1997): 225-30; D. Soldatovic, D. Vujanovic, V. Matovic, et al., "Compared Effects of High Oral Mg Supplements and of EDTA Chelating Agent on Chronic Lead Intoxication in Rabbits," *Magnesium Research* 10, no. 2 (June 1997): 127-33; and D. Soldatovic, V. Matovic, and D. Vujanovic, "Prophylactic Effect of High Magnesium Intake in Rabbits Exposed to Prolonged Lead Intoxication," *Magnesium Research* 6, no. 2 (June 1993): 145-8.

34.   E. Erdem, N. Karapinar, and R. Donat, "The Removal of Heavy Metal Cations by Natural Zeolites, *Journal of Colloid and Interface Science* 280, no. 2 (December 15, 2004): 309–314; H. M. Baker, A. M. Massadeh, and H. A. Younes, "Natural Jordanian Zeolite: Removal of Heavy Metal Ions from Water Samples Using Column and Batch Methods," *Environmental Monitoring and Assessment*

157, no. 1-4 (October 2009): 319-30, doi:10.1007/s10661-008-0537-6; and A. R. Elmore, "Final Report on the Safety Assessment of Aluminum Silicate, Calcium Silicate, Magnesium Aluminum Silicate, Magnesium Silicate, Magnesium Trisilicate, Sodium Magnesium Silicate, Zirconium Silicate, Attapulgite, Bentonite, Fuller's Earth, Hectorite, Kaolin, Lithium Magnesium Silicate, Lithium Magnesium Sodium Silicate, Montmorillonite, Pyrophyllite, and Zeolite," *International Journal of Toxicology* 22, no. 1 (2003): 37-102.

35.   Magdalena Karamać, "Chelation of Cu(II), Zn(II), and Fe(II) by Tannin Constituents of Selected Edible Nuts," *International Journal of Molecular Science* 10, no. 12 (2009): 5485-5497, doi:10.3390/ijms10125485.

36.   M. Meydani, S. N. Meydani, and J. N. Hathcock, "Effects of Dietary Methionine, Methylmercury, and Atrazine on Ex-Vivo Synthesis of Prostaglandin E1 and Thromboxane B2," *Prostaglandins, Leukotrienes, and Medicine* 14, no. 2 (May 1984): 267-78; M. Waly, H. Olteanu, R. Banerjee, et al., "Activation of Methionine Synthase by Insulin-Like Growth Factor-1 and Dopamine: A Target for Neurodevelopmental Toxins and Thimerosal," Molecular Psychiatry 9, no. 4 (April 2004): 358-70; and J. Mutter, J. Naumann, and R. Schneider et al., "Mercury and Autism: Accelerating Evidence?" *Neuro Endocrinology Letters* 26, no. 5 (October 2005): 439-46.

37.   S. Hussain, D. A. Rodgers, H. M. Duhart, and S. F. Ali, "Mercuric Chloride-Induced Reactive Oxygen Species and Its Effect on Antioxidant Enzymes in Different Regions of Rat Brain," *Journal of Environmental Science and Health* 32, no. 3 (May 1997): 395-409.

38.   Philip A. Rea. "Phytochelatin Synthase, Papain's Cousin, in Stereo," *Proceedings of the National Academy of Sciences of the United States of America* 103, no. 3 (January 17, 2006): 507-508, doi:10.1073/pnas.0509971102 and Philip A. Rea, Olena K. Vatamaniuk, and Daniel J. Rigden, "Weeds, Worms, and More. Papain's Long-Lost Cousin, Phytochelatin Synthase," *Plant Physiology* 136, no. 1 (September 2004): 2463-2474, doi:10.1104/pp.104.048579

39.   Morton Walker, *The Chelation Way: The Complete Book of Chelation Therapy* (Garden City Park, NY: Avery Publishing Group, 1990): 245.

40.   *Translational Stroke Research from Target Selection to Clinical Trials*, eds. Paul A. Lapchak and John H. Zhang (New York: Springer, 2012): 514.

41.   S. Hussain, D. A. Rodgers, H. M. Duhart, and S. F. Ali, "Mercuric Chloride-Induced Reactive Oxygen Species and Its Effect on Antioxidant Enzymes in Different Regions of Rat Brain," *Journal of Environmental Science and Health* 32, no. 3 (May 1997): 395-409.

42.   M. V. Rao and B. Chhunchha, "Protective Role of Melatonin Against the Mercury Induced Oxidative Stress in the Rat Thyroid," *Food and Chemical Toxicology* 48, no. 1 (January 2010): 7-10, doi:10.1016/j.fct.2009.06.038.

43.   Walker, *The Chelation Way: The Complete Book of Chelation Therapy*, 178.

44.	M. Walker and H. Shah, *Everything You Should Know About Chelation Therapy* (New York: McGraw Hill, 1998): 158-61.

45.	Fruit juice consumption lowered lead and homocysteine levels. M. Yakub and M. P. Iqbal, "Association of Blood Lead (Pb) and Plasma Homocysteine: A Cross Sectional Survey in Karachi, Pakistan," *Public Library of Science One* 5, no. 7 (July 21, 2010): e11706.

THE RIVER OF LIFE AND THE RHYTHM OF SLEEP

1. Ya Li, Sha Li, Yue Zhou, et al., "Melatonin for the Prevention and Treatment of Cancer," *Oncotarget* 8, no. 24 (June 13, 2017): 39896–39921, doi:10.18632/oncotarget.16379; Carlos Martínez-Campa, Javier Menéndez-Menéndez, Carolina Alonso-González, et al., "What Is Known About Melatonin, Chemotherapy and Altered Gene Expression in Breast Cancer," *Oncology Letters* 13, no. 4 (April 2017): 2003–2014, doi:10.3892/ol.2017.5712; and A. Kapinova, P. Kubatka, O. Golubnitschaja, et al., "Dietary Phytochemicals in Breast Cancer Research: Anticancer Effects and Potential Utility For Effective Chemoprevention," *Environmental Health and Preventative Medicine* 23 (2018): 36, doi:10.1186/s12199-018-0724-1.

2. "Inspire: Sleep Apnea Innovation," last modified 2021, https://www.inspiresleep.com/?gclid=EAIalQobChMI-PDR9-Pg_AIV-PLijBx3svQhIEAAYASAAEgLvdfD_BwE.

3. James J. DiNicolantonio, James H. O'Keefe, and William Wilson, "Subclinical Magnesium Deficiency: A Principal Driver of Cardiovascular Disease and a Public Health Crisis," *Open Heart* 5, no. 1 (2018): e000668, doi:10.1136/openhrt-2017-000668.

4. Morteza Taheri and Elaheh Arabameri, "The Effect of Sleep Deprivation on Choice Reaction Time and Anaerobic Power of College Student Athletes, *Asian Journal of Sports Medicine* 3, no. 1 (March 2012): 15–20, doi:10.5812/asjsm.34719 and P. Philip, P. Sagaspe, J. Taillard, et al., "Fatigue, Sleep Restriction, and Performance in Automobile Drivers: A Controlled Study in a Natural Environment," *Sleep* 26, no. 3 (May 1, 2003): 277-80.

5. L. Torsvall and T. Akerstedt, "Sleepiness on the Job: Continuously Measured EEG Changes in Train Drivers," *Electroencephalogram Clinical Neurophysiology* 66 (1987): 502-511.

6. Björn Rasch and Jan Born, "About Sleep's Role in Memory," *Physiological Reviews* 93, no. 2 (April 2013): 681-766, doi:10.1152/physrev.00032.2012.

7. Kristen L. Knutsona and Eve Van Cauterb, "Associations Between Sleep Loss and Increased Risk of Obesity and Diabetes," *Annals of the New York Academy of Sciences* 1129 (2008): 287–304, doi:10.1196/annals.1417.033.

8. S. M. Schmid, M. Hallschmid, K. Jauch-Chara, et al., "A Single Night of Sleep Deprivation Increases Ghrelin Levels and Feelings of Hunger in Normal-Weight Healthy Men," *Journal of Sleep Research* 17, no. 3 (September 2008): 331-4 and S. Taheri, L. Lin, D. Austin, et al., "Short Sleep Duration Is Associated with Reduced Leptin, Elevated Ghrelin, and Increased Body Mass Index," *Public Library of Science Medicine* 1, no. 3 (2004): e62, doi:10.1371/journal.pmed.0010062.

9. Rachel Leproult and Eve Van Cauter, "Role of Sleep and Sleep Loss in Hormonal Release and Metabolism," *Endocrine Development* 17 (2010): 11-21, doi:10.1159/000262524.

10. Ibid., 139.

11. F. S. Ruiz, M. L. Andersen, A. Zager et al., "Sleep Deprivation Reduces the Lymphocyte Count in a Non-Obese Mouse Model of Type 1 Diabetes Mellitus," *Brazilian Journal of Medical and Biological Research* 40, no. 5 (May 2007): 633-7.

12. Vikesh Khanijow, Pia Prakash, Helene A. Emsellem, et al., "Sleep Dysfunction and Gastrointestinal Diseases," *Gastroenterology and Hepatology* 11, no. 12 (December 2015): 817–825.

13. Harvard Mental Health Letter, "Sleep Deprivation Can Affect Your Mental Health," last modified March 18, 2019, https://www.health.harvard.edu/newsletter_article/sleep-and-mental-health.

14. Ibid., 32.

15. Michael Ash, "Sleep and Its Detoxing Effect on The Brain and Body," ClinicalEducation.org, last modified April, 6 2017, https://www.clinicaleducation.org/news/sleep-and-its-detoxing-effect-on-the-brain-and-body/.

16. Jane E. Ferrie, Martin J. Shipley, Tasnime N. Akbaraly, et al., "Change in Sleep Duration and Cognitive Function: Findings from the Whitehall II Study," *Sleep* 34 (2011): 565-573.

17. National Sleep Foundation, "School Start Time and Sleep," accessed December 4, 2019, https://www.sleepfoundation.org/articles/school-start-time-and-sleep.

18. Kirsten Weir, "The Science of Naps," *Monitor on Psychology* 47, no.7 (2016): 48.

19. Roger Ekirch, "Segmented Sleep in Preindustrial Societies," *Sleep* 39, no. 3 (March 2016): 715-716, https://doi.org/10.5665/sleep.5558.

20. James Perl, *Sleep Right in Five Nights: A Clear and Effective Guide for Conquering Insomnia* (New York: William Morrow, 1993): 30-31.

21. Ibid., 35.

1.   Timothy Scott, *America Fooled: The Truth About Antidepressants, Antipsychotics And How We've Been Deceived* (Victoria, TX: Argo Publishing, 2006), 330-31.

2.   Scott, *America Fooled*, 170 and M. Babyak, J. A. Blumenthal, S. Herman, et al., "Exercise Treatment for Major Depression: Maintenance of Therapeutic Benefit at 10 Months," *Psychosomatic Medicine* 62, no. 5 (September-October 2000): 633-8 and John J. Ratey, *Spark: The Revolutionary New Science of Exercise and the Brain* (New York: Little, Brown Spark, 2008), 299.

1.   Laurie Barclay, "Mortality Greater for Hip Fracture Than Breast Cancer in Elderly Women," *AGS 2007 Annual Scientific Meeting: Abstract* (last modified May 18, 2007), 28, https://www.medscape.com/viewarticle/556768.

2.   N. Charoenngam, A. Shirvani, T. A. Kalajian, et al., "The Effect of Various Doses of Oral Vitamin D3 Supplementation on Gut Microbiota in Healthy Adults: A Randomized, Double-blinded, Dose-response Study," *Anticancer Research* 40, no. 1 (January 2020): 551-556, doi:10.21873/anticanres.13984; A. B. Hassan, R. F. Hozayen, R. A. Alotaibi, and Y. I. Tayem, "Therapeutic and Maintenance Regimens of Vitamin D3 Supplementation in Healthy Adults: A Systematic Review," *Cellular and Molecular Biology* 64, no. 14 (November 2018): 8-14; M. Jalili, H. Vahedi, H. Poustchi, and A. Hekmatdoost, "Soy Isoflavones and Cholecalciferol Reduce Inflammation, and Gut Permeability, without any Effect on Antioxidant Capacity in Irritable Bowel Syndrome: A Randomized Clinical Trial," *Clinical Nutrition ESPEN* 34 (December 2019): 50-54, doi:10.1016/j.clnesp.2019.09.003; and H. Heidari, R. Amani, A. Feizi et al., "Vitamin D Supplementation for Premenstrual Syndrome-Related Inflammation and Antioxidant Markers in Students with Vitamin D Deficient: A Randomized Clinical Trial," *Scientific Reports* 9, no. 1 (October 2019): 14939, doi:10.1038/s41598-019-51498-x.

3.   Deanna M. Minich, *The Rainbow Diet: A Holistic Approach to Radiant Health Through Foods and Supplements* (Newburyport, MA: Red Wheel/ Weiser, 2018).

4.   Darrell Miller, "Lutein—The Antiordinary Antioxidant," *Vitanet* (February 27, 2008) http://vitanetonline.com/forums/1/Thread/868.

1. Marci Shimoff, *Happy for No Reason: 7 Steps to Being Happy from the Inside Out* (New York: Free Press, 2008), 83-85.

2. Bruce H. Lipton, *The Biology of Belief: Unleashing the Power of Consciousness, Matter & Miracles* (Santa Rosa: Mountain of Love/Elite Books, 2005), 162-172.

3. Thich Nhat Hanh and Dr. Lilian Cheung, *Savor: Mindful Eating, Mindful Life* (New York: Harper One, 2010), 88.

4. Elitsa Dermendzhiyska, "How You Attach to People May Explain a lot about Your Inner Life," *The Guardian* (January 10, 2020).

5. Amir Levine and Rachel S.F. Heller, *Attached: The New Science of Adult Attachment and How it can Help You Find—And Keep—Love* (New York: Jeremy P. Tarcher/Penguin, 2010), chap. 7.

6. Ibid., chap. 7.

7. Ibid., chap. 3.

8. Ibid., chap. 7.

9. Thich Nhat Hanh, *Peace is Every Step: The Path of Mindfulness in Everyday Life* (New York: Bantam Books, 1992), 74.

10. Hanh, *Savor*, 88.

11. Karol Kuhn Truman, *Feelings Buried Alive Never Die . . .* (St. George, UT: Olympus Distributing, 2015).

12. Ibid., 87.

13. Ibid., 86-87.

14. Elitsa Dermendzhiyska, "How You Attach to People May Explain a Lot About Your Inner Life" *The Guardian* (January 10, 2020).

15. Ibid.

16. Ibid.

17. Ibid.

18. Ibid.

19. Mosiah 3:19 (*Book of Mormon*).

20. John 3:3.

21. 1 Peter 1:23.

22. Hanh, *Peace Is Every Step*, 73-74.

23. Hanh, *Savor*, 89.

24. Ibid., 90.

25. R. Kevin Hennelly, "The Heart Chakra and the Kingdom of God," (last modified July 5, 2015), https://www.christianityandthechakras.com/heart-chakra-kingdom-god-jesus-revelation/.

1. Bruce Lipton, *The Biology of Belief: Unleashing the Power of Consciousness, Matter & Miracles* (New York: Hay House, 2015).
2. Norman Cousins, *Anatomy of an Illness* (New York: Open Road Media, 2016).
3. Joel F. Wade, *Mastering Happiness: Ten Principles for Practicing a More Fulfilling Life* (Rolling Hill Estates: Vervante, 2007), 19.
4. M. P. Seligman, T. A. Steen, N. Park, et al., "Positive Psychology Progress: Empirical Validation of Interviews," *The American Psychologist* 60, no. 5 (July-August 2005), 410-21.

1.   Jonny Bowden and Stephen Sinatra, *The Great Cholesterol Myth: Why Lowering Your Cholesterol Won't Prevent Heart Disease-and the Statin-Free Plan That Will* (Beverly, MA: Fair Winds Press, 2012).

2.   A. L. Geers, S. G. Helfer, K. Kosbab, et al., "Reconsidering the Role of Personality in Placebo Effects: Dispositional Optimism, Situational Expectations, and the Placebo Response," *Journal of Psychosomatic Research* 58 (2005): 121–7 and R. P. Greenberg, S. Fisher, and J. A. Riter, "Placebo Washout Is Not a Meaningful Part of Antidepressant Drug Trials" *Perceptual and Motor Skills* 81, no. 2 (October 1995): 688-90, doi:10.2466/pms.1995.81.2.688.

3.   John P. A. Ioannidis, "Effectiveness of Antidepressants: An Evidence Myth Constructed from a Thousand Randomized Trials?" *Philosophy, Ethics, and Humanities in Medicine* 3, no. 14 (2008), doi:10.1186/1747-5341-3-14.

4.   M. Moscucci, L. Byrne, M. Weintraub, and C. Cox, "Blinding, Unblinding, and the Placebo Effect: An Analysis of Patients' Guesses of Treatment Assignment in a Double-Blind Clinical Trial," *Clinical Pharmacology and Therapeutics* 41, no. 3 (March 1987): 259-65, doi:10.1038/clpt.1987.26.

5.   Adriaan Louw, Ina Diener, César Fernández-de-las-Peñas, et al., "Sham Surgery in Orthopedics: A Systematic Review of the Literature," *Pain Medicine*, 18, no. 4 (April 24, 2017): 736–750, doi.10.1093/pm/pnw164.

6.   Adrian Cho, "Quantum Experiment in Space Confirms that Reality Is What You Make It," *Science* (October 27, 2017), https://www.sciencemag.org/news/2017/10/quantum-experiment-space-confirms-reality-what-you-make-it-0.

7.   Ron Eccles, "The Power of the Placebo," *Current Allergy and Asthma Reports* 7, no. 2 (May 2007): 100-4, doi:10.1007/s11882-007-0006-2; Novera Herbert Spector, "Neuroimmunomodulation: A Brief Review: Can Conditioning of Natural Killer Cell Activity Reverse Cancer and/or Aging?" *Regulatory Toxicology and Pharmacology* 24, no. 1 (August 1996): S32-S38, https://doi.org/10.1006/rtph.1996.0074; and D. Spiegel, J. R. Bloom, H. C. Kraemer, and E. Gottheil, "Effect of Psychosocial Treatment on Survival of Patients With

Metastatic Breast Cancer," *Lancet* 14, no. 2 (October 14, 1989): 888-91, doi:10.1016/s0140-6736(89)91551-1.

8.   Bruce H. Lipton, *The Biology of Belief: Unleashing the Power of Consciousness, Matter and Miracles* (London: Hay House, 2008), xv and Aravinda Chakravarti and Peter Little, "Nature, Nurture and Human Disease," *Nature* 421 (January 23, 2003): 412–414.

9.   Allen C. Bowling, *Complementary and Alternative Medicine and Multiple Sclerosis* (New York: Demos Health, 2006), 20.

10.   Ibid., 16-21.

11.   Bruce H. Lipton, *The Biology of Belief: Unleashing the Power of Consciousness, Matter and Miracles* (London: Hay House, 2008).

1. Michael Fowler, "The Michelson-Morley Experiment," *Galileo and Einstein: Lectures from the University of Virginia Physics*, http://galileoandeinstein.physics.virginia.edu/lectures/michelson.html.
2. Richard Milton, *Shattering the Myth of Darwinism: A Rational Criticism of Evolution Theory* (New York: Bowater Books, 2015).
3. E. Demirkaya, S. Lanni, F. Bovis, et al., "A Meta-Analysis to Estimate the Placebo Effect in Randomized Controlled Trials in Juvenile Idiopathic Arthritis," *Arthritis & Rheumatology* 68 no. 6 (June 2016): 1540-50, doi:10.1002/art.39583 and V. Yeung, L. Sharpe, N. Glozier, et al., A Systematic Review and Meta-Analysis of Placebo Versus No Treatment for Insomnia Symptoms," *Sleep Medicine Reviews* 38 (April 2018): 17-27, doi:10.1016/j.smrv.2017.03.006.
4. Gina Kolata, "Dashing Hopes, Study Shows a Cholesterol Drug Had No Effect on Heart Health," *New York Times,* April 3, 2016, https://www.nytimes.com/2016/04/04/health/dashing-hopes-study-shows-cholesterol-drug-has-no-benefits.html.
5. David Hoffmann, *Medical Herbalism: The Science and Practice of Herbal Medicine* (Rochester: Healing Arts Press, 2003), 11.
6. Matthew Wood, *The Practice of Traditional Western Herbalism: Basic Doctrine, Energetics, and Classification* (Berkley: North Atlantic Books, 2013), 31.
7. K. K. Ray, S. R. K. S. Seshasai, S. Erqou, et al., "Statins and All-Cause Mortality in High-Risk Primary Prevention," *Archives of Internal Medicine* 170 (2010): 1024–1031, doi:10.1001/archinternmed.2010.182 and John Abramson, "Cholesterol-Lowering Statin Therapy for Healthy People Is Not as Simple as 'Yes' Or 'No,'" last modified March 7, 2017, *Clinical Pharmacist* 9 no. 3 (March 7, 2017), https://www.pharmaceutical-journal.com/news-and-analysis/opinion/insight/cholesterol-lowering-statin-therapy-for-healthy-people-is-not-as-simple-as-yes-or-no/20202407.article.
8. "WHO Technical Document of the Use of Non-Pharmaceutical Forms of Artemisia," *World Health* Organization, October 2019, https://www.who.int/malaria/mpac/mpac-october2019-session3-non-pharmaceutical-use-artemisia.pdf.
9. Stephen Harrod Buhner, *Herbal Antibiotics: Natural Alternatives for Treating Drug-resistant Bacteria* (North Adams: Storey Publishing, 2012).

1.   Heinz Pagels, *The Cosmic Code: Quantum Physics as the Language of Nature* (New York: Simon and Schuster, 1982), 13.

2.   Ervin Laszlo and Jude Currivan, *Cosmos: A Co-Creator's Guide to the Whole-World* (Carlsbad: Hay House, 2008), xiii.

3.   L. Mason, R. Patterson, and D. Radin, "Exploratory Study: The Random Number Generator and Group Meditation," *Journal of Scientific Exploration* 21 (2007).

4.   "The Quantum Mechanical Model of the Atom," *Khan Academy*, last modified 2022, https://www.khanacademy.org/science/physics/quantum-physics/quantum-numbers-and-orbitals/a/the-quantum-mechanical-model-of-the-atom.

5.   Ethan Siegel, "It's The Power of Quantum Mechanics That Allows The Sun To Shine," *Forbes* (June 22, 2015), https://www.forbes.com/sites/ethansiegel/2015/06/22/its-the-power-of-quantum-mechanics-that-allow-the-sun-to-shine/?sh=3335afa643f7.

6.   A. Lohreya and B. Boreham, "The Nonlocal Universe," *Communicative & Integrative Biology* 13, no. 1 (2020): 147–159, doi:10.1080/19420889.2020.1822583.

7.   "Nonlocality," *The Quantum Physics Lady*, last modified January 10, 2020, http://www.quantumphysicslady.org/glossary/quantum-nonlocality/.

8.   J. Yin, Y. Cao, and Y. H. Li, "Satellite-Based Entanglement Distribution Over 1200 Kilometers," *Science* 356, no. 6343 (2017): 1140-1144, doi:10.1126/science.aan3211.

9.   A. Lohrey and B. Boreham, "The Nonlocal Universe," 147–159.

10.   Joseph Selbie, *The Physics of God* (Newburyport: New Page Books, 2021), xvi.

11.   A. Lohreya and B. Boreham, "The Nonlocal Universe," 147–159.

12.   Amit Goswami, *Self-Aware Universe: How Consciousness Creates the Material World* (New York: Tarcher/Putnam, 1995), 10.

13.   Matthew 17:20-21.

14.   Stanley Wolpert, *Gandhi's Passion: The Life and Legacy of Mahatma Gandhi* (Oxford: Oxford University Press, 2002), 14, 25–27.

15.   Selbie, *The Physics of God*, 26.

16.   S. Hameroff and R. Penrose, "Consciousness in the Universe: A Review of the 'Orch OR' Theory," *Physics of Life Reviews* 11, no. 1 (March 11, 2014): 39-78, doi:10.1016/j.plrev.2013.08.002.

17.   Lohreya and Boreham, "The Nonlocal Universe," 147–159.

www.ingramcontent.com/pod-product-compliance
Lightning Source LLC
Chambersburg PA
CBHW070049030426
42335CB00016B/1837